DISABILITY AND CHRONIC DISEASE

DISABILITY STUDIES

JOAV MERRICK - SERIES EDITOR –

NATIONAL INSTITUTE OF CHILD HEALTH AND HUMAN DEVELOPMENT,
MINISTRY OF SOCIAL AFFAIRS, JERUSALEM, ISRAEL

DISABILITY AND CHRONIC DISEASE

JOAV MERRICK
SHOSHANA ASPLER
AND
MOHAMMED MORAD
EDITORS

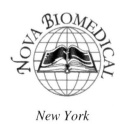

New York

NOTICE TO THE READER

Library of Congress Cataloging-in-Publication Data

ISBN: 978-1-62948-288-0

Library of Congress Control Number: 2013950456

Published by Nova Science Publishers, Inc. † New York

CONTENTS

INTRODUCTION

Acute coronary syndrome (ACS) refers to a group of symptoms attributed to obstruction of the coronary arteries with the most common symptom presented as chest pain. In this book, the authors discuss current research in the study of the symptoms, treatment and prevention of ACS. Topics include antiplatelet therapy in ACS and novel antiplatelet agents; ACS in patients with prior coronary artery bypass graft; the incidence, impact on morbidity and mortality on atypical presentation in ACS; statins use in acute coronary syndrome; dietary assessment and cardiovascular disease risk estimation scores; the importance of renal insufficiency in ischemic heart disease; the relationship between acute coronary syndrome and leukocyte count; and ischemic heart disease in the elderly.

In: Disability and Chronic Disease
Editors: J. Merrick, S. Aspler and M. Morad

ISBN: 978-1-62948-288-0
© 2014 Nova Science Publishers, Inc.

Chapter 1

DISABILITY AND CHRONIC DISEASE

Joav Merrick, MD, MMedSc, DMSc [*,1,2,3,4], *Shoshana Aspler, RN, BScN, MPH* [1,2] *and Mohammed Morad, MD, FRCP (Edin), MRCPS(Glasg)* [1,4,5]

[1]National Institute of Child Health and Human Development, Jerusalem
[2]Office of the Medical Director, Health Services, Division for Intellectual and Developmental Disabilities, Ministry of Social Affairs and Social Services, Jerusalem
[3]Division of Pediatrics, Hadassah Hebrew University Medical Center, Mt Scopus Campus, Jerusalem, Israel
[4]Kentucky Children's Hospital, University of Kentucky, Lexington, US
[5]Yaski Medical Center, Clalit Health Services, Department of Family Medicine, Faculty of Health Sciences, Ben Gurion University of the Negev, Beer-Sheva, Israel

ABSTRACT

Once upon a time pediatrics was involved with infectious disease and acute disorders, but a new pattern of morbidity has emerged. Social difficulties, behavioral problems, developmental difficulties, disabilities and chronic disease have become a main part of the scope of pediatric practice. Among adults multiple chronic disease is increasingly prevalent, whereas the prevalence of impairment and disability remain stable, but substantial and therefore present day health professionals must be aware of disability and chronic disease.

INTRODUCTION

Before birth through young adulthood there is a wide range of health issues that affect our children, such as general childhood illnesses, eating and obesity, accidents and injuries, and

[*] Correspondence: Professor Joav Merrick, MD, MMedSci, DMSc, Medical Director, Health Services, Division for Intellectual and Developmental Disabilities, Ministry of Social Affairs and Social Services, POBox 1260, IL-91012 Jerusalem, Israel. E-mail: jmerrick@zahav.net.il.

particular stages of life, such as teenage independence. Child health and pediatrics focus on the well-being of children from conception through adolescence, but human development is a life span issue, so research in childhood does not stop with the end of adolescence, but we need a long-term and life long study to observe and understand the development process. Pediatrics is vitally concerned with all aspects of children's growth and development and with the unique opportunity that each child has to achieve their full potential as a healthy adult.

Pediatrics or child health was once not a specific entity, just as adolescence really did not exist as a concept, since all were part of adult medicine. This field emerged in the 19th and early 20th century as a medical specialty, because of the gradual awareness that the health problems of children were different from those of adults and children's response to illness, medications and the environment is very depending upon the age of the child.

This uniqueness of children, along with diseases that are particular to this age group, has been responsible for the development of pediatrics as a specialty and for the creation of children's hospitals for the care of children.

ONCE UPON A TIME

Once upon a time pediatrics was involved with infectious disease and acute disorders, but a new pattern of morbidity has emerged. Social difficulties, behavioral problems, developmental difficulties, disabilities and chronic disease have become a main part of the scope of pediatric practice and recognition of the importance of these areas has increased (1).

CS Mott Children's Hospital at the University of Michigan in Ann Arbor conducted a National Poll on Children's Health in order to monitor the future. In their collaboration with Knowledge Networks in this nationally representative household survey they administer to a randomly selected, group of adult with and without children of about 2,000 persons that closely resembles the United States population. In 2010 the following overall health concerns for US children in 2010 and the percentage of adults who rate each as a "big problem" included (2):

- Childhood obesity, 38 percent
- Drug abuse, 30 percent
- Smoking, 29 percent
- Internet safety, 25 percent
- Stress, 24 percent
- Bullying, 23 percent
- Teen pregnancy, 23 percent
- Child abuse and neglect, 21 percent
- Alcohol abuse, 20 percent
- Not enough opportunities for physical activity, 20 percent
- Chemicals in the environment,18 percent
- Sexting,16 percent
- Depression, 15 percent
- Sexually transmitted infections, 15 percent
- School violence, 13 percent

- Asthma. 10 percent
- Neighborhood safety, 8 percent
- Autism, 8 percent
- Suicide, 8 percent

Just a few decades ago, children born with significant congenital anomalies or genetic and metabolic diseases perished at an early age and very few survived into their teens and even less into adulthood. Congenital heart disease, major errors in metabolism, cancer, cystic fibrosis and many other major diseases were fatal. Because of that many physicians in adult primary care did not have the opportunity to see patients with these problems and thus were unable to learn how to care for them.

With major advancements in medical knowledge, technology, imaging techniques, surgical skills and pharmaceutical products as well as prosthetic devices, many of these patients now live much longer life and sometimes even close to the average life expectancy for the country at least in the developed world. With that, a new medical care challenge has been created and we have to take a life span approach.

CHRONIC DISEASE

Chronic diseases, such as heart disease, stroke, cancer, diabetes and arthritis are among the most common, costly and preventable of all health problems in the Western World.

Chronic diseases are the leading causes of death and disability in the United States with 7 out of 10 deaths among Americans each year from chronic diseases. Heart disease, cancer and stroke account for more than 50% of all deaths each year (3) and in 2005, 133 million Americans – almost 1 out of every 2 adults – had at least one chronic illness (4).

In a recent research from the United States (5) the 1998, 2004 and 2008 waves of the Health and Retirement Study, a nationally representative survey of older adults in the United States, were analyzed. 31,568 community dwelling adults aged 65 years and over were included and the following measurements were conducted: prevalence of chronic diseases including hypertension, heart disease, stroke, diabetes, cancer, chronic lung disease and arthritis; prevalence of impairments, including impairments of cognition, vision, hearing, mobility, and urinary incontinence; prevalence of disability, including activities of daily living (ADLs) and instrumental activities of daily living (IADLs) (5).

The proportion of older adults reporting no chronic disease decreased from 13.1% in 1998 to 7.8% in 2008, whereas the proportion reporting one or more chronic diseases increased from 86.9% in 1998 to 92.2% in 2008. People reporting four or more diseases increased from 11.7% in 1998 to 17.4% in 2008. The proportion of older adults reporting no impairments was 47.3% in 1998 and 44.4% in 2008, whereas the proportion of respondents reporting three or more was 7.2% in 1998 and 7.3% in 2008. The proportion of older adults reporting any ADL or IADL disability was 26.3% in 1998 and 25.4% in 2008. This study must therefore conclude that multiple chronic disease is increasingly prevalent among older adults, whereas the prevalence of impairment and disability remain stable.

Health professionals today must therefore be aware of this changing pattern of disease in order to provide better care, prevention and intervention to improve the quality of life and well-being of the current population

REFERENCES

[1]   American Academy of Pediatrics. The new morbidity revisited: A renewed commitment to the psychosocial aspects of pediatric care. Pediatrics 2001;108(5):1227-30.

[2]   CS Mott Children's Hospital National Poll on Children's Health. Monitoring the Future Study. Accessed 2013 Jul 22. URL: www.med.umich.edu/mott/npch

[3]   Kung HC, Hoyert DL, Xu JQ, Murphy SL. Deaths: Final data for 2005. National Vital Statistics Reports 2008;56(10).

[4]   Wu SY, Green A. Projection of chronic illness prevalence and cost inflation. Santa Monica, CA: RAND Health, 2000.

[5]   Hung WW, Ross JS, Boockvar KS, Siu AL. Recent trends in chronic disease, impairment and disability among older adults in the United States. BMC Geriatrics 2011;11:47. doi:10.1186/1471-2318-11-47.

SECTION ONE: DEVELOPMENTAL ISSUES

In: Disability and Chronic Disease
Editors: J. Merrick, S. Aspler and M. Morad
ISBN: 978-1-62948-288-0
© 2014 Nova Science Publishers, Inc.

Chapter 2

TEACHING YOUNG MOTHERS TO IDENTIFY DEVELOPMENTAL MILESTONES

Katelyn M Guastaferro, MPH, John R Lutzker, PhD, Julie J Jabaley, MS MPH, Jenelle R Shanley, PhD and Daniel B Crimmins, PhD*

Center for Healthy Development, Georgia State University, Atlanta, Georgia, US

ABSTRACT

Early identification of a developmental delay may allow for early intervention, a strategy shown to improve child outcomes. Often, pediatricians rely on parent observations to share concerns about development. The purpose of this research was to examine whether a combination of line-art drawings and discussion framed within SafeCare® increases a mothers' identification of developmental milestones. Thus, we examined the tDevelop, a tool designed to increase parent identification of developmental milestones and age-appropriate activities. Two high-risk families with children approximately 24-months of age were recruited from a residential program for young mothers. The mothers were presented with the tDevelop along with standard SafeCare® Parent-Child Interaction (PCI) information, including Planned Activities Training and age-appropriate activities. Data from a multiple-probe, single-case experimental design, suggest that mothers are able to recognize developmental milestones with increased accuracy upon intervention with the tDevelop. The enhanced PCI protocol may enhance parental identification of developmental milestones and may have significant implications for the early identification of developmental delays.

---

* Correspondence: Professor John R Lutzker, PhD, Director, Center for Healthy Development, Professor and Dean, School of Public Health, Georgia State University, P.O. Box 3995, Atlanta, GA 30302-3995 United States. E-mail: jlutzker@gsu.edu.

INTRODUCTION

Developmental milestones are used to monitor social and behavioral growth in multiple aspects of child development: language and communication, motor skills, cognitive processing, and social/emotional skills. Proper stimulation and interactions in early childhood are critical in promoting optimal brain development. Disadvantaged parents may not have the resources or knowledge to provide the stimulation to foster this optimal brain development in their children (1). Mothers at high risk, especially teen parents, typically wane in providing developmental stimulation as their children age, specifically after the first six months of life (2).

Identification, intervention and surveillance

Developmental milestones are typically separated into four categories to capture the spectrum of child development. Language and communication milestones deal with the child's understanding and response to language stimulation in addition to progress toward independent communication. Milestones relating to motor skills, or physical movement, include gross motor and fine motor control. Cognitive processing milestones deal with problem-solving abilities. For infants, this might include learning to self- soothe, whereas with young, ambulatory children, it could mean finding a hidden toy during a game of hide and seek. Finally, milestones in the social-emotional category concerns the socialization of children, including temperament development

Early identification of delays in these four developmental areas can lead to early intervention to optimize development and minimize delays (3). It is estimated that early intervention yields positive effect sizes of nearly one-half to three-quarters of a standard deviation (4). The earlier a delay is identified, the greater the likelihood a disability is prevented, or minimized, and thus minimizing the negative impact on the child and family (5). Mild developmental delays can be identified by age two (6). However, despite the utility of early detection, it is estimated that in the global west, fewer than 30% of children with developmental and behavioral problems are identified prior to the child entering school (7).

Developmental surveillance is a continual process during which a health professional performs skilled observations of the child during routine well-child visits. Thus, pediatricians are often involved in early identification (8). Developmental surveillance is not a means of diagnosis; rather, it is a tool to identify children who need to be evaluated further. Continued surveillance is also essential as a child's risk factors may change or develop over time. The emphasis placed on parent-reported concerns has been controversial, and while parents should not be the sole screening source, research indicates that parental observations and concerns about language, fine motor, and cognitive and emotional-behavior development are highly predictive of a subsequent diagnosed delay (9). While parental concerns have been shown to be as accurate as professional screening, varying levels of parents' health literacy and access to care, in addition to motivation for screening need be considered. The lack of parental concern does not confirm the absence of a developmental delay (10). Thus, parents must be educated and provided with the tools to detect and assess developmental milestones, and must be enabled to discuss concerns with physicians.

Development and child maltreatment

Parents' unrealistic understanding of developmentally appropriate behaviors increases a child's risk for maltreatment (11). The U.S. National Child Abuse and Neglect Data System (NCANDS) estimated that 3.6 million referrals of alleged maltreatment were received by Child Protective Services (CPS) in 2010, of which 78.3% experienced neglect (12). Sequelae of child maltreatment include impaired physical health, impeded emotional/mental health, social difficulties, cognitive dysfunction, high-risk behaviors, and behavioral problems (13).

Child maltreatment is viewed as an "extreme traumatic insult" to a child's developmental trajectory (14) with direct impact on neurodevelopment and lasting effects on the structure and functioning of the brain (15). Continual exposure to stress alters the neurophysiology and neuro-anatomy of the brain through the persistent activation of the hypothalamic-pituitary-adrenal (HPA) axis and the catecholamine stress system.

Intervention for child maltreatment

Evidence-based home visiting models, such as SafeCare (16), work with high-risk parents to prevent child maltreatment and prevent recidivism in those with substantiated child maltreatment cases. Further, home visiting models have been determined effective by the by the United States Task Force on Community Preventative Services and the American Academy of Pediatrics. Early participation in these prevention programs help parents to manage stress and create an optimal development environment before negative behavior patterns emerge (1). SafeCare is delivered to parents with children between birth to five years, five and targets three areas associated with child physical abuse and neglect: 1) parent-child interaction, 2) child health, and 3) home safety. The curriculum is particularly well suited to address neglect, the most common form of child maltreatment. In a statewide, seven-year randomized controlled trial in Oklahoma, SafeCare was shown to be effective in lowering risk for both physical abuse and neglect (17).

The participants of this study received only the Parent-Child Interaction (PCI) module of SafeCare. A core component of PCI is Planned Activities Training, which involves teaching parents strategies for structuring daily activities to prevent challenging behaviors. The curriculum encourages age-appropriate behaviors and activities so that the child understands what is expected and acceptable. It presents developmental milestones in a checklist format to parents intended as a screener, but no research has examined mothers' acquisition of the material.

Because of the increased prevalence of developmental disabilities, the Centers for Disease Control and Prevention (CDC) developed the *Learn the Signs. Act Early.* (LTSAE) campaign, which was launched nationally in 2004 disseminated through social media. The LTSAE campaign provides parents with information on developmental milestones from birth through age five, activities to encourage development, and indicators of when to speak with the child's pediatrician. The materials are presented in a text heavy format written at a 10th grade reading level. The multi-stage, audience-centered campaign was targeted for parents, healthcare educators, and early childhood educators (18). The primary target is parents of children under four-years-old as they are at the highest risk for child maltreatment and developmental disabilities, such as Autism Spectrum Disorder, are able to be diagnosed under age three (19). Parents at high-risk for child maltreatment often have low literacy skills, so reduction of the literacy level of the LTSAE material could be beneficial for them.

Thus, to address these issues, our research question was: "Can a combination of line-art drawings and discussion increase mothers' identification of developmental milestones?" We believed that the introduction of these milestones in a pictoral format would facilitate the mother's identification of developmental milestones for their 24-month-old children. A multiple-probe, single-case research design across two mothers was used to assess the efficacy of a tool created to enhance parental recognition of developmental milestones. The goal was to enhance the mothers' ability to detect milestones, detect delays, and to be alert to developmentally appropriate activities from her child while encouraging monitoring of her child's development, knowing when to contract the child's physician.

OUR STUDY

The research presented here received approval from the Georgia State University Institutional Review Board. Participants were recruited with the help of the Parents as Teachers state leader. Mothers recruited met the following eligibility criteria: consented to participation; had a child between 19 and 30-months-old so that by the final follow-up session, the child would be at a minimum of 2-years-old, or would not have yet reached the next stage of developmental milestones (36-months); and, had an interest in enhancing parent-child interactions.

The state leader connected the researcher (hereafter referred to as Home Visitor) to parent educators at an affiliate organization who had received basic information regarding the research and the eligibility criteria. Families A and B were recruited from this affiliate program aimed at empowering families to be self-sufficient also provides rent-free housing to mothers between the ages of 13 to 26 with children under pre-school age. The mothers attend parenting classes and complete their education.

A residence coordinator initiated recruitment by screening participants using the eligibility criteria and introducing the study those eligible. The coordinator then invited the Home Visitor (HV) to attend an individual meeting with the families where the HV introduced herself, the SafeCare program, and briefly reviewed what being a participant would entail. A copy of the informed consent was given to the mothers to review before their first individual sessions. At the start of the first session, the HV reviewed the informed consent with the participant and the forms were signed. A copy of the informed consent was given to the mother. The mothers received $10 at the end of each session (six intervention sessions and first follow-up) and $30 at the end of the second follow-up (the total compensation was $100).

Demographic information for each family is presented in Figure 1. Family A, a 20-year-old mother and her 25-month-old daughter, had lived at the facility since the child was 7-months-old. The mother was enrolled in vocational classes, but was otherwise unemployed, earning an annual income under $10,000. The mother came from the foster care system due to a history of violence in her family of origin and a personal history in the criminal justice system. Family B, a 17-year-old mother and her 29-month-old daughter, were new to the facility. The mother found the program through Internet searches as a means of avoiding a turbulent home environment and the foster care system. Prior to moving into the residence, she was living in another state while her daughter stayed with a family friend. The day they moved into the facility was the first time they had seen each other in two months. She worked part-time as an administrative support and teachers' aide in the daycare that her daughter attended.

Family	Marital Status	Age of Child(ren)	Highest Level of Education	Employment Status	Average Annual Income
A	Single, Never Married	25 month (daughter)	Some College	Unemployed	Under $10K
B	Single, Never Married	29 month (daughter)	Some High School	Part-Time Employment/ Looking	Under $10K

Figure 1. Demographic Description of Participants.

Setting

All training and observations were conducted at the participants' residence at the facility. SafeCare sessions are typically conducted in the parent's home environment to maximize generalization of skills. Because these two families resided in a residential center, sessions were conducted in convenient locations within the center and often involved role-playing daily routine activities, such as bath time and bedtime, as proxies to real-life situations. Sessions for Family A were conducted in the facility conference room or the caseworker's office. Initially, the HV met Family B in the conference room, but after seeking approval from the facility staff, the Family B mother invited the HV to conduct sessions 3-6 in her room.

Materials

Demographic form. A deidentified demographic survey was delivered to the mothers at the conclusion of the sixth visit. The demographic form was presented to the mother as a useful tool when discussing the relevance of the findings to a wider population.

Consumer satisfaction survey. Utilizing a Likert Scale, the mother rated the program and the HV so that improvements and modifications could be made for future participants.

Intervention materials. Throughout the course of training the mothers were provided with traditional PCI materials. As this research utilized an adaptation of the curriculum, please note that the 't' in material titles was used to indicate a toddler age. The mothers received 'tCards,' handouts emphasizing the skills taught by the HV including the PCI specific Planned Activities Training. Additionally, the mother was provided with the Daily Activities Checklist used to identify challenging parent-child interactions. This checklist is completed prior to training and after training to measure improvement in the ease of interactions. As an enhancement specific to this study, the mothers were presented with the tDevelop that the HV added to throughout the intervention. The tDevelop consisted of a series of 8.5" x 5.5" cards, with milestones segmented into the four categories delineated in the LTSAE campaign. It is based closely on this campaign and was designed as a parent aide to integrate developmental milestones and corresponding developmentally appropriate activities into the SafeCare curriculum. Prior to this development, SafeCare materials presented participants with developmental milestones and age-appropriate activities separately.

The materials reflected an average of an 8th grade reading level. As the tDevelop was based closely on the LTSAE campaign, we sought to make the materials more accessible. The reading level was lowered, utilizing the Flesch-Kincaid Grade Level readability function of Microsoft Word®. Representational pictures, those that have a close physical resemblance to the concept the picture is conveying, guided modifications and were created for each individual milestone (20). Line drawings, a more abstract, highly detailed version of representational pictures that rely on realism in visualization were the most effective and helpful to adult learners (20).

The front side of each card contained a verbal description of two to three developmental milestones, such as "Gets excited with other children," and a line art scenario depicting each developmental milestone, such as a girl smiling and raising her arms when she sees children her age.

On the backside of each card were activities that support corresponding development through interaction between child and parent. Additionally, the cards provided guidance and recommendations should the mother be concerned about missed developmental milestones. The tDevelop cards were designed to be given to the mother one at a time, so as to control the amount of materials and information. Each session, the HV added more cards to the tDevelop until all 27-milestones specific to 2-years-old were represented. The order of cards presented to the mothers was randomized and the number of cards presented to each mother during a given session varied due to individual learning levels.

Home visitor materials. The HV created a score sheet to assess progress in the mothers' identification of developmental milestones. Each score sheet consisted of 10 sections, each for one of the randomly pre-selected milestones on which the mother would be assessed each session. In these sections, the HV had space to document the milestone asked, the mothers' verbal response, and any gestures accompanying her answer. There was a space where the HV would designate if the mother was correct or incorrect. An unscored copy of assessments was provided to the reliability observer (RO).

Observation system

Data Collection. Data were collected by the HV using the score sheet. The milestones for the assessments were randomized with replacement. Thus, the families were likely to have the same prompts repeated any number of times during the course of all the sessions. The HV documented the mothers' response verbatim on the score sheet as well as any gestures or movements that accompanied their responses. For each response reflecting an example of a child behavior that corresponded to the milestone prompt, a checkmark was placed in the score box on the score sheet. Answers that did not provide an example of a child behavior corresponding to the milestone prompt were recorded with an X. The mothers were given the assessment at the beginning of each session.

Data were collected during Condition A, during which the HV prompted the mother to provide an example of a child behavior that corresponded to a milestone prior to any intervention and without any reference materials. For example, if the milestone read: "Says sentences with 2 to 4 words," the mother needed to supply an answer such as, "More milk!" for a correct score to be recorded. An incorrect answer might have been "I'd like to go to the zoo tomorrow and wear my new dress" or "mmmmm milk" or "I don't know."

During condition B, the mother responded to the prompt after having received training with the tDevelop. The mother responded to the same prompt from the HV, but was able to consult the tDevelop that was received and reviewed with the HV during a prior session. When prompted by the HV, the mother had to provide a novel behavior, meaning one different from that was depicted in the line art scenarios, in order to receive a correct score. If the milestone read: "Says sentences with 2 to 4 words," and the line art scenario depicted a child saying "More milk!" the mother had to supply a different response indicating a novel concept such as "Let's go!" for a checkmark to be recorded. If an example extremely similar to that depicted in the line drawing is supplied, such as "More Water!", an X was recorded. Mastery criteria were specified as correctly identifying 8 out 10 correct responses during a given session.

Reliability

The RO, a graduate research assistant, repeatedly reviewed the materials with the HV using a bank of sample responses to the probes provided in advance by a sample of students, staff, and faculty.

The RO completed the score sheet with the HV to create operational definitions and guidelines that were used as a guide for reliability scoring. The HV and RO practiced scoring until reliability agreement consistently reached a minimum of 80%. Reliability was calculated by the following equation: number of agreements divided by the sum of all agreements plus all disagreements multiplied by 100. Reliability observations were conducted a minimum of 25% of each condition for each mother. The HV provided the unscored completed score sheet electronically to the RO. Gestures and all verbal responses were recorded on the score sheet.

Experimental procedure

Design. Multiple probe designs are used to validate the functional relationship between an intervention and outcomes, and in doing so, establish internal validity of the intervention (21). A multiple-probe design across mothers was employed to evaluate the effects of the tDevelop intervention on parents' acquisition of milestones. Milestone training was introduced sequentially such that after two probes showing the lack of requisite knowledge (baseline), tDevelop cards were introduced. The staggered introduction of the interventions between mothers indicates that mastery of milestones occurs upon the introduction of the tDevelop and not other external factors, thus establishing internal validity. Not only are these designs robust, but they are clinically relevant in that parents do not become overwhelmed with lengthy baselines.

Dependent variables. Mothers were prompted by the HV to provide examples of behaviors corresponding to developmental milestones for the referent child during baseline and training conditions. Intervention implementation, the introduction of the tDevelop, taught the mothers developmental milestones using line art scenarios to facilitate comprehension and generalization. The HV prompted mothers the same way in each condition: "One milestone for a two- year old is _____. Can you give me an example of a 2-year old _____?" For example, "One milestone for a 2-year-old is copying others. Can you give me an example of a 2-year old copying others?"

Intervention

In order to contextualize the milestones, the HV integrated the milestone discussion into the Planned Activities Training of PCI. First, the mother would read the milestone with the HV, pointing out important components of the accompanying line-art scenario, for instance, noting the smile and arms raised for the "Gets excited when with other children" milestone. The HV and mother then selected the related activity on the opposite side of the tDevelop card and asked the mother to go through the planned activities training steps as applicable to the specified milestone. Milestones were discussed in a random order.

Baseline. The mother's existing knowledge regarding behaviors that depict developmental milestones was assessed during baseline in which the mother was provided no instruction, materials or feedback from the HV.

Training. If the data showed a descending or stable baseline trend for Mother A, training was implemented. When the data showed skill acquisition with Mother A and baseline showed stability with Mother B, the intervention was implemented with Mother B.

The Mothers were presented with a two to five tDevelop cards and the HV reviewed the critical components of the milestone with the mother. The HV presented possible ways of considering the milestone, emphasizing what elements were important following the example provided in the line art scenario. The Mother was then asked to choose corresponding activities to practice for homework. At the beginning of each training session, the HV prompted the mother for responses to the 10 pre-selected milestones. The HV assessed the responses quickly in situ and then modeled with the mother considerations for how to identify the milestones, if necessary, while introducing the subsequent round of milestones.

The mother was permitted to refer to the cards she had previously received during subsequent assessments. Assessment questions were randomly pre-selected as were the tDevelop cards the mother received during each session. Thus, the mothers may or may not have had the tDevelop card specifically addressed in the assessment at her disposal even though she was allowed to refer to her cards at any time. The tDevelop cards were left with the mother to review and practice corresponding age-appropriate activities for homework at the conclusion of every session.

Follow-up. At one-month and two-months post intervention the HV returned to the residential facility to assess the mothers' retention of 24-month developmental milestones. The mothers were permitted to refer to the tDevelop cards if they wanted to do so; however, neither mother referred to the cards during either follow-up session.

FINDINGS

Figure 2 shows that there was a considerable improvement after introduction of the discussion of developmental milestones with the tDevelop cards. Each mother received six sessions and two follow-up sessions at one and two months post intervention. The duration of visits ranged from 30 mins to 1.5 hrs.

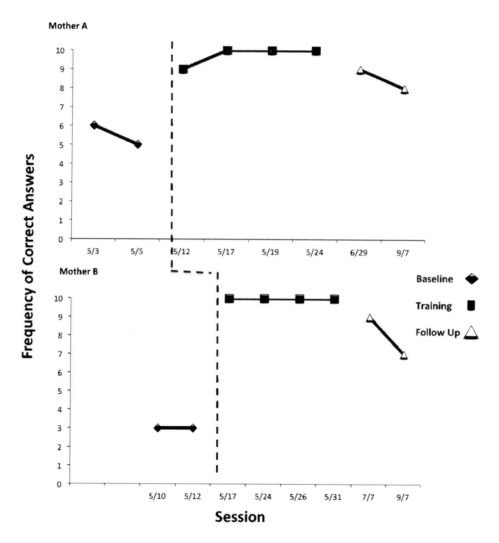

Figure 2. Results.

Outcomes for both mothers during baseline sessions were below the identified mastery criterion(8 correct responses). Mother A's data indicated a decreasing trend. Mother B's data remained stable at three correct answers during her first two sessions. Intervention began with Mother A at the conclusion of the session 2 because the descending baseline trend. She was given several tDevelop cards to review and practice corresponding activities until the next home visit. Upon receiving training, which included a subset of tDevelop cards and discussion with the HV, Mother A's scores increased to 9 correct answers. Thus, intervention began with Mother B who then displayed 10 out of 10 correct responses. Both mothers subsequently showed 100% mastery. The duration of sessions for each mother is presented in Table 2. Session duration was not longer than typical PCI sessions without the tDevelop enhancement.

At one-month post intervention, Mothers A and B showed a high level of retention. At the two-month post intervention follow-up, Mother A again showed a high level of retention, correctly identifying 8 out of 10 milestones. Mother B's scored 7 out of 10 correct.

Reliability

Reliability sessions were conducted in three of the six sessions with each mother. Two reliability sessions occurred for each family during baseline and once during intervention. Reliability observation means for the two families were 90% and 93.3%, respectively. Given the high level of reliability during intervention, reliability was not conducted during follow-up sessions.

Consumer Satisfaction Results

The mothers completed a consumer satisfaction survey during the sixth session. Overall, the mothers' responses showed a general satisfaction with the HV and SafeCare, including the tDevelop. Both mothers indicated they had learned new or useful skills and that they believed the training and materials would be useful to other parents. When asked about providing age-appropriate activities to their children following the PCI training, both mothers 'strongly agreed' that they had more ideas and felt comfortable in engaging in the activities.

Both mothers agreed that the pictures on the tDevelop were clear; however, they disagreed on whether they actually made it easier to understand the milestones. Each mother was positive in response to her use of the cards to follow her child's development. There was a discrepancy with regard to the use of the cards to decide to speak to the child's pediatrician; one mother indicated 'neutral' and the other 'agree'.

DISCUSSION

The purpose of the present study was to increase a mothers' ability to identify developmental milestones, observe delays, and provide developmentally appropriate activities to her child. The introduction of the tDevelop and discussion to the SafeCare PCI module yielded an increase in each mother's identification of developmental milestones for her two-year-old child. The multiple-probe design demonstrated that it was the intervention that caused the improvement in identification rather than extraneous factors. The findings confirm that these mothers were able to identify developmental milestones and generalize milestones to their own child's behaviors once trained. This finding has the potential to inform modifications to the SafeCare curriculum and future research endeavors.

Prior to intervention, neither mother was able to translate a standard milestone to her own child's development. Mother A scored moderately well during baseline, indicating some familiarity with the material. Mother B displayed less familiarity during baseline. Upon introduction of the tDevelop tool, a marked increase in correctly identified developmental behaviors indicates that when provided proper training, mothers can be successful in this task. Both mothers surpassed the mastery criterion immediately and sustained it throughout the intervention. The one-month post intervention follow-up data showed a slight decrease in correct responses, although remaining above mastery criteria. At the follow-up two-months post intervention, both mothers dropped below mastery criterion. The decreases in correctly identified responses may be indicative of a loss of retention of the materials or other factors. During the second follow-up session, both mothers commented to the HV that the task was challenging given their child's progression towards milestones more typical of a 36-month-old. They stated it was challenging to give an example of a milestone that their child had surpassed. Additionally, the HV observed the mothers appeared to face challenges in providing abstract examples of a milestone; that is, their remarks focused exclusively on their own children's development.

The tDevelop tool utilized the findings of prior research in an effective manner. Turner and colleagues(22) showed that pediatricians use simple language, repetition and the limiting of materials presented per session and Parker's (23) finding that health educators "teach back" was a successful strategy employed by the HV in having the mothers discuss the important aspects of the milestones. The success of the line drawings confirms Dwyer's research showing these pictures that relied on realism in visualization were the most helpful to adult learners (20).

The mothers were told that they were allowed to refer to the milestone cards as they needed during assessments, however, the HV observed Mother A do this only once and Mother B did not actively refer to her cards during assessment, although they were in a visible location each time the HV was in the family's room. This speaks to their level of comprehension of the material, but may also suggest that it was the discussion played a critical role in retention. Additionally, the randomization of the milestones during each assessment supports this speculation.

The consumer satisfaction survey results indicated an affinity for the program, materials, and home visitor. The mothers were generally positive in their perception of the tDevelop material. However, one mother suggested the cards be 'updated'. Although she did not elaborate, her feedback is useful when considering making large-scale modifications to the SafeCare curriculum. The overall positive attitude toward the tDevelop is evident in its positive effect on assessment outcomes.

Parents should be provided the opportunity to learn developmental milestones, recognize them in their children, and receive guidance on when to seek medical opinion. Additionally, these findings also indicate that particularly high-risk mothers succeed when provided individual support and modeling.

Given what is known about the barriers high-risk parents face while raising their children, it could not have been predicted that these mothers would do so well. These young mothers are atypical given the structured, parent-centered environment in which they reside, however, the mother's age, education level, income, and marital status highly represent a typical child welfare parent sample. The success of the tDevelop in this population bodes well for other mothers at varying degrees of risk.

The introduction of the tDevelop into standard PCI sessions did not prolong session duration. The variation in session duration is perhaps attributable to information overload as the longest sessions for the Mothers included the most amount of new material. Additionally, varied session duration could be attributable to the child being in the same room during the session and occasionally requiring a shift in the mothers attention. To be a sustainable, effective intervention, the more concrete and succinct the material is, the better suited it is for dissemination (24).

While these findings are promising, several limitations are apparent. Only two high-risk young mothers with low incomes and levels of education limit the generalizability of these findings to other populations at risk. It would be beneficial to see how the materials are received and interpreted by a wider range of participants. Additionally, the present research does not examine whether typical SafeCare Home Visitors can produce similar results. Also, we did not assess whether or not these parents would follow-through with seeking medical consultation when a delay or missed milestone is detected. Thus, another limitation assessing whether the intervention translates into action by the parent. For Mother B, changing the setting from baseline (conference room) and intervention (her room) sessions may have introduced or eliminated distractions. By design, the present research sought to evaluate the effects of discussion supported by the tDevelop. It is thus not possible to determine whether it was the discussion alone, the tDevelop aide alone, or the pairing of the two that had the positive effect on identification of developmental milestones.

In future research, it would be beneficial to include a broader range of milestones to examine the validity of the materials with other ages. Also, putting the tDevelop in an electronic format, such as a Smartphone App, would be of interest as prior research has indicated the introduction of technology increase adherence to treatment in physical and mental health interventions (25).

Despite the recognized limitations, the present research suggests that the integration of developmental milestones and age appropriate activities in the SafeCare curriculum is effective in increasing parental identification of developmental milestones. Moreover, this research shows that high-risk mothers can be taught to utilize the tDevelop tool. This may be beneficial in the long-term in preventing instances of child maltreatment, and aiding parents in making early decisions to seek intervention for a child whom they determine may have a developmental delay.

ACKNOWLEDGMENTS

The publication is funded in part by the Centers for Disease Control and Prevention (CDC), National Center on Birth Defects and Developmental Disabilities (NCBDDD) under Cooperative Agreement U01DD000231 to the Association of University Centers on Disabilities (AUCD). The content of this material does not necessarily reflect the views and policies of CDC, NCBDDD nor AUCD.

REFERENCES

[1] Hawley T, Gunner M. Starting smart: How early experiences affect brain development. Washington: Zero To Three, Ounce Prevention Fund, 2000.

[2] Pomerleau A, Scuccimarri C, Malcuit G. Mother-infant behavioral interactions in teenage and adult mothers during the first six months postpartum: Relations with infant development. Infant Ment Health J 2003;24(5):495-509.

[3] Majnemer A. Benefits of early intervention for children with developmental disabilities. Semin Pediatr Neurol 1998;5(1):62-9.

[4] Sonnander K. Early identification of children with developmental disabilities. Acta Paediatr Suppl 2000;434:17-23.

[5] Geeraert L, Van den Noortgate W, Grietens H, Onghena P. The effects of early prevention programs for families with young children at risk for physical child abuse and neglect: A meta-analysis. Child Maltreat 2004; 9(3):277-91.

[6] Glascoe FP. Screening for developmental and behavioral problems. Dev Disabil Res Rev 2005;11:173-9.

[7] Williams N, Mughal S, Blair M. 'Is my child developing normally?': A critical review of web-based resources for parents. Dev Med Child Neurol 2008;50:893-7.

[8] Committee on Children with Disabilities. Developmental surveillance and screening of infants and young children. Pediatr 2001;108(1): 192-5.

[9] Committee on Children with Disabilities. Role of pediatrician in family-centered early intervention service. Pediatrics 2001;107(5): 1155-7.

[10] American Academy of Pediatrics, Council on Children With Disabilities, Section on Developmental Behavioral Pediatrics, Bright Futures Steering Committee, Medical Home Initiatives for Children with Special Needs Project Committee (AAP). Identifying infants and young children with developmental disorders in the medical home: An algorithm for developmental surveillance and screening. Pediatrics 2006;118(1): 405-20.

[11] Azar ST, Weinzierl KM. Child maltreatment and childhood injury research: A cognitive behavioral approach. J Pediatr Psychol 2005;30(7): 598-614.

[12] US Department of Health and Human Services, Administration for Children and Families, Administration on Children, Youth and Families, Children's Bureau. Child maltreatment 2010. Accessed 2012 Apr 02. URL: http://www.acf.hhs.gov/programs/cb/stats_research/index.htm#can.

[13] Chapman DP, Dube SR, Anda RF. Adverse childhood events as risk factors for negative mental health outcomes. Psychiatric Ann 2007;37(5): 359-64.

[14] Hagele DM. The impact of maltreatment on the developing child. NC Med J 2005;66(5):356-9.

[15] Cicchetti D, Rogosch FA. Adaptive coping under conditions of extreme stress: Multilevel influences on the determinants of resilience in maltreated children. In: EA Skinner, MJ Zimmer-Gembeck, eds. Coping and the development of regulation. New directions for child and adolescent development. San Francisco: Jossey-Bass, 2009:47-59.

[16] Edwards-Gaura AE, Whitaker DJ, Lutzker JR, Self-Brown S, Lewis E. SafeCare: Application of an evidence-based program to prevent child maltreatment. In: Rubin A, ed. A clinician's guide to evidence-based practice. Hoboken, NJ: John Wiley, 2011:259-72.

[17] Chaffin M, Hecht D, Bard D, Silovsky JF, Beasley WH. A statewide trial of the SafeCare home-based serviced model with parents in child protective Services. Pediatrics, in press.

[18] Daniel KL, Prue C, Taylor MK, Scales TM. Learn the signs. Act early: A campaign to help every child reach his or her full potential. Public Health 2009;123:e11-6.

[19] Corsello CM. Early intervention in autism. Infants Young Child 2005; 18(2):74-85.

[20] Alesandrini KL. Pictures and adult learning. Instr Sci 1984;13:63-77.

[21] Barlow DH, Nock MK, Hersen M. Single-case experimental design: Strategies for studying behavior change. Boston, MA: Pearson Allyn Bacon, 2009.

[22] Turner T, Cull WL, Bayldon B, Klass P, Sanders LM, Frinter MP, et al. Pediatricians and health literacy: Descriptive results from a national survey. Pediatrics 2009;124(Supp 3):S299-S305.

[23] Parker R. Health literacy: a challenge for American patients and their health care providers. Health Promot Int 2000;15(4):277-83.

[24] Fixsen DL, Naoom SF, Blase KA, Friedman RM, Wallace F. Implementation research: A synthesis of the literature. Tampa, FL: University of South Florida, Louis de la Parte Florida Mental Health Institute, The National Implementation Research Network (FMHI Publication #231), 2005.

[25] Kazdin AE. Evidence-based treatments and delivery of psychological services: Shifting our emphases to increase impact. Psychol Serv 2008;5(3):201-15.

In: Disability and Chronic Disease
Editors: J. Merrick, S. Aspler and M. Morad

ISBN: 978-1-62948-288-0
© 2014 Nova Science Publishers, Inc.

Chapter 3

CATEGORIZATION ACTIVITIES PERFORMED BY CHILDREN WITH AN INTELLECTUAL DISABILITY AND TYPICALLY DEVELOPING CHILDREN

Olga Megalakaki[*] and Hanan Yazbek

Université de Picardie, Faculté de Philosophie,
Sciences Humaines et Sociales,
Chemin du Thil, Amiens, France

ABSTRACT

The purpose of this chapter was to explore the use of categorization strategies and the mobilization of knowledge by children with intellectual disability, compared with typically developing children matched on mental or chronological age, with regard to three knowledge domains (animals, plants and artifacts). Method: To this end, we administered a match-to-sample task, where children had to make choices and justify them. Results and conclusion: Results revealed that children with intellectual disability performed similarly to typically developing children with regard to thematic categories, but had greater difficulty mobilizing and explicitly processing taxonomic categories. Concerning the type of knowledge were mobilized to justify the choices that were made, our results suggest that the deficits observed in individuals with intellectual disability vary according to the knowledge domain, as the participants in our study had greater difficulty with the animal and artifact domains than with plants.

INTRODUCTION

Research has shown that individuals with intellectual disability have lower performances than typically developing people of the same chronological or mental age. Moreover, the greater

---

[*] Correspondence: Olga Megalakaki, Université de Picardie, Faculté de Philosophie, Sciences Humaines et Sociales, Équipe CRP-CPO EA 7273, Chemin du Thil, 80025 Amiens Cedex 1, France. E-mail: olga.megalakaki@u-picardie.fr.

the complexity of the cognitive processing required to complete a task, the greater the difficulty encountered by people with intellectual disability. The results of different studies tally with the idea that knowledge is organized in memory in the same way, whether or not the person has a deficiency, but that people with intellectual disability have difficulty making effective use of their knowledge in tasks that require explicit processes. Furthermore, this deficit would appear to contribute to the emergence and maintenance of their difficulty in the course of development (1, 2).

It has been observed that when a task requires automatic processing of the information, the performances of people with intellectual disability are equivalent to those of people without any such intellectual disability, whereas the former perform less well when the task needs controlled attentional processing, be it verbal or strategic (1-4).

Research on categorical organization looks at the structure or function of semantic memory, and how this differs across populations. Studies have shown that individuals with intellectual disability have difficulty exploiting the categorical links between stimuli, thereby preventing them from successfully performing recall and recognition tasks (5), developing metacognitive recall strategies (6) and understanding the semantic strategies that are proposed (7). The extent of this difficulty depends on the typicality of the material used (8, 9). McFarland and Sandy (7) compared the performances of adolescents with intellectual disability with those of a group of chronological age-matched, intellectually average individuals on a task in which they had to memorize semantic information using three kinds of encoding (semantic, phonetic, no indication). Adolescents with intellectual disability performed similarly to the intellectually average participants in the phonetic and no indication conditions, but less well in the semantic condition. The authors concluded that semantic representations of concepts are less elaborated in people with intellectual disability. Similarly, the results reported by Glidden et al. (6) and Winters and Semchuk (5) illustrated the difficulty that people with intellectual disability have in effectively exploring semantic links and accessing information in immediate and delayed recall tasks. Results of studies by Winters and Hoats (8) highlighted equivalent semantic memory structures when items were relatively close to the prototype and difficulties for less frequent items. More recently, Hayes and Conway (9) noticed that, in short-term memorization, the ability to encoding and storage of exemplar characteristics (based on the retrieval and activation in memory of exemplars with the greatest overall similarity to the concept being categorized) were consistently less efficient in children with intellectual disability, whatever their mental age. By way of contrast, the ability to process prototypical categories, based on the proximity of the characteristics of the element being categorized to those of the categorization prototype, seem not to depend on intellectual efficiency. In short, people with intellectual disability possess categorical knowledge, but its elaboration may be impaired.

Other authors postulate that the differences observed between individuals with and without intellectual disability arise not from the organization of knowledge in memory but rather from the assessment procedures that are used, which require too many verbal and strategic skills. This position is defended by studies reporting better performances on tasks which do not directly draw on verbal or metacognitive skills (4, 10-12). For example, Landau and Hage (10) found that children with intellectual disability performed similarly on picture sorting but less well on verbal tasks. The research by Sperber et al. (11) involving adolescents with or without intellectual disability highlighted differences in performances when participants had to verbalize semantic links between items. In a semantic priming task where the categorical relations were automatically activated, participants with intellectual disability performed similarly to their intellectually average counterparts. However, when the task required them to explicitly retrieve and use categorical knowledge to justify the categories they had produced, the adolescents with intellectual disability performed less well. According to these authors, differences in the performances of people with intellectual disability should be attributed not to the organization of knowledge in memory, but rather to difficulty mobilizing that knowledge. Gavornikova-Baligand and Deleau (13) and Gavornikova-Baligand (14) also highlighted a dissociation between the categorical organization of knowledge and its mobilization. The authors observed similar performances by participants with and without intellectual disability on a forced-choice categorization task requiring no intentional processing (pointing to items), but poorer performances by the former on a task that did require intentional processing (justification of associations and a sorting task).

The above-mentioned studies show that although people with intellectual disability have semantic information stored in memory, they also have a deficit in the way that information is accessed and processed. However, they tell us little about either the nature of this deficit or the areas of knowledge that are affected by it. The present study therefore set out to investigate the categorization strategies (15, 16) that are used by children and the nature of the knowledge they mobilize in semantic memory for different knowledge domains, rather than the type of processing that is undertaken.

We chose to administer a categorization task because of the important role played by this cognitive activity in the organization of the conceptual world, and because of the opportunities it offers for manipulating the structural and functional characteristics of this organization. Research on conceptual development has shown that intellectually average children categorize information using several types of categories: perceptual (objects grouped together according to their appearance, shape/color), thematic (heterogeneous objects grouped together because they belong to a particular scene or event) and taxonomic (objects of the same kind grouped according to different types of shared properties, such as name, function, etc.). However, there are different theoretical conceptions concerning the development of these different categories. The first conception views the development of categories as a succession of hierarchical steps, with a shift from thematic to slot-filler (members of the same taxonomic category for example the foods eggs and cereal are part of the eating breakfast script) and taxonomic categories (17). According to the second theoretical conception, the acquisition of categories is neither hierarchical nor age-related. Thus, children are able to access all categories at a very early age (15), but favor different categories according to the nature of the task, individual characteristics and their own familiarity with the items in the experiment (15, 16). According to Rosch (18), meanwhile, taxonomic categories are formed at a very early stage, on the basis of perceptual similarity and shared properties. Thus, basic-level categories are the ones that are learned most rapidly in the course of development.

These theoretical approaches refer to intellectually average children. However, we were interested in finding out which categorization strategies are implemented by children with intellectual disability and which types of knowledge they mobilize compared with typically developing children matched on mental or chronological age. To this end, we administered a forced-choice matching test in which children had to make a first choice and justify it, then make a second choice and again justify it. We elicited two choices in order to observe the children's cross-classification abilities. We systematically manipulated three ontological domains (animals, plants and artifacts) to underscore the distinction between living and nonliving things, which plays an important role in children's conceptual organization (19). Insofar as previous studies had shown that basic-level categories are the ones that are learned most rapidly (18), we focused on the superordinate level in our study.

We sought to answer two questions: How do children with intellectual disability categorize items? and Are they able to make effective use of categories in a task involving explicit recourse to them? We compared the performances of children with mild intellectual disability with those of typically developing children matched on mental or chronological age, in terms of 1) the types of choices they made (taxonomic or thematic) for the three ontological domains (animals, plants and artifacts), 2) their cross-classification abilities, and 3) the justifications they gave for these choices in relation to the three domains.

OUR SAMPLE

Our sample comprised 90 children, divided into three groups. A group of 30 children with mild intellectual disability (13 girls and 17 boys), but no organic intellectual disability was recruited from a special school in Amiens (in the north of France) and matched with typically developing children on mental and chronological age (13 girls and 17 boys) in each group, recruited from schools in Amiens. The participants with intellectual disability had a mean chronological age (CA) of 12.2 years (standard deviation (SD) = 2.3), a mean IQ of 62.4 (SD = 7.3) and a mental age (MA) of 6.2 (SD = 1.3). Their diagnosis of mild intellectual disability was based on French national criteria and those of the World Health Organization (WHO). The IQ and MA measures had been made of these children within the previous 12 months, based on the Wechsler Intelligence Scale for Children (WISC-IV) (20).

The 30 typically developing children matched on chronological age had a mean CA of 12.3 (SD = 0.9) and the 30 children matched on mental age had a mean CA of 5.11 (SD =1.3). Care was taken to ensure that they had no particular delay or advance. We deemed that their mental age was equivalent to their real age. The groups were established with the preliminary agreement, teachers, parents and children.

Material

We administered a match-to-sample task, contrasting a target item with a taxonomic associate, a thematic item and a perceptual item, namely a geometric figure that was the same color as the target item (see figure 1 for an example of the picture board and appendix 1 for the list of items). We used a geometric figure associated with the target item on the basis of color as our third item in order to make it easier to distinguish between the taxonomic and thematic items, and thus observe the children's cross-classification (taxonomic and thematic) abilities. The color (or predominant color) of the target item was copied using Paint software to fill in the geometric shape. Target items belonged either to the living or the nonliving world more specifically, to one of three ontological domains: animals, plants or artifacts. We used six items for each domain, basing our selection of taxonomic associates on a superordinate level.

We began constructing the experimental material by selecting items from two databases, looking for the most familiar items for 6-year-old children. We took identification and naming frequency into account for the BD2I database (21) and lexical frequency for MANULEX (22). The target items and their taxonomic associates in the animal domain were mammals (e.g., a dog and a giraffe). In the plant domain, they were flowers and trees (e.g., a daffodil and a tulip), and in the artifact domain, they were pieces of furniture (e.g., a bed and a bench). The thematic items were artifacts, places (e.g., a zoo and a circus) or natural things (a forest). We then tested the set of taxonomic and thematic associates we had chosen in order to make sure that the children would recognize them. In the pretest, each potential target was presented with either a taxonomic or a thematic associate, plus two items that were unrelated to the target. For each potential target, we therefore constructed eight boards (four with taxonomic associates and four with thematic associates) and the children (fifteen 5-6 year-olds and 15 children with intellectual disability of a different structure from the one we investigated in our experiment) had to say which item "went" with the target on each board. We then selected the associations that received the highest number of correct responses (approx. 75%). In order to determine the strength of association between targets and associates (taxonomic or thematic), we carried out an assessment task. Each target item was presented alongside three different taxonomic or thematic associates (those which had most often been recognized as associates by the children in the pretest). In random order, 30 first-year psychology students were asked to rate the strength of association of each pair on a 7-point scale ranging from 1 (no association at all) to 7 (very strong association). We retained those items that had been given equivalent ratings (4 to 6 points) as our taxonomic and thematic associates. A repeated-measures analysis of variance (ANOVA) was conducted (based on MANULEX lexical frequencies) to check the homogeneity of the target items and their taxonomic and thematic associates. This analysis failed to reveal any significant difference between the items. The resulting material consisted of 18 picture boards. The order of presentation of the target items was counterbalanced. The location of the taxonomic associates on the boards was also counterbalanced, resulting in the construction of six sets of 18 boards. For each version of the game, we used a separate form to record the items that were selected, together with their respective justifications.

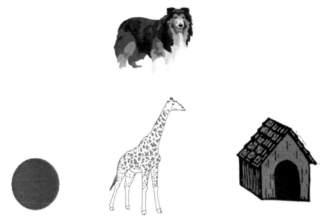

Figure 1. An example of the match-to-sample task.

Procedure

We conducted individual interviews lasting approximately 20 minutes. Interviews were recorded and transcribed, with the addition of the experimenter's notes. Children were tested in a quiet room at their school. One of the six versions, with its corresponding form for noting the choices, was selected at random. The experimenter asked the child to name the target item, then decide which of the other three pictures ''went best'' with the target item, emphasizing that there was no wrong answer. We deliberately used neutral instructions in order to avoid influencing the children's choices. The child was then asked to justify his or her choice: "Why did you put them together?" Once the first choice had been made, the experimenter asked the child to choose between the two remaining pictures and once more justify his or her choice.

Coding criteria and data analysis

The children's first choices were coded according to whether the matches were taxonomic, thematic or perceptual. We coded the second choices in the form of response patterns, which simultaneously took both choices into account. There were therefore six possible patterns: Taxonomic-Thematic, Taxonomic-Perceptual, Thematic-Taxonomic, Thematic-Perceptual, Perceptual-Taxonomic and Perceptual-Thematic. We created a number of categories for coding the justifications (for coding categories, see Table 1). Our data were coded by two independent examiners and interrater agreement was 95%. All disagreements were discussed and resolved. For the statistical analysis, we conducted a repeated-measures ANOVA to compare the children's first choices and response patterns, and a chi-square analysis to compare their justifications.

Table 1. Data coding categories and criteria for attribution

Coding categories	Criteria for category attribution	Examples
Other	The child does not justify his or her choice, or the justification does not fit any of our coding categories.	*Because...*
Perceptual	The justification refers to color, shape and/or physical attributes.	*They are the same color.* *They both have leaves.* *They both have paws.*
Spatiotemporal	Items are matched on the basis of a spatial and/or temporal link.	*The dog lives in the house.* *We can see horses and bears at the zoo.*
Functional	Items are linked by their functionality (what they are for).	*The bed goes with the little boy because the bed is for sleeping.*
Category membership	The child names the category to which the chosen items belong (animals, plants, artifacts).	*The dog goes with the giraffe because they are both animals.*
Biological Properties	The items share the same biological property.	*The dog goes with the giraffe because they both eat.* *The daffodil goes with the tulip because they both grow.* *The plant goes with the watering can because it needs water to grow.*

FINDINGS

Type of first choice (taxonomic, thematic or perceptual)

For the first choice, when all three ontological domains were taken together, there was an interaction effect between type of choice and group, $F(4, 174) = 11.211$, $p < .05$. Overall, the typically developing children in the chronological age (CA) group made more taxonomic choices, $F(1, 87) = 26.757$, $p < .05$, and fewer perceptual choices, $F(1, 87) = 40.277$, $p < .05$, than the children in the other two groups. We did not observe any difference between the children with intellectual disability (IDC) and the typically developing children in the mental age (MA) group on taxonomic and perceptual choices. In general, the majority of choices made by the three populations were thematic and did not differ significantly (see figure 2).

When ontological domains were considered separately, we found an interaction between type of first choice and group for each of the three domains (Animal: $F(4, 174) = 4.267$, $p < .05$, Plant: $F(4, 174) = 14.173$, $p < .05$, Artifacts: $F(4, 174) = 7.186$, $p < .05$). For all three domains, the children in the CA group made more taxonomic choices than the children in the other two groups, who did not differ significantly (Animal: $F(1, 87) = 10.776$, $p < .05$, Plant: $F(1, 87) = 32.159$, $p < .05$, Artifacts: $F(1, 87) = 11.361$, $p < .05$). All three groups made equivalent numbers of thematic choices for the animal and plant domains. For the artifact domain, however, the children in the CA group made more thematic choices than the children in the other two groups, $F(1, 87) = 6.898$, $p < .05$). The CA group also made fewer perceptual choices for the animal and artifact domains than the other two groups, who did not differ significantly (Animal: $F(1, 87) = 14.765$, $p < .05$, Artifacts: $F(1, 87) = 21.578$, $p < .05$). For the plant domain the MA group made more perceptual choices than the other two groups, who did not differ significantly ($F(1, 87) = 49.174$, $p < .05$) (see figure 3).

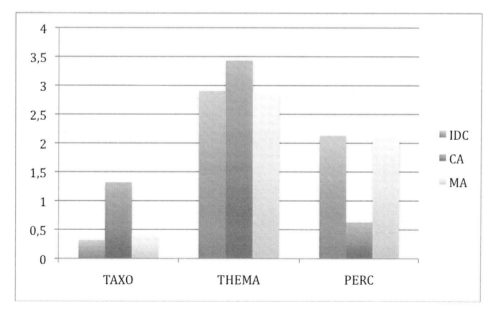

Figure 2. Mean number of Choice 1 matches made by children with intellectual disability (IDC) and children matched on mental age (MA) or chronological age (CA).

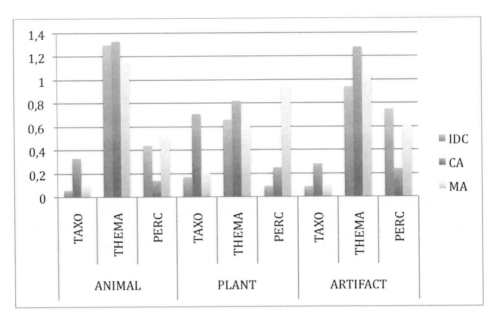

Figure 3. Mean number of Choice 1 matches made by children with intellectual disability (IDC) and children matched on mental age (MA) or chronological age (CA), according to ontological domain.

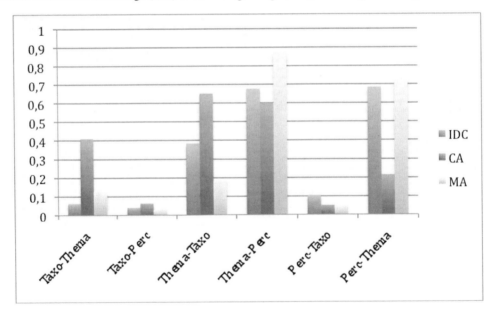

Figure 4. Mean number of patterns produced by children with intellectual disability (IDC) and children matched on mental age (MA) or chronological age (CA).

Type of second choice in relation to the first one

An analysis of results revealed an interaction between response pattern and group, $F(5, 435) = 9.09$, $p < .05$. Generally speaking, the Taxonomic-Thematic and Thematic-Taxonomic patterns, which showed that the children were capable of undertaking cross-classification for a given target, were less frequently observed in the IDC and MA groups, who produced more Perceptual-Thematic patterns than the CA group (see figure 4). When ontological domain was taken into account, there was a triple interaction between domain, response pattern and group, $F(20, 870) = 3.06$, $p < .05$. For each of the three domains (animals, plants, artifacts), the Taxonomic-Thematic and Thematic-Taxonomic patterns were less frequent among the children in the IDC and MA groups, who tended to produce the Thematic-Perceptual and Perceptual-Thematic patterns, than among those in the CA group (see figure 4).

Nature of the justifications given by children for the three ontological domains

The children's justifications were analyzed in order to see whether there was any coherence between choices and justifications. For the taxonomic choices we consider the categories: ''category membership'' and ''biological properties'' as more advanced than others and showing the coherence between choices and justifications. To this end, we coded justifications given for taxonomic and thematic choices separately, according to each of our coding categories (see table 1 for a description of coding categories).

The justifications given for first and second choices were considered together (see table 2). We did not analyze the justifications for perceptual choices, as most of them concerned color.

We found a significant difference between the groups in the justifications they gave for taxonomic choices in the Animal domain, $X^2(8) = 123.189$; $p < .0001$. To justify their taxonomic choices, the children with intellectual disability made more frequent references to biological properties (IDC: 35%, CA: 8%, MA: 11.5%) and to the shared perceptual characteristics of the selected items (30%), whereas the two groups of typically developing children mainly cited category membership (CA: 78.4%, MA: 49.2%, IDC: 15%). All three groups alluded to spatiotemporal links (IDC: 16.6%, CA: 8% and MA: 27.5%). In justifications of thematic choices in the Animal domain, we again found significant differences between the groups, $X^2(4) = 50.502$; $p < .001$. Thematic choices were justified mainly by item functionality by the children with intellectual disability (IDC: 67.6%, CA: 35.7%, MA: 39.3%) and mainly by spatiotemporal links by the typically developing children (CA: 64.1%, MA: 58.9%, IDC: 29.4%).

The analysis of justifications of taxonomic choices for the Plant domain revealed a significant effect of group, $X^2(6) = 39.162$; $p < .001$. Children matched on mental age justified their taxonomic choices mainly by referring to category membership than the two other groups (who did not differ significantly) (CA: 90.8%, IDC: 80.6%, MA: 64.1%). Children in all three groups also cited biological properties (IDC: 14.7%, CA: 9.17%, MA: 9.7%). We did not find any significant differences between the groups for justifications of thematic choices in the Plant domain, $X^2(6) = 10.817$; ns. In all three groups, thematic choices were justified mainly by item functionality (approximately 84%). For the Artifact domain, there was a significant different between the groups in their justifications for taxonomic choices, $X^2(8) = 108.571$; $p < .0001$. These were mainly justified by item functionality by the children with intellectual disability and children matched on mental age (55.3% and 58.8%, respectively) and by category membership by the children matched on chronological age (77.9%).

Table 2. Frequency and percentage (in parentheses) of justifications given for the taxonomic and thematic choices (Choices 1+2) by children with intellectual disability (IDC) and children matched on mental age (MA) or chronological age (CA), for each ontological domain (animals, plants, artifacts)

JUSTIFICATIONS of TAXONOMIC CHOICES (1+2)

Categories	ANIMALS IDC	CA	MA	PLANTS IDC	CA	MA	ARTIFACTS IDC	CA	MA
Other	2 (5)	7 (5.6)	8 (11.5)	1 (1.1)	-	14 (15.2)	9 (13.8)	-	5 (7.3)
Perceptual	18 (30)	-	-	3 (3.4)	-	6 (6.5)	4 (6.1)	-	2 (2.9)
Spatiotemporal	10 (16.6)	10 (8)	19 (27.53)	-	-	-	7 (10.7)	9 (6.6)	6 (8.8)
Function	-	-	-	-	-	-	36 (55.3)	21 (15.4)	40 (58.8)
Category membership	9 (15)	98 (78.4)	34 (49.2)	71 (80.6)	99 (90.8)	59 (64.1)	9 (13.8)	106 (77.9)	15 (22)
Biological property	21 (35)	10 (8)	8 (11.5)	13 (14.7)	10 (9.17)	13 (9.7)	-	-	-
TOTAL	60/360*	125/360	69/360	88/360	109/360	92/360	65/360	136/360	68/360

JUSTIFICATIONS of THEMATIC CHOICES (1+2)

Categories	ANIMALS IDC	CA	MA	PLANTS IDC	CA	MA	ARTIFACTS IDC	CA	MA
Other	5 (2.8)	-	9 (6.1)	8 (5.4)	3 (1.59)	9 (6.1)	4 (2.5)	-	10 (6.1)
Spatiotemporal	51 (29.4)	111 (64.1)	99 (58.9)	4 (2.7)	10 (5.3)	10 (6.8)	27 (16.8)	66 (39.5)	21 (12.9)
Function	117 (67.6)	62 (35.8)	66 (39.2)	126 (85.1)	169 (89.8)	122 (83.5)	129 (80.6)	101 (60.4)	131 (80.8)
Biological property	-	-	-	10 (6.7)	6 (3.1)	5 (3.4)	-	-	-
TOTAL	173/360	173/360	168/360	148/360	188/360	146/360	160/360	167/360	162/360

* 6 animals x 30 children x 2 choices = 360.

For justifications of thematic choices, we also observed a significant difference between the groups, $X^2(4)= 46.28; p < .001$). The majority of children in the IDC and MA groups referred to item functionality (80% for both groups), whereas the children in the CA group justified their choices on the basis of either item functionality (60.4%) or spatiotemporal links (39.5%).

DISCUSSION

The aim of this research was to study categorization strategies and mobilization of knowledge in relation to three ontological domains (animals, plants, artifacts), by analyzing the types of matching choices (taxonomic and thematic) and their justifications given by children with intellectual disability, comparing the latter with typically developing children matched on mental or chronological age.

The results for first choices showed that children with intellectual disability performed similarly to both groups of typically developing children for thematic choices (the predominant choice). The IDC and MA groups performed similarly, but less well, than the CA group for taxonomic choices, making more perceptual choices instead.

An analysis of the response patterns that simultaneously took both the first and second choices into account showed that all the children were capable of undertaking cross-classification for a given target as all of them were able to make two choices, albeit in different proportions. However, if we consider the patterns taxonomic/thematic and thematic/taxonomic, as the most developed, we observe that the IDC group performed similarly to the MA group but less well than the CA group. The patterns thematic/perceptual and perceptual/thematic are the most present in the IDC group and in the MA group.

The analysis of justifications for taxonomic and thematic choices revealed differences between the three groups of children. The CA group cited category membership to justify their taxonomic choices for the animal and artifact domains more often than the other two groups. However, there were no differences between the IDC and CA groups in their justifications of taxonomic choices for the plant domain, with both groups mainly citing category membership. The IDC group tended to use item functionality to justify their thematic choices for the animal and artifact domains, whereas the typically developing children also mentioned spatiotemporal links. In the case of the plant domain, all the children justified their thematic choices by referring to item functionality.

In line with previous studies, we observed lower performances by children with intellectual disability when they were required to explicitly retrieve and use categorical knowledge to justify the taxonomic choices they had made (10, 13). This suggests that they had greater difficulty extracting the conceptual invariants needed to mobilize the categories. If we assume that taxonomic categories are abstractions from the perceived world and are based on interpretive representations of relations between objects, mobilizing high-level cognitive processes, our results suggest that children with intellectual disability have difficulty mobilizing these categories, which require a higher level of abstraction and conceptualization than thematic categories. Thus, the present results corroborate previous findings showing that people with intellectual disability have difficulty processing semantic information (7) or perform less well when tasks are explicit or controlled (1, 3, 11, 14).

The higher number of taxonomic choices made by the CA group and their use of category membership to justify these choices showed that they had fully mastered these categories and found it easy to mobilize them in a task involving explicit recourse to them.

The fact that the children matched on mental age were able to make taxonomic choices shows that these categories are available even to young children and thus supports the pluralist theory of categorical development for typically developing children (15, 16). The preference for thematic choices displayed by all three groups has already been reported in studies with typically developing children and has been attributed either to individual preferences or to task characteristics (16, 23) and strength of association (24).

Our analysis of justifications yielded additional information about the nature of the differences we had observed. Results showed that there was often no coherence between choices and justifications, especially in the case of taxonomic choices. Like other authors (25) we noticed that a choice classified as "taxonomic" could be justified "thematically", by referring to spatiotemporal links between the chosen items (e.g., "we see horses and bears at the zoo"). In this case, we can conclude that the choice was not a genuine taxonomic one. Similarly, a "thematic" choice could be justified by citing the item's biological properties (e.g., "the flower goes with the watering can because it needs water to grow"). This lack of coherence between choices and justifications shows that, in the absence of justifications, we cannot know the true nature of a choice. It is therefore difficult to identify the basis on which children categorize and, consequently, to draw inferences about the underlying mobilization of their knowledge. Furthermore, according to Tulving's model of semantic memory (26), the organization of knowledge relies on abstract semantic links between the concepts, and the quality of these links depends directly on the quality of the processing.

Thus, the analysis of justifications of taxonomic choices yielded more specific information concerning the verbalization of the semantic links between the items and highlighted differences between the justifications given by the three groups, though more so for the animal and artifact domains than for plants. For the latter, the responses of the children with intellectual disability were similar to those of the typically developing children matched on chronological age. For the Animal domain, the IDC group relied more on observable biological properties or physical attributes to justify matching ("the dog and the giraffe both eat" or "the mouse goes with the rabbit because they both grow", or "they both have paws"), whereas the typically developing children mentioned category membership ("the dog goes goes with the giraffe because they are both animals"). It may be that children with intellectual disability more readily mobilize information based on visible properties and find it harder to make the abstractions needed to mobilize taxonomic categories, as defined by Nelson (17). This would make memory retrieval more costly and could partly explain the difficulties they encounter in tasks requiring the explicit processing of information. For their part, typically developing children can more readily mobilize overall concepts, by performing the abstractions needed to include several exemplars within the same category. This interpretation would appear to support previous results showing that the differences observed between people with intellectual disability and intellectually average individuals concern the way in which knowledge is organized in memory (5-9). Similarly, for Artifacts, the analysis of justifications showed that the CA group mainly cited category membership to justify their taxonomic choices, whereas the IDC and MA groups justified all their choices thematically, whether they were taxonomic or thematic, citing item functionality. These results are in line with those reported by other authors for typically developing young children, showing that artifacts are viewed in terms of their functional characteristics and living things in terms of their biological properties (27). We also noticed differences between the populations in their justifications of thematic choices for the animal domain. The IDC group referred more often to the functionality of the items they had chosen, explaining the purpose of each object, whereas both groups of typically developing children took a more general view, basing their justifications on spatiotemporal links.

For Plants, there were fewer differences in the justifications given by the three populations for taxonomic and thematic choices. Children with intellectual disability and children matched on chronological age provided similar justifications for their taxonomic choices, mainly citing the items' category membership ("the daisy and the lily-of-the-valley are plants"). In the same way, all the children tended to justify their thematic choices by referring to item functionality. Accordingly, our results suggest that semantic links in the Plant domain were mobilized in a similar way by both children with intellectual disability and typically developing children. In this particular instance, the need for verbal skills and explicit processing proved less of a hindrance to the mobilization of information. These results contradict previous findings suggesting that poor verbal and strategic skills can, in themselves, explain deficits observed in people with intellectual disability (4, 11, 12, 14). Thus, our observations suggest that the deficit varies according to the knowledge domain being studied. This is an interesting finding, especially as we know that it is difficult to acquire the Plant domain because of it particular status (perceptual markers for attributing biological mechanisms, such as movement, breathing, etc., are not directly accessible) (28).

CONCLUSION

On the basis of previous studies showing that people with or without intellectual disability perform similarly on tasks calling for automatic retrieval processes, it has been inferred that knowledge is organized in a relatively similar way in both populations. The difficulties displayed by children with intellectual disability have thus been attributed to attentional processes governing access to knowledge and the way in which this knowledge is then mobilized (8, 12). Our results support this interpretation and go one step further, by showing that these differences vary according to category (taxonomic or thematic) and knowledge domain. Our study recorded equivalent performances by children with intellectual disability and typically developing children matched on mental or chronological age on the mobilization and processing of thematic categories. Insofar as this type of conceptual organization is based on contextual information that is readily available in the environment, our results suggest that the knowledge subtending thematic classification is mobilized in a similar way by both populations. Throughout the experiment, however, the children with intellectual disability had greater difficulty justifying their taxonomic choices, revealing a deficit in mobilizing and explicitly processing taxonomic categories, which reflect the organization of semantic information in memory. In line with previous findings (5-9), this result suggests that people with intellectual disability have difficulty implementing efficient information processing strategies. Our results show that the extent of this deficit depends on the knowledge domain being probed, as the participants in our study had greater difficulty with the animal and artifact domains than with plants. For animals, children with intellectual disability more readily mobilized shared biological properties and physical attributes, whereas the typically developing children cited category membership more often. However we have to mention the limitations of our study as we have not control the verbal ability of the participants. Nonetheless, we believe that the introduction of categorization activities in different knowledge domains would allow for more tailored interventions, drawing on recipients' potential in order to help them to construct more abstract knowledge which could then be transferred to other domains and other situations. This is the goal we are currently pursuing, through the design of categorization activities intended to promote the learning of a certain number of concepts and help children with intellectual disability realize their full potential.

APPENDIX: LIST OF ITEMS IN THE MATCH-TO-SAMPLE TASK

	Target items	Taxonomic	Thematic	Perceptual
ANIMALS	Brown dog	Giraffe	Kennel	Brown circle
	White horse	Bear	Saddle	White lozenge
	Orange lion	Cow	Circus	Orange parallelogram
	Gray rabbit	Mouse	Cage	Gray square
	Brown monkey	Cat	Zoo	Brown trapezoid
	Gray elephant	Pig	Forest	Gray triangle
PLANTS*	White and orange daisy	Houseplant	Vase	Orange parallelogram
	Daffodil	Tulip	Garden spade	Yellow square
	Pink rosebush	Poppy	Watering can	Pink square
	Cherry tree	Lemon tree	Basket	Red triangle
	Appletree	Fir tree	Ladder	Red trapezoid
	Banana palm	Oak	Rake	Yellow lozenge
ARTIFACTS	Yellow bed	Bench	Boy	Yellow parallelogram
	Green bookcase	Armchair	Book	Green circle
	Brown desk	Sideboard	Notebook	Brown triangle
	Gray table	Shelf	Plate	Gray square
	Blue wardrobe	Stool	Coat hanger	Blue trapezoid
	Pink sofa	Chair	Cushion	Pink lozenge

* The fruit trees were shown bearing fruit.

REFERENCES

[1]   Vicari S, Bellucci S, Carlesimo GA. Implicit and explicit memory: A functional dissociation in persons with Down's syndrome. Neuropsychologia 2000;38:240–51.

[2]   Atwell JA, Conners FA, Merrill EC. Implicit and explicit learning in young adults with mental retardation. Am J Ment Retard 2003;108, 56–68.

[3]   Ellis NR, Woodley-Zanthos P, Dulaney CL. Memory for spatial location in children, adults, and mentally retarded persons. Am J Ment Retard 1989;93:521-7.

[4]   Bebko JM, Luhaorg H. The development of strategy use and metacognitive processing in mental retardation: Some sources of difficulty. In: Burack JA, Hodapp RM, Zigler E, eds. Handbook of mental retardation and development Cambridge: Cambridge University Press, 1998:382–407.

[5]   Winters JJ, Semchuk MT. Retrieval from long-term store as a function of mental age and intelligence. Am J Ment Deficiency 1986;90:440-8.

[6]   Glidden LM, Bilsky LH, Mar HH, Judd TP, Warner DA. Semantic processing can facilitate free recall in mildly retarded adolescents. J Exp Child Psychol 1983;36:510-32.

[7]   McFarland CE, Sandy JT. Automatic and conscious processing in retarded and nonretarded adolescents. J Exp Child Psychol 1982;33:20-38.

[8]   Winters JJ, Hoats DL. Comparison of verbal typicality judgments of mentally retarded and nonretarded persons. Am J Ment Deficiency 1986;90:335-41.

[9]   Hayes BK, Conway RN. Concept acquisition in children with mild intellectual disability: Factors affecting the abstraction of prototypical information. J Intellect Dev Disabil 2000;25:217-34.

[10]   Landau BL, Hage JW. The effect of verbal cues on concept acquisition and retention in normal and educable mentally retarded children. Child Dev 1974;45:643-50.

[11]   Sperber RD, Ragain RD, McCauley C. Reassessment of category knowledge in retarded individuals. Am J Ment Deficiency 1976;81:227-34.

[12]   Sperber RD, McCauley C. Semantic processing efficiency in the mentally retarded. In: Brooks P, Sperber R, McCauley C, eds. Learning and cognition in the mentally retarded, Hillsdale, NJ: Erlbaum, 1984:141–63.

[13]   Gavornikova-Baligand Z, Deleau M. La catégorisation chez les adultes déficients intellectuels: Déficit de structuration ou de mobilisation? Revue Francophone de la Déficience Intellectuelle 2004;15 :5-21. [French]

[14]   Gavornikova-Baligand, Z. Catégories implicites, catégories explicites et déficience intellectuelle. Enfance 2005;57:253-60. [French]

[15]   Bauer PJ, Mandler JM. Taxonomies and triads: Conceptual organization in one-to two-year-olds. Cogn Psychol 1989;21:156-84.

[16]   Kalénine S, Garnier C, Bouisson K, Bonthoux F. Le développement de la catégorisation: L'impact différencié de deux types d'apprentissage en fonction des catégories d'objets, naturels ou fabriqués. Psychologie et Éducation 2007;1:33-45. [French]

[17]   Nelson K. Making sense: The acquisition of shared meaning. New York: Academic Press, 1985.

[18]   Rosch E. Principles of categorization. In: Rosch E, Lloyd BB, eds. Cognition and categorization. Hillsdale, NJ, Erlbaum, 1978:21-48.

[19]   Gelman SA, Opfer JE. Development of the animate-inanimate distinction. In: Goswami U, ed. Handbook of childhood cognitive development. Malden, MA: Blackwell, 2002:151-66.

[20]   Wechsler D. Wechsler Intelligence Scale for Children (WISC IV). Paris: ECPA, 2005.

[21]   Cannard C, Bonthoux F, Blaye A, Scheuner N, Schreiber AC, Trinquart J. BD2I: Normes sur l'identification de 274 images d'objets et leur mise en relation chez l'enfant français de 3 à 8 ans. L'Année Psychologique 2006;106:375-96. [French]

[22]   Lété B, Sprenger-Charolles L, Colé P. Manulex: A grade-level lexical database from French elementary-school readers. Behav Res Methods Instruments Computers 2004;36:166-76.

[23]   Megalakaki O, Yasbek H, Fouquet N. Activités de catégorisation chez les enfants déficients intellectuels légers et les enfants tout-venant appariés par âge mental. Neuropsychiatrie de l'Enfance et de l'Adolescence 2010;58:317-26. [French]

[24]   Scheuner N, Bonthoux F, Cannard C, Blaye A. The role of associative strength and conceptual relations in matching tasks in 4- and 6-year-old children. Int J Psychol 2004;39:290-304.

[25]   Lucariello,J, Kyratzis A, Nelson K. Taxonomic knowledge: What kind and when? Child Dev 1992;63:978–98.

[26]   Tulving, E. Episodic and semantic memory. In: Tulving E, Donaldson W, eds. Organization of memory. New York: Academic Press, 1972:381-403.

[27]   Grief ML, Kemler Nelson DG, Keil FC, Gutierrez F. What do children want to know about animals and artifacts? Psychol Sci 2006;17:455-9.

[28]   Inagaki K, Hatano G. Young children's recognition of commonalities between animals and plants. Child Dev 1996;67:2823–40.

In: Disability and Chronic Disease
Editors: J. Merrick, S. Aspler and M. Morad

ISBN: 978-1-62948-288-0
© 2014 Nova Science Publishers, Inc.

Chapter 4

DON'T TAG ME MENTALLY RETARDED AS I AM NORMAL

Munir Moosa Sadruddin, PhD Scholar and Zaira Wahab, PhD*

Hamdard Institute of Education and Social Sciences (HIESS),
Hamdard University, Karachi, Pakistan and Faculty of Education and Learning Sciences
and Faculty of Business Administration, Iqra University, Karachi, Pakistan

ABSTRACT

The purpose of this chapter is to understand the emotional development of persons with mild intellectual disability. We are primarily interested in understanding the feelings, emotions and fears of persons with mild intellectual disability and how they perceive social relations. This chapter also deals with social and emotional problems faced by persons with mild intellectual disability. In this case study, a single descriptive (providing narrative accounts) case study methodology was carried out. A male with mild intellectual disability was selected for the case study. The data was collected through multiple sources with in-depth interviews and direct observation. We found that the selected person was expressive, cooperative, supportive, kind-hearted, intelligent and understandable. He was peace loving and expressed emotions and fears like a normal person would, however his wishes were of a different nature. The respondent for this particular case was not socially active due to fears and anxiety. He has minor communication and physical movement problems, but his expressions were mature. The respondent was emotionally disturbed, insecure about his future and exhibited mild behavior problem mainly due to rejection by society. The barrier of society norms and family attitudes towards the respondent resulted in negative feelings towards people and life. The respondent needed courage and moral support in order to face these realities. Finally, the respondent wanted people to stop labelling him mentally retarded.

* Correspondence: Munir Sadruddin, Hamdard University, Institute of Education and Social Sciences, Pakistan. E-mail: munirmoosa@yahoo.com.

INTRODUCTION

Humans have a unique nature, traits and different types of personalities. We consider ourselves an important part of society and mostly interact with socially active people, but we often look down upon people, who are unable to adapt to basic social skills or have some kind of cognitive or mental disabilities. People with intellectual disability (formerly called mental retardation) have difficulties with society, because other people have a hard time understanding their feelings and emotions.

According to AAIDD (1), intellectual disability (ID) refers to limitations in intellectual functioning in two or more adaptive skills areas from the following areas: communication, self-care, home living, social skills, community use, self-direction, health and safety, functional academics, leisure, and work. Manjunatha et al. (2) defined mental retardation (MR) as sub-average general intellectual functioning, associated with disability in adaptive behavior. Intellectual disability may occur as part of a syndrome or a broader disorder (3), while the Arizona Revised Statutes as cited in Smith and Strick (4) defined mental retardation as a disability associated with development rather than a mental disease. Intellectaul disability is caused by multiple factors, such as genetics causes, infections during pregnancy, infectious diseases during infancy or drug abuse by the mother during pregnancy among others.

Pelegano and Healy (5) categorized intellectaul disability into five general categories: borderline, mild, moderate, severe and profound. The categorical divisions are based on the scores obtained though standardized tests of cognitive ability. The IQ of mild intellectaul disability is between 50-70. They show no unusual physical signs, but are slow in all developmental areas. They can integrate themselves in society, but need practical and vocational skills. Moderate intellectual disability shows noticeable delay, particularly physically or in speech. Their IQ is between 35-49. They learn simple skills like communication, self-care, safety habits and perform simple tasks easily. Severe intellectual disability shows marked delay in physical development. Their IQ is between 20-34. They have communication barriers and require supervision to learn simple tasks such as self-care or daily routines, while profound intellectaul disability shows marked delay in all the areas of their development. Their IQ is below 20 and they can only perform physical tasks under close supervision.

According to Daily et al. (6) both children and adults with an intellectaul disability may also exhibit some or all of the following characteristics like delay in the development of adaptive behaviors and oral language development; difficulty in learning basic skills; problem solving skills and social rules.

People with an intellectual disability have the same emotional illnesses as people with normal intellectual abilities. The full range of personality disorders, behavior disorders that are noted in the normal population are also noticeable in people with intellectual disability (7).

In the diagnostic studies by Webster (8), it was revealed that intellectaul disability included an impairment in emotional as well as intellectual development. Children with an intellectual disability were less proficient in recognizing emotions, in responding to others' emotions, and in pro-social behaviors. Longitudinal studies on children with intellectual disability below the age of 12 years reported a 20% to 35% frequency of emotional disturbances (9-11).

In the view of Scheerenberger (12), mild intellectual disability is one of the classifications of mental disability. Daily et al. (13) defined mild intellectaul disability as those with intelligence test scores between 70 and 85. They are capable of improving their mathematics and reading skills to the level of a typical child aged 9 to 12 year old and they can learn basic skills besides performing basic tasks easily.

People with an intellectual disability have difficulty in communication. They find it difficult to communicate besides learning skills at a slower pace. However those with mild/borderline intellectual disability are often able to lead independent lives as adults and learn adaptive behaviors through peers (14).

Unfortunately, children with a mild intellectual disability are mostly rejected by their peers (15). According to Zigler et al. (16) and Eaton et al. (17) people with intellectual disability have greater sensitivity and fewer interpersonal coping skills and therefore such rejection greatly hampers their mental and social development.

According to Reynolds and Dombeck (18), individuals with mild intellectual disability are less emotionally immature. Contrary to that Olley (19) suggested that people with intellectual disability knows love, anger, fear and joy and feel the same emotions as the others.

According to Kumar et al. (20), due to low intellectual growth and limited functions, the people with intellectual disability are less socially active. These children vary greatly in their social skills. The nature and degree of social impairment may vary depending on the diagnostic condition associated with intellectual disability (21).

This case study is concerned with exploring the emotional development, dreams and insecurities of people with a mild intellectual disability. The research questions arising from the case-study are as follows:

- Are people with mild intellectual disability emotional? Do they think in a similar pattern as we do?
- Are people with mind intellectual disability socially active?
- What are their dreams and insecurities?
- How do they perceive other people?
- How do they react in different situations?

CASE STUDY RESEARCH

Case study research has been used across many disciplines. Hamel (22) traced the origin of modern social science case studies through anthropology and sociology. Merriam (23) advocated a general approach to qualitative case studies in the field of education, while Stake (24) used systematic procedures for case study research.

Feagin et al. (25) viewed the case study as an ideal methodology when an in-depth investigation is required. Clifford (26) considered it as a method, which gives reflection on reality and provides 'detailed description' of the participants' experiences of thoughts about and feeling for a given situation.

According to Yin (27) one of the reasons to consider a case study design is when the focus of the study is to answer "how" and "why" questions. In case-study method, Crabtree and Miller (28) believed that there is a close bonding between the researcher and the participant, while enabling participants to tell their stories (29, 30) and they believed that through these stories the participants are able to describe their opinions, close to reality.

In this research, holistic single qualitative case study methodology was carried out (31). According to Alvarez et al. (32), the descriptive type of case study is used to develop critical thinking and to describe an intervention or phenomenon of the real-life context in which it occurred.

Since we wanted to understand the multi-layered emotions and feelings of people with mild intellectual disability, a single male with mild intellectaul disability was selected for the study.

The potential participant was informed about the nature and purpose of the research and about the expected benefits to society. Informed consent was signed by the respondent on a voluntary basis. Field and Morse (33) and Munhall (34) referred to consent as a negotiation of trust, and it requires continuous renegotiation. The name was kept confidential throughout the research paper and the final outcomes were also shared with the respondent.

The data was collected through multiple sources, like in-depth interviews and direct observation. In the final interpretative phase, we refer to the lesson learned from the case (35).

A CASE STUDY

Joseph is a tall, fair and handsome man with a presentable personality. He is 30 years of age and has a mature attitude. He thinks, analyzes and observes each situation before expressing his opinions. It is hard for anyone to recognize that he is labelled as "mental" by other people. Though, medical sciences have proved that he has a mild intellectaul disability, but the tagged stigma has disturbed him emotionally.

This case study is unique, because a person with mild intellectual disability never inquires the creator about his problems associated with communication and movement. He only blames people for treating him bad and for recalling his disabilities. He has a few joyous memories like us, and he dreams to achieve his goals. He worries about his future like we all do. He is intelligent and no one can beat him in counting. His cognitive abilities are very sharp. He wants to get pleasure from life to the fullest, but he is emotionally disturbed. He thinks hundreds of time before expressing his emotions and often curses his fate as he believes that no one give him importance. He wants to socialize, but has many fears in the community, where people often treat him like a kid and at times, people totally ignore him. He thinks he is living in a cage and considers himself a robot, operated by the owners of a remote control. He wants the world to avoid calling him "mental". According to him

> "I am living a miserable life, because I can't express my feelings to others. Most of the people consider my comments as unripe dialogues; but I want the world to understand and my views and opinions."

He was informed to meet me at the mosque regularly after the religious service. He was punctual and excited throughout the sessions. In one of the very first meeting he inquired

"I am very much excited. You want to take my interview right? Please publish it around the world to let others know that I am a NORMAL human being. I want others to know that I am not mental. I walk, speak, talk, and think like others. Though I have minor physical disability and can't communicate clearly; that doesn't mean that I am abnormal. ... don't forget to publish about my decorated handmade bottles, as I really want to boost my business."

No one would believe that the above mentioned comments were communicated by a person with mild intellectual disability. When asked to give a brief introduction, he told me that he is 30 years of age and has three siblings. Routinely, he wakes up early in the morning, brushes teeth, eats breakfast and then goes to a vocational centre with a social worker. He returns back home at 1 pm, eats lunch and then rest for two hours. Later, he attends religious service. After returning home, he eats dinner and before going to bed, he routinely watch TV. He makes decorative bottles on the weekends and also spend some time rendering community services. He loves to play bocce and wish to travel by plane. He wants to earn an income in order to support his family and wants to be independent in his life.

He lives with his family, but his social activities are very limited. He is not allowed to go anywhere alone, except to the religious place for services. Though he visited several places with vocational centre volunteers and students, he was not permitted to enjoy the beauty of nature.

At times, it was difficult to understand his speech. He stooped his head when he was unable to speak a few words clearly, but he was given moral support to speak-up with confidence without thinking of communication barriers.

Spradlin (36) found that individuals with intellectual disability have more speech-related problems. Dunn (37) noted that as they mature, language differences between normal people and persons with mild intellectaul disability become more pronounced. Kirk and Gallagher (38) reported that persons with mild intellectual disability encounter problems communicating effectively. In this case, Joseph was facing some articulation and speech problems, however his thoughts and ideas were clear.

Joseph was unable to recall his childhood clearly, but he informed us that he was enrolled in a rehabilitation centre for disabled children by one of the family members. When the news was presented to him, he was shocked and wept a lot. He inquired one of his family members in order to know the reasons behind enrolling him in a rehabilitation center. He was informed that since he is uneducated and has communication problems, he has to attend classes at the rehabilitation centre. During our conversation, he looked really disappointed and his voice was very cold. For a few minutes he was quiet and refused to give further comments. Later he informed us that he cried a lot, because he wanted to learn with normal children, and that it was difficult for him to adjust in a new environment. He said

"I wish I could attend a main stream school... I have to live my whole life like a mental person, because I am of no worth to anyone. No one values my opinion. Why do people call me scary? Am I really scary?"

The life of persons with an intellectaul disability has not been as easy as we think. Joseph's personality was underdeveloped, because he faced many critical incidents and challenges in his life, but was unable to share it with others. His thinking was a bit constructed in a negative way, as the society made him realize that he is alien on this earth. His mood also swung multiple times during our interview sessions.

Mood disorders are also common amongst individuals with intellectual disability. This view was further strengthened by Marston, Perry and Roy (39) by revealing the facts that several studies found very high rates of depression in individuals with intellectual disability. When asked about his three most demanding wishes, he thought and replied

"I want to travel by bus and want to experience a journey by plane and want to earn lots of money."

When asked about the places he had travelled so far, his eyes sparkled with tears. We found him upset and felt as if something was going on in his mind. For a few minutes, he looked here and there and was quiet, but later he broke the ice to inform us about the false promises and talks made by the management of the rehabilitation centre to take him to Islamabad (Capital of Pakistan) via plane to participate in games, but that day has not yet arrived. Once he asked his parents to go for an outing, but he was totally de-motivated. Moreover, a social worker wanted to take him for an outing, but also faced rudeness and slur from his family side. He shared

"I am a controlled robot. I can't go anywhere. I heard and learnt about the places through TV, because I can't go anywhere alone; I'm bound. I only go to attend religious services on my own, but people overlook me. I am confined not to travel without permission. My siblings went to international destinations during holidays, but I was never offered to accompany them. I want to experience the thrill, but I know, this would always remain a dream, because I am MENTAL. The rehabilitation centre lied about taking me to Islamabad by plane, but I was very much disappointed, when I realized that it was nothing more than idle talk."

Something was going on in Joseph's mind. He later asked about our experience of travelling by public bus and airplane. While sharing this experience, he listened with anticipation, though interrupted multiple times due to excitement, and also expressed his wish to experience the same. Mikkelsen (40) believed that people with intellectual disability experience the full range of human emotions. In this case study, the same was observed by the researcher as Joseph shared both happy and gloomy emotions during detailed interviews.

Turkington and Harris (41) wrote that many people with a mild intellectual disability are able to live and work independently. When asked, what sort of work he wants to do, he informed that he is already earning by selling decorative handmade bottles and earns around 10-15$ per month. He shared with us that he always wanted to earn, but was discouraged by XYZ during his adolescence; however at the age of 21 years, he started selling rosary at public places through the support of a social worker, but was highly discouraged by the volunteers of rehabilitation centre. When his family was informed, he was disregarded. He informed that he was also threatened that if he worked at a public place, he would face severe consequences. Things changed for him at the age of 27 years, when a team of social workers supported him to make decorative bottles.

He was dissatisfied with the reaction of society. According to him, a few people bought decorative bottles, because they consider him mental. Few even offer him money without buying bottles, because they feel pity over his condition, while there are some people, who keep a distance from him as they consider him insane. At times, Joseph gets frustrated and aggressive by recalling his past, but his behavior and aggression is under control. The only reason behind such aggressive behavior was an immature attitude of society towards him.

Aggressive behavior is commonly found among people with intellectual disability. Crocker and Hodgins (42) mentioned research that documented high rates of aggressive behavior and violence. A model was developed by Gardner and Graeber (43) that suggested that aggressive behavior was determined by a number of factors including genetic disorders, personality traits, anti-social personality disorder or depression. When asked whether his family is happy to know about his work, he gave a positive gesture. He believed that his siblings are now giving him importance. He said

> "…I know XYZ consider me mental, but I have to adjust or else XYZ might take me out of the house and I have nowhere to go. I earn very little, but my family has now started giving me some importance and encourages me to sell and earn more."

According to Bedrosian and Prutting (44), research was conducted with four adults with an intellectual disability to analyze the communicative performances and social interactions. The results indicated that they were capable of expressing the same types of control as normal adults. In this particular case study, it was observed and realized that the social interaction of the respondent was limited; however the respondent was capable to express his views to trustworthy people.

He informed his fears of sharing his ideas with many people, because several times, he tried to ask people to help him getting a job, but the people just calmed him and made false promises. Once he approached a shop to sell his bottle, but the owner called him names, which abandoned him to further express his views.

The respondent was close to his father. He cried a lot when his father expired, because he felt all alone. Since the day his father died, he is insecure and lives a life full of fears and worries. In his opinion, although he has a family, no one can fill that alien feeling within him. He shared

> "…though I have my mother and siblings, but dad is dad. No one can fill that gap. I feel insecure about what would happen after my mother dies? Who will take care of me? I can do things on my own but I can't."

According to Blodgett (45), people with intellectual disability do have feelings and emotions, but they do not develop their emotional capacity to the same degree or with the same differentiation as do normal children. Throughout the discussions, I found him emotionally disturbed. His facial gestures were clear and supported his conversation, but at times, he was drowned in perplexity.

Begun (46) found that there was less bonding in the sibling relationship, when one had a disability. When inquired about his relations with siblings, he informed that he is close to his sister; however he is often ignored by his brothers. He also added that since his brothers are educated, they are given more privileges and favor from his family.

He asked me several flabbergast questions like, if a person can't read or write, should we tag them mental? If a person has a speech problem, does that mean that he is mental? Why do people keep a distance from me in society? Is it possible that I can earn more to become rich?

His questions were mature enough to ponder why he constructed such questions in his mind? Does that really mean that he is still confused about his status in society or is he dissatisfied with the kind of reaction he is getting from people?

Moral support was provided to him throughout the interviews. We also cherished happy moments. He informed about the most unfavorable incident that XYZ always calls him mental in front of others and his relatives also taunt him the same, that's why he keep himself detached from society as he fears experiencing the same from others.

The mentally challenged people face the same emotional challenges which other adults face, but don't always receive the same levels of attention and understanding from family members and caregivers. Their emotions and feelings are often overlooked. He said

> "I have emotions but when others call me MENTAL, it sometimes force me to commit suicide, because I can't tolerate such comments. It is more of an allegation than a gesture. No one cares for me. My feelings are baseless for everyone."

He attempted to commit suicide thrice in his life. The reason he gave me for taking such step was due to the pressure of society and restrictions from the family side. Once he tried to cut his hand; the second time he wanted to eat tablets, but was unable to eat them, while for third time, he tried to run away from home, but was caught red- handed.

Mulick et al. (47) mentioned that the research indicated that intellectual disability is frequently accompanied by personality disorder, notably problems of aggression. In this particular case anxiety, aggressive attitude and fear were observable during interactions with the respondent. I found him gloomy when he told me that he has not achieved anything in his life, which he wanted to achieve, that's why he had negative feelings about his life.

According to American Academy of Child and Adolescent Psychiatry [AACAP] (48), adolescents and young adults with intellectual disabilities may become depressed. They might not have enough language skills to express their feelings. In this case study, it was revealed that persons with mild Intellectual disability do have language skills to talk about their feelings, but are limited to share their views to everyone.

He was interested in knowing about my hobbies and education. When he learnt about my interest in playing piano and singing, he informed about his similar interest. He also sung a song for me. He loves to play piano and he is crazy about computers. Unfortunately, he cannot touch a computer at home as he is not allowed. He shared that he used the computer for the very first time at the age of 27 years, when the rehabilitation centre provided him with a platform to learn it for a few days. He wants to learn computers to prove others that he is not illiterate. Moreover, he wants to market his decorative bottles worldwide though the internet.

When asked about his social interaction with friends and community members, he informed me that no one is close to him in the community. He loves to live in isolation, because he has observed people keeping a distance with him. He shared that once he visited the Office of National Identity Card with his family members, where he was asked for the signature. The man on the counter rejected his signature and suggested him to print thumb on the paper and tagged him mental in front of others. This discrimination led him to think about his identity in this world.

Gresham and MacMillan (49) conducted an empirical research to examine the social competence (social skills, adaptive behavior, peer relationship) and affective functioning of children with mild disabilities. The review showed that children with mild disabilities had poorer social skills, exhibited more interfering problem behaviors, and were poorly accepted or rejected by peers.

Sigafoos et al. (50) viewed mentally challenged people as those with poorly socialized behavior that is expressed in a variety of ways, including aggression or conduct disorders. In this case, the respondent lacked social interactions and also exhibited mild behavior problem, mainly because of being rejected by society.

Joseph heard people calling him mental. He has seen parents keeping their children away from him. Moreover, he has observed and heard negative comments about his personality. Sometimes, children also make fun of him. He feels bad, when people reject him. He sits alone in religious service and keeps distance from the people. Joseph informed us that since he is labelled mental due to difficulties in physical and oral speech, he feels shame to face people, because people sometimes find it difficult to understand him.

A study was conducted by the Institute of Psychiatry (51), where adolescents and young adults with intellectual disability, together with children without disability were individually matched for verbal mental age, given tasks to understand their comprehension about emotions. The results suggested that individuals with intellectual disability may have specific deficits in recognizing how bodily expressions of emotion are coordinated with each other. This case study proofed that people with mild intellectual disability are emotionally expressive. A similar pattern of activity was conducted. Throughout the activity, he performed well and there was no specific deficit in recognizing bodily expressions of emotions.

He informed me that his future plan was to sell more decorative bottles and wants to earn his living by starting his business on a national and international platform. He repeatedly asked for moral support.

Several questions were asked to assess the feelings and emotions, situation tackling capabilities, intelligence, besides knowing how people with mild intellectual disability respond at different situations. The gathered answers were quiet mature. He shared that he feels happy, when he earns money, but wants people not call him mental. He considers the world as a place of living for rude people, but he never hates human beings. He is willing to help his family members in the future, but he wants to demagnetize himself from the other people. He keeps his savings in the bank as he is well aware about the risk of keeping money at home. He provides financial support to his mother and also buys her dresses from his own earning. He does not want to begin his own family, because people consider him mental and that label has emotionally disturbed him, besides all his other social barriers. He expressed his wish to travel by plane. He expressed his insecurity as he has fears that no one would keep him after the death of his mother. Whenever he feels loneliness, he watches TV. Once he fought with someone as he was unable to control his temper over intolerable situation. He knows basics of first aid and knows how to tackle different situations. He considers his life as a precious gift from the Creator, but often curse his fate. He keeps himself up-to-date about world affairs and replied to all general IQ answers correctly. He also understands the sensitive terms like terrorism. He recalls all the phone numbers, dates, times and performed well in the calculation test. Few general knowledge questions were also asked like: who the current president of the United States is and what is the capital of India? He replied correct to most of the questions. Many objects were exposed to him and he successfully identified objects through names. When a task was given to compare things, he chose respect over disrespect, love over scold, family over world, love over hate, peace over war, sister over brothers, money over poverty, money over friendship, and opted for an airplane ride over a bus ride.

CONCLUSION

In this presented case, a male person with a mild intellectual disability showed expressive, cooperative, supportive, kind-hearted, intelligent and understandable behavior. He was peace loving and evaluated things closely. He had no specific deficit in recognizing bodily expressions of emotions; however, he was somewhat emotionally disturbed and insecure about the future and life. He lacked social interactions and also exhibited mild behavior problems, mainly because of being rejected by society. Anxiety, mood swings and fear were observable. He had minor communication and physical movement problems, but his expressions were mature.

He wanted to lead a normal life and wanted to experience different moments of joy. He had positive views about his family, but negative feelings from the local society and for his own life. He dreams like us, but with some limitations. He wants motivation and support from society and wants the world to accept him with an open arm. This case study taught us to correct our behavior towards all mentally challenged people. To change their views about us, we must socialize with them and value their opinions. Parents should never underestimate their emotions. Parents should love and provide them support to follow their dreams. At the same time, we must avoid rude remarks and stop labelling them mental. They are like any other human being and nothing is different about them. They need courage and moral support to face the world and reality. They are willing to share their experiences with us, but they need time to correct our attitudes towards them. They should get opportunities to turn their dreams into realities for which awareness is the most powerful tool to integrate them into society.

REFERENCES

[1]   Schalock RL, Borthwick-Duffy SA, Bradley VJ, Buntinx WHE, Coulter DL, Craig EM, et al. Intellectual disability: Definition, classification, and systems of supports, 11th ed. Washington, DC: American Association Intellectual Developmental Disabilities, 2010.

[2]   Manjunatha KR, Chetan GK, Arathi R, Bhaskara GV, Latha P, Padma S, et al. Frequency, association and genetic implications of chromosomal fragile sites in mental retardation. Int J Health Geogr 2002;2:33-9.

[3]   Donna K, Holly H, Grace E. Identification and evaluation of mental retardation. Am Fam Physician 2000;61(4):1059-67.

[4]   Smith C, Strick L, eds. Learning disabilities: A to Z: A parent's complete guide to learning disabilities from preschool to adulthood. New York: Simon Schuster, 1999.

[5]   Pelegano JP, Healy A. Mental retardation Part II- Seeing the child within. Fam Pract Recertification 1992;14:58-71.

[6]   Daily DK, Ardinger HH, Holmes GE. Identification and evaluation of mental retardation. Am Fam Physician 2000;61(4):1059-67.

[7]   Bertelli M, Scuticchio D, Ferrandi A, Lassi S, Mango F, Ciavatta C, et al.

[8]   Reliability and validity of the SPAID-G checklist for detecting psychiatric disorders in adults with intellectual disability. Res Dev Disabil 2012;33(2):382-90.

[9]   Webster TG. Problems of emotional development in young retarded children. Am J Psychiatry 1963;20(1):37-43.

[10]   Chess S. Emotional problems in mentally retarded children. In: Menolascino FJ, ed. Psychiatric approaches to mental retardation. New York: Basic Books, 1970:55–67.

[11]   Menolascino FJ, Bernstein NR. Psychiatric assessment of the mentally retarded child. In: Bernstein NR, ed. Diminished people. Boston: Little Brown, 1970:201-22.

[12]   Phillips I, Williams N. Psychopathology: A study of 100 children. Am J Psychiatr 1975;132:1265-73.

[13]   Scheerenberger RC. A history of mental retardation: A quarter century of promise. Baltimore: Paul Brookes, 1987.

[14]   Daily DK, Ardinger HH, Holmes GE. Identification and evaluation of mental retardation. Am Fam Physician 2000;61(4):1059-67.

[15]   Mental retardation. Human diseases and conditions. Accessed 2012 Jan 01. URL: http://www.humanillnesses.com/Behavioral-Health-Fe-Mu/Mental-Retardation.html

[16]   Taylor AR, Asher SR, Williams GA. The social adaptation of mainstreamed mildly retarded children. Child Dev 1987;58:1321-34.

[17]   Zigler E, Burack JA. Personality development and the dually diagnosed person. Res Dev Disabil 1989;10:225-40.

[18]   Eaton LF, Menolascino FJ. Psychiatric disorders in the mentally retarded: types, problems, and challenges. Am J Psychiatry 1982;139: 1297-1303.

[19]   Reynolds T, Dombeck M. Mental retardation (intellectual disabilities). Accessed 2012 Jan 01. URL: http://www.mentalhelp.net/poc/view_doc

[20]   Olley JG. Mental retardation. Nature, cause and development. Philadelphia, PA: Brunner Mazel, 1999.

[21]   Kumar I, Singh AR, Akhtar S. Social development of children with mental retardation. Ind Psychiatry J 2009;18:56-59.

[22]   Kasari C, Bauminger N. Social and emotional development in children with mental retardation. In: Burack JA, Hodapp RM, Zigler E, eds. Handbook of mental retardation and development. Cambridge: University of Cambridge, 1998.

[23]   Hamel J, Dufour S, Fortin D. Case study methods. Newbury Park, CA: Sage, 1993.

[24]   Merriam SB. Qualitative research and case study applications in education. San Francisco: Jossey-Bass, 1998.

[25]   Stake R. The art of case research. Thousand Oaks, CA: Sage, 1995.

[26]   Feagin J, Orum A, Sjoberg G, eds. A case for case study. Chapel Hill, NC: University North Carolina Press, 1991.

[27]   Clifford G. Thick description: Toward an interpretive theory of culture. In: Clifford G, ed. The interpretation of cultures: Selected essays. New York: Basic Books, 1973:3-30.

[28]   Yin RK. Case study research: Design and methods. Newbury Park, CA: Sage, 1984.

[29]   Crabtree BF, Miller WL. Doing qualitative research, 2nd ed. Thousand Oaks, CA: Sage, 1999.

[30]   Lather P. Critical frames in educational research: Feminist and post-structural perspectives. Theory Pract 1992;31(2):87-99.

[31]   Robottom I, Hart P. Research in environmental education: Engaging the debate. Australia: Deakin University Press, 1993.

[32]   Yin RK. Case study research: Design and methods, 3rd ed. Thousand Oaks, CA: Sage, 2003.

[33]   Alvarez M, Binkley E, Bivens J, Highers P, Poole C, Walker P. Case-based instruction and learning: An interdisciplinary project. Proceedings 34th Annual Conference, College Reading Association, 1990:2-18.

[34]   Field PA, Morse JM. Nursing research. The application of qualitative approaches. London: Chapman Hall, 1992.

[35]   Munhall P. Ethical considerations in qualitative research. Western J Nurs Res 1988;10(2):150-62.

[36]   Lincoln YS, Guba EG. Naturalistic inquiry. Newbury Park, CA: Sage, 1985.

[37]   Spradlin JE. (1963). Language and communication of mental defectives. In Ellis, N. R. (Ed.) Handbook of mental deficiency. New York: McGraw-Hill, 1963.

[38]   Dunn LM. Exceptional children in the schools: Special education in transition. New York: Holt Rinehart Winston, 1973.

[39]   Krik SA, Gallagher JJ. Educating exceptional children, 3rd ed. Boston: Houghton Mifflin, 1979.

[40]   Marston GM, Perry DW, Roy A. Manifestations of depression in people with intellectual disability. J Intellect Disabil Res 1997;41:476–80.

[41]   Mikkelsen E. Is psychotherapy useful for the mentally retarded? Harvard Mental Health Letter 1994;11(2):8.

[42]   Turkington C, Harris J. The encyclopedia of the brain and brain disorders, 3rd ed. New York: Infobase, 2002

[43]   Crocker AG, Hodgins S. The criminality of noninstitutionalized mentally retarded persons. Evidence from a birth cohort followed to age 30. Criminal Justice Behav 1997;24(4):432-54.

[44]   Gardner WI, Graeber JL. Treatment of severe behavioral disorders in persons with mental retardation: A multimodal behavioral treatment model. In: Fletcher R, Dosen A, eds. Mental health aspects of mental retardation. New York: Lexington Books, 1993.

[45]   Bedrosian JL, Prutting C. Communicative performance of mentally retarded adults in four conversational settings. J Speech Hearing Res 1978;21:79-95.

[46]   Blodgett HE. Mentally retarded children. What parents and others should know. Minnesota: University Minnesota, 1971.

[47]   Begun AL. Sibling relationships involving developmentally disabled people. Am J Ment Retard 1989;93: 566–574.

[48]   Mulick JA, Hammer D, Dura JR. Assessment and management of antisocial and hyperactive behavior. In: Matson JL, Mulick JA, eds. Handbook of mental retardation. New York: Pergamon Press, 1991.

[49]   AACAP. Children who are mentally retarded. Washington, DC: American Academy Child Adolescent Psychiatry, 2004.

[50]   Gresham FM, MacMillan DL. Social competence and affective characteristics of students with mild disabilities. Rev Educ Res 1997;67(4):377-415.

[51]   Sigafoos J, Elkins J, Kerr M, Attwood T. A survey of aggressive behaviour among a population of persons with intellectual disability in Queensland. J Intellect Disabil Res 1994;38(4):369-81.

[52]   Hobson RP, Ouston J, Lee A. Recognition of emotion by mentally retarded adolescents and young adults. Am J Ment Retard 1989;93(4): 434-43.

In: Disability and Chronic Disease
Editors: J. Merrick, S. Aspler and M. Morad

ISBN: 978-1-62948-288-0
© 2014 Nova Science Publishers, Inc.

Chapter 5

THE THERAPEUTIC INTERVENTIONS IN CEREBRAL PALSY

Helayne Feferman, MPH, BS[1], Janell Harro, BS[1],
Dilip R Patel, MD[1]*
and Joav Merrick, MD, MMedSci, DMSc[2,3,4,5]

[1]Department of Pediatrics and Adolescent Medicine,
Western Michigan University School of Medicine, Kalamazoo,
Michigan, US
[2]National Institute of Child Health and Human Development, Jerusalem
[3]Office of the Medical Director, Health Services,
Division for Intellectual and Developmental Disabilities,
inistry of Social Affairs and Social Services, Jerusalem
[4]Division of Pediatrics, Hadassah Hebrew University Medical Center,
Mt Scopus Campus, Jerusalem, Israel
[5]Kentucky Children's Hospital, University of Kentucky College of Medicine,
Lexington, Kentucky, US

ABSTRACT

Various other philosophies or approaches of treatment have been advocated for children with cerebral palsy. Many such interventions are based on personal observations and their usefulness has not been clearly established by well controlled studies, while many have supporting evidence for their application in the treatment of cerebral palsy. This chapter provides an overview of salient aspects of neurodevelopmental treatment, sensory integration, electrical stimulation, body-weight support treadmill training, conductive education, patterning, constraint-induced therapy, hippotherapy, hyperbaric oxygen therapy, acupuncture, Vojta method, gait training and dorsal rhizotomy.

* Correspondence: Professor Dilip R Patel, MD, Department of Pediatric and Adolescent Medicine, Western Michigan University School of Medicine, 1000 Oakland Drive, D48G, Kalamazoo, MI 49008-1284, United States. E-mail dilip.patel@med.wmich.edu.

INTRODUCTION

Management of children with cerebral palsy (CP) requires an interdisciplinary approach that draws on the expertise of many specialists in different disciplines (1-3). Numerous therapeutic interventions, including non-traditional or complementary and alternative medicine are used widely by families and professionals alike for their children with cerebral palsy (4-6). Early intervention, interdisciplinary team approach, and family focused intervention strategies are essential. Traditional physiotherapy and occupational therapy have been shown to be efficacious in improving functional capabilities of children with cerebral palsy. Although not within the scope of this article, other essential and integral components of management of children with CP include: braces, appliances, orthotics, various orthopedic interventions, speech and language therapy, treatment of spasticity, and general medical management of various associated problems (1-3).

PHYSIOTHERAPY

Traditional physiotherapy used in children with cerebral palsy (CP) has been shown to improve muscle strength, local muscular endurance, and overall joint range of motion (2, 6, 7). Physiotherapy is routinely used as part of an interdisciplinary treatment approach for children with CP, who are school aged and above, because of the need for certain degree of cooperation and active participation on the part of the child (7, 8). A program of progressive resistive exercises is used to improve muscle strength (3, 9). A program that uses low resistance and more repetitions will enhance local muscular endurance. The physical therapist carries out repetitive passive range of motion exercises to improve and maintain joint mobility. Passive, static, gentle stretches are performed on individual joints to decrease and prevent joint contractures. Such stretches should be performed within a pain free joint range of motion. The physical therapist, working with the orthopedic surgeon and orthotist also assists in designing and implementing exercises to improve balance, posture control, gait, mobility, and ability to transfer (for instance from bed to wheel chair).

OCCUPATIONAL THERAPY

Occupational therapy is a recommended component of an interdisciplinary team approach to the treatment of children with CP (10, 11). Occupational therapist (OT) works with children with CP in improving fine motor abilities, especially the use of upper extremity in performing activities of daily living. OT has been shown to be effective in improving and maintaining adaptive fine motor activities of children with CP. In addition to focusing on specific fine motor movements, the OT also works on organizing play areas, providing adaptive equipment for self care and learning, and to modify the learning environment to facilitate attention and information processing.

NEURODEVELOPMENTAL TRAINING (NDT)

This therapeutic approach was developed by Berta (1907-1991 and Karel Bobath (1906-1991) in the 1940s, based on their personal observations working with children with cerebral palsy (6, 12). It is one of the more popular therapeutic interventions for the treatment of children with CP. There are thousands of trained therapists all over the world using this approach, who are trained at various NDT training centers and NDT courses (6). The basis of NDT approach as conceptualized by Bobaths is that the motor abnormalities in children with CP are due to failure of normal development of postural control and reflexes because of the underlying dysfunction of the central nervous system (4, 12). The aim of the NDT approach is to facilitate normal motor development and function and to prevent development of secondary impairments due to muscle contractures and joint and limb deformities.

Originally, the Bobath approach used various techniques to inhibit and control abnormal tone, reflexes and movement patterns (12). This was postulated to facilitate normal postural and righting reflexes, and movement patterns. The normal developmental sequence of child development is used as the underlying guiding principle. It was postulated that such normal therapeutic experience in automatic movements and reflexes will translate into the child developing normal tone and volitional movements with improved functional capabilities. With further experience, the Bobaths noted that there was a lack of such carry over effects, and modified their approach so as to allow the child to take over more control of balance and movement, treat children in natural play environments, and not necessarily to follow rigid developmental sequence.

There is a wide variation in the expertise and training of therapists who use NDT approach with various modifications (6). There is also significant differences in the NDT application in different countries. Typically most sessions are of one hour duration each, and given at least two times per week (12). Intensive NDT has been practiced by some with one hour per day for five days per week and reported to be more effective (13). The parents and caregivers are also trained to continue the therapy at home during daily activities and play. Various therapeutic aides such as orthotics, and balls are used as necessary. NDT approach takes long term view recognizing the need for continued intervention to maintain functional capabilities and prevent deformities and contractures. Although the effectiveness of NDT in CP has been questioned by some published reports, there are some studies suggesting its effectiveness (4, 7, 12, 13).

SENSORY INTEGRATION (SI)

The theory of sensory integration was originally developed by Anna Jean Ayres (1920-1989) in the 1970s (14). The principles of SI theory are used by occupational therapists in developing treatment approaches for children with sensory processing difficulties, including CP. As conceived by Ayres, the SI model was developed to treat learning disabilities. SI theory is based on the hypothesis that in order to develop and execute a normal adaptive behavioral response, the child must be able to optimally receive, modulate, integrate, and process the sensory information (14, 15). Many children with learning disabilities, cerebral palsy and other neurodevelopmental disabilities have associated sensory difficulties. The SI approach attempts to facilitate the normal development and improve the child's ability to process and integrate sensory information (visual, perceptual, proprioceptive, auditory, etc.) (14). It is proposed that this will allow improved functional capabilities in daily life activities.

As originally described by Ayres, the objective of SI approach is not to teach specific skills but "to enhance the brain's capacities to perceive, remember, and motor plan" (14). A therapeutic environment is created in which the child gains rich sensory motor experience. The therapist engages the child in challenging play activities in such a way, that the child is able to overcome the challenge, and adapts to subsequently face more challenging stimulus (14, 15). The therapist takes cues from child's behavior and provides appropriate sensory rich play environment.

The occupational therapist works closely with other members of the interdisciplinary team, so that an appropriately challenging sensory-motor experience can be provided for the child in daily life settings, and functional capabilities can be monitored.

Three classic patterns of SI disorders have been proposed, namely, sensory modulation disorders, sensory discrimination disorders, and sensory based motor disorders (14). Such grouping is intended to guide formulation of specific intervention for homogeneous disorders. Overall some studies find SI as a useful treatment approach in children with CP while others do not find any functional benefit (14, 15).

ELECTRICAL STIMULATION

The goal of the electrical stimulation is to increase muscle strength and motor function. Electrical stimulation is provided by TENS (transcutaneous electrical nerve stimulation) unit, which is portable, non-invasive and can be used in the home setting by parents or the patient (16).

Neuromuscular electrical stimulation (NMES) involves application of transcutaneous electrical current that results in muscle contraction (16). NMES has been postulated to increase muscle strength by increasing the cross-sectional area of the muscle and by increased recruitment of type 2 muscle fibers. Functional electrical stimulation (FES) refers to the application of electrical stimulation during a given task or activity when a specific muscle is expected to be contracting (16, 17).

Threshold electrical stimulation (TES) is also applied transcutaneously, is of low intensity, and does not elicit actual muscle contraction. TES is supposed to act by increasing the muscle blood flow and bulk (16, 18).

Typically the electrical stimulation is used in children older than 4-5 years old with diplegic or hemiplegic CP. Each session of NMES typically lasts from 15 to 30 minutes, with varying frequencies of half hour to up to 21 hours per week, for duration that ranges from 1 month to 1 year (17). Electrical stimulation is typically used for lower extremity muscles. TES is generally give for 8-12 hours during sleep at home, and used for up to 1 year (17, 18).

There is evidence to support the use and effectiveness of NMES in children with CP. However, studies are limited by many confounding variables including concomitant use of other therapies, wide variation in methods of application, heterogeneity of subjects, difficulty in measuring functional outcomes and lack of control subjects.

BODY WEIGHT SUPPORT TREADMILL TRAINING

Stepping movements (or reflex stepping reactions) are normally present in newborns and infants, before the infant starts to bear weight, stand and walk (8). In treadmill training, the child is supported in a harness on the treadmill in an upright posture limiting weight bearing (8, 19, 20). The child then attempts to walk on the slowly moving treadmill eliciting the stepping movements. Treadmill training, thus allows development of stepping movements needed for ambulation. Studies using 3-4 sessions per week lasting for 3-4 months have shown improvement in lower extremity movements and gait patterns in children with cerebral palsy (8, 20, 21).

CONDUCTIVE EDUCATION

CE was developed by András Pető (1893-1967) in the 1940s (4, 6). It is based on the concept that children with motor disabilities learn the same way as those with no disability (22). CE is carried out by trained "conductors" who use repeated verbal reinforcement to promote and facilitate intended motor activity by the child (6, 22). Participation in CE requires reasonable cognitive abilities to comprehend the verbal instructions. The idea is to develop independence in daily activities by the child by facilitating all aspects of child's development. The child is encouraged to participate and practice all daily activities to the best of his or her abilities (22, 23). CE is typically carried out in separate group sessions for school age children. The effectiveness of CE in improving functional capabilities of children with CP has not been established by any controlled clinical trials (4, 6, 22, 23).

PATTERNING

The concept of patterning is based on theories developed by Fay, Delacato, and Doman in the 1950s and 1960s (6). Patterning is based on the principle that typical development of the infant and child progresses through a well established, pre-determined sequence; and failure to normally complete one stage of development therefore impairs or inhibits the development of the subsequent stage (4, 6, 24).

It was hypothesized that typical motor development can be facilitated in the brain injured children by passively repeating the sequential steps of typical development, a process called patterning (4, 6). Parents and other care givers are taught to carry out patterning at home. This approach is labor intensive and time consuming as it requires multiple sessions every day. Effectiveness of patterning has not been established and its use in children with CP is not recommended (24).

CONSTRAINT-INDUCED THERAPY

Constraint-induced therapy is used to improve the use of affected upper extremity in a child with hemiplegic CP (8, 25, 26). The normally functioning or stronger upper extremity is immobilized for a variable duration in order to force the use of the affected or weaker upper extremity over time. The efficacy of this approach has not been established, and adverse effects of prolonged immobilization of the normally developing upper extremity are a significant concern (8, 25, 26).

HIPPOTHERAPY

Therapeutic horse-back riding has been shown to improve muscle tone, balance, and postural control in children with CP (27, 28, 29, 30). Children with CP enjoy horse riding and it also provides a setting for increased social interaction and psychosocial development.

HYPERBARIC OXYGEN THERAPY

Use of hyperbaric oxygen therapy (HBOT) in children with CP is based on the hypothesis that HBOT will increase the oxygen available to the neurons surrounding the injured area of the brain and revive these dormant neurons (4, 31, 32). Additionally, HBOT is postulated to decrease brain edema by inducing cerebral vasoconstriction. Typically, HBOT is administered at 1.75 atmospheres pressure, each session lasing about an hour, given 1-2 time per day for 5-6 days per week, initially for 40 treatments (4, 6, 31, 32).

Potential complications of HBOT include ear pain, bleeding from ears, tympanic membrane perforation, myopia, pneumothorax, and seizures (1, 32). At present there is insufficient evidence to determine whether the use of HBOT improves the functional outcome of children with CP (32).

ACUPUNCTURE

Acupuncture has been used in children with CP for over two decades. There is some evidence that acupuncture may be of benefit in some children with CP to reduce painful muscle spasms and overall motor function (4, 33, 34).

VOJTA METHOD

Vojta approach is based on the observation that children with CP exhibit many of the reflexes seen in normal newborns (4, 6, 8). According to Václav Vojta (1917-2000), the persistence of these newborn reflex patterns in a child with CP interferes with postural development. It is postulated that with appropriate stimulation, the newborn reflex pattern can be provoked and activated in a child with CP, thereby facilitating the development of reflex locomotion (4, 6). No controlled studies are available supporting Vojta approach in the treatment of children with CP (4, 6, 7, 8,).

LOCOMOTOR GAIT TRAINING

The methods behind locomotor gait training are based off of the promising treatment option of treadmill training, mentioned above. The difficulty with treadmill training was the physical strain and amount of labor time needed by physical therapists, and therefore locomotor gait training was implemented. Locomotor gait training involves a robotic-assisted device that is placed on the treadmill and can be easily installed and removed. The device harnesses the patient appropriately and uses levers and a uniform stride length to simulate normal gait (35, 36). The eventual goal of the machine is to restore independent, normal gait and walking ability. In randomized control trials, locomotor gait training has been shown to have a lasting improvement in gait velocity, spatiotemporal station, and endurance in CP patients, as compared to control participants (36).

VIDEO GAIT ANALYSIS OR 3-D GAIT ANALYIS

Video Gait Analysis provides an informative method in the analysis of gait in cerebral palsy patients. Markers are applied to bony landmarks of the patient, and cameras and computers calculate the trajectory of those landmarks. This makes it possible to observe a pathological gait in a cerebral palsy patient. Additionally, most gait analysis laboratories have transducers in the floors that can measure the amount of pressure being distributed when the patient walks. The use of this information gives insight into which muscle groups are being used in the patient's gait. The ultimate outcome of this technology is the interventions that can be performed based on this information (42, 43). Options for the treatment of cerebral palsy include muscle lengthening, Botox injection into spastic muscle groups, and attachment or detachment of certain muscle tendons.

DORSAL RHIZOTOMY

Selective dorsal rhizotomy (SDR) is a surgical procedure used to limit the amount of spasticity in children with neuromuscular conditions, namely spastic diplegia and spastic forms of cerebral palsy. The procedure hopefully eliminates the halt in motor skill development, and alleviates orthopedic complications (38). At the time of the operation, the patient lies flat down while the neurosurgeon separates out groups of 3-5 afferent nerve rootlets of the spinal cord and stimulates them. The muscle responses are recorded via electromyography (EMG) and nerves causing muscle spasticity are selectively cut. This reduces the amount of abnormal activity resulting from the spinal cord, and hopefully reduces spasticity, improves mobility and function in selected patients (37, 39).

Studies indicate that there is a concordance between age and SDR procedure. It was found that the younger the patient when receiving the procedure, the better the outcome in reducing spasticity and improved function. In another study, SDR showed significant improvement in reduction in tone, quality of gait, stride length, and gait velocity (37-39).

STEM CELL THERAPY

The idea of stem cell therapy in infants born with cerebral palsy has had increasing potential over the past years due to the rising survival of premature infants born with the chronic motor disability. The majority of hypoxemia in cerebral palsy patients occurs in the oligodendrocyte cell-line, as well as the cerebral white matter. It has been proposed to inject this cell line into the vasculature of cerebral palsy patients or infants who have suffered neonatal hypoxic ischemia. There are currently no controlled trials of stem cell therapy in cerebral palsy patients, and only a few in neurologically disabled patients; however, there are studies of the therapy being done in stroke-induced animals. In expert opinion, however, the use of stem cell therapy in chronic brain injury is not well enough understood, and more animal trials and translational controlled human trials must be completed (40, 41).

CONCLUSION

Management of children and adults with cerebral palsy requires a team based approach that draws on the expertise of professionals in different disciplines. Use of braces, appliances, orthotics and other orthopedic interventions are well supported and accepted interventions for the treatment of musculoskeletal complications of cerebral palsy. Other treatment modalities with wide acceptability include speech and language therapy, pharmacologic treatment of spasticity, and general medical management of associated or secondary medical conditions. Many other interventions have minimal or equivocal supporting evidence and are used with a wide variability. Some of these include sensory intergration, conductive education, patterning, constraint-induced therapy, and Vojta method. Some newer approaches being explored include gait training and stem cell therapy.

ACKNOWLEDGMENT

Sections of this article are partly adapted and updated from author's previous work: Patel DR. Therapeutic interventions in the treatment of children with cerebral palsy. Indian J Pediatr 2005;72(11):979-83.

REFERENCES

[1] Koman LA, Smith BP, Shilt JS: Cerebral palsy. Lancet 2004;363:1619-31.
[2] Singhi PD: Cerebral palsy management. Indian J Pediatr 2004;71(7):635-9.
[3] Mathews DJ, Wilson P. Cerebral palsy, In: Monnar G, Alexander MA, eds. Pediatric rehabilitation, 3rd edition. Philadelphia, PA: Hanley Belfus, 1999:193-218.
[4] Liptak GS: Complementary and alternative therapies for cerebral palsy. Ment Retard Dev Disabil Res Rev 2005;11:156-63.
[5] Hurvitz EA, Leonard C, Ayyangar R, et al: Complementary and alternative medicine use in families of children with CP. Dev Med Child Neurol 2003;45:364-70.

[6]   Mayston M. Physiotherapy management in cerebral palsy: an update on treatment approaches. Clin Dev Med 2004;161:147-60.

[7]   Taggart P, Aguilar C: Therapeutic exercise. In: Monnar G, Alexander MA, eds. Pediatric rehabilitation, 3rd edition. Philadelphia, PA: Hanley Belfus, 1999:125-38.

[8]   Stanger M, Oresic S. Rehabilitation approaches for children with cerebral palsy: overview. J Child Neurol 2003;18:S79-S88.

[9]   Dodd KJ, Taylor NF, Damiano DL: A systematic review of the effectiveness of strength-training programs for people with cerebral palsy. Arch Phys Med Rehabil 2002;83:1157-64.

[10]   Palisano RJ, Snider LM, Orlin MN: Recent advances in physical and occupational therapy for children with cerebral palsy. Seminars Pediatri Neurol 2004;11(1):66-77.

[11]   Steultjens EM, Dekker J, Boulter LM, et al: Occupational therapy for children with cerebral palsy: a systematic review. Clin Rehabil 2004;18:1-14.

[12]   Butler C, Darrah J: Effects of neurodevelopmental treatment (NDT) for cerebral palsy: an AACPDM evidence report. Dev Med Child Neurol 2001;43:778-90.

[13]   Tsorlakis N, Evaggelinou C, Grouios G, Tsorbatzoudis C: Effect of intensive neurodevelopmental treatment in gross motor function of children with cerebral palsy. Dev Med Child Neurol 2004;46:740-5.

[14]   Schaaf R, Miller LJ: Occupational therapy using a sensory integrative approach for children with developmental disabilities. Ment Retard Dev Disabil Res Rev 2005;11:143-8.

[15]   Vargas S, Camilli G: A meta-analysis of research on sensory integration treatment. Am J Occup Ther 1999;53:189-98.

[16]   Kerr C, McDowell B, McDonough S: Electrical stimulation in cerebral palsy: a review of effects on strength and motor function. Dev Med Child Neurol 2004;46:205-13.

[17]   Johnston TE, Finson RL, McCarthy JJ, et al: Use of functional electrical stimulation to augment tradtitional orhopaedic surgery in children with CP. J Pediatr Orthop 2004;24:283-91.

[18]   Dali C, Hansen FJ, Pedersen SA, et al: Threshold electrical stimulation in ambulant children with CP: A randomized double-blind placebo-controlled clinical trial. Dev Med Child Neurol 2002;44:364-9.

[19]   Thelan E: Treadmill-elicited stepping in seven month old infants. Child Dev 1986;57:1498-1506.

[20]   Schindl MR, Forstner C, Kern H, et al: Treadmill training with partial body weight support in nonambulatory patients with cerebral palsy. Arch Phys Med Rehabil 2000;81:301-6.

[21]   Richards CL, Malouin F, Dumas F, et al: Early and intensive treadmill locomotor training for young children with cerebral palsy: A feasibility study. Pediatr Phys Ther 1997;9:158-65.

[22]   Darrah J, Watkins B, Chen L, et al: Conductive education intervention for children with CP: An AACPDM evidence report. Dev Med Child Neurol 2004;46:187-203.

[23]   Reddihough DS, King J, Coleman G, et al: Efficacy of programmes based on conductive education for young children with cerebral palsy. Dev Med Child Neurol 1998;40:763-70.

[24]   American Academy of Pediatrics: Committee on Children with Disabilities. The treatment of neurologically impaired children using patterning. Pediatrics 1999;104:1149-51.

[25]   Willis JK, Maello A, Rice JL, el: Forced use treatment of childhood hemiparesis. Pediatrics 2002;110:94-6.

[26]   Echols K, DeLuca SC, Ramey SL, et al: Constraint-induced movement therapy versus traditional therapy services for young children with CP. Dev Med Child Neurolo Suppl 2002;91:44.

[27]   Meregillano G: Hippotherapy. Phys Med Rehabil Clin N Am 2004;15(4):843-54.

[28]   Cherng R, Liao H, Leung HWC, et al: The effectiveness of therapeutic horseback riding in children with spastic CP. Adapt Phys Activ Q 2004;21:103-21.

[29]   Casady RL, Nichols-Larsen DS: The effectiveness of hippotherapy on ten children with CP. Pediatr Phys Ther 2004;16:165-72.

[30]   Benda W, McGibbon NH, Grant KL: Improvements in muscle symmetry in children with CP after equine-assisted hippotherapy. J Altern Complement Med 2003;9:817-25.

[31]   Collet JP, Vanasse M, Marois P, et al: Hyperbaric oxygen for children with CP: A randomized multicentre trial. HBO-CP Research Group. Lancet 2001;357:582-6.

[32]   McDonagh M, Carson S, Ash J, et al: Hyperbaric oxygen therapy for brain injury, cerebral palsy, and stroke. Evid Rep Technol Assess (Summ). 2003;85:1-6.

[33]   Kaptchuk TJ: Acupuncture: Theory, efficacy, and practice. Ann Intern Med 2002;136:374-83.

[34]   Shi B, Bu H, Lin L: A clinical study on acupuncture treatment of pediatric CP. J Tradit Chin Med 1992;12:45-51.

[35]   Freivogel S, Schmalohr D, Mehrholz J. Improved walking ability and reduced therapeutic stress with an electromechanical gait device. J Rehabil Med 2009;41(9):734-9.

[36]   Smania N, Bonetti P, Gandolfi M, Cosentino A, Waldner A, Hesse S, Werner C, Bisoffi G, Geroin C, Munari D. Improved gait after repetitive locomotor training in children with cerebral palsy. Am J Phys Med Rehabil 2011 Feb;90(2):137-49.

[37]   Illum NO, Torp-Pedersen L, Midholm S, Selmar PE, Simesen K. Rhizotomy for children with severe spastic cerebral palsy. Ugeskr Laeger 2006;168(8):785-9. [Danish]

[38]   Oki A, Oberg W, Siebert B, Plante D, Walker ML, Gooch JL. Selective dorsal rhizotomy in children with spastic hemiparesis. J Neurosurg Pediatr 2010;6(4):353-8.

[39]   Hodgkinson I, Bérard C, Jindrich ML, Sindou M, Mertens P, Bérard J. Selective dorsal rhizotomy in children with cerebral palsy. Results in 18 cases at one year postoperatively. Stereotact Funct Neurosurg 1997;69(1-4 Pt 2):259-67.

[40]   Carroll, James E., Mays, Robert W. Update on stem cell therapy for cerebral palsy. Expert Opin Biol Ther 2011;11(4):463-71.

[41]   Bartley J, Carroll JE. Stem cell therapy for cerebral palsy. Expert Opin Biol Ther. 2003;3(4):541-9.

[42]   Harvey A, Gorter JW. Video gait analysis for ambulatory children with cerebral palsy: Why, when, where and how! Gait Posture 2011;33(3):501-3.

[43]   Dobson F, Morris ME, Baker R, Graham HK. Gait classification in children with cerebral palsy: a systematic review. Gait Posture 2007;25(1):140-52.

In: Disability and Chronic Disease
Editors: J. Merrick, S. Aspler and M. Morad

ISBN: 978-1-62948-288-0
© 2014 Nova Science Publishers, Inc.

Chapter 6

USING VML (VERBAL MOTOR LEARNING) METHOD TECHNIQUES IN TREATMENT OF PROSODY DISORDER DUE TO CHILDHOOD APRAXIA OF SPEECH

*Elad Vashdi, BPT, MPE, DPT**
Yael Center, Aloney Aba, Israel

ABSTRACT

Childhood apraxia of speech (CAS) is a motor deficit phenomenon that affects the child's ability to communicate verbally with his environment and has a wide spectrum of classifications. One of these classifications is a prosody deficit which has a pragmatic manifestation. In this case study we examine the influence of a manual VML techniques on prosody. In this chapter the subject is a 14 years old teenager diagnosed with severe CAS and limb apraxia. The subject was treated for years for prosody with no success. We applied a new manual technique as an experiment for a month involving daily sessions. Results showed reduced volume, differentiation between high and low pitch and improved control over word lengths. This is one step in creating a wide inventory of manual techniques to treat prosody among CAS patients.

INTRODUCTION

Communication among people can be expressed in several ways such as through written correspondence, body language picture exchange or visual signals. However, the most powerful communication tool is speech which is unique to humans. Speech is build from verbal structures such as words and sentences and from non verbal structures. A non-verbal communicative element of speech is the intonation which is produced by a combination of Vocal cord frequency, duration and intensity (1). Intonation is an ability that a child starts to control and develop in the first year of his life. This case study will describe the absence of

---
* Correspondence: Vashdi Elad, BPT, MPE, DPT, Yael Center, POBox 197, Aloney Aba, Israel. E-mail: Center@yaelcenter.com.

intonation control in a child with childhood apraxia of speech (CAS) and a VML intervention for intonation control and prosody.

The origin of CAS is debated. Researchers have several approaches to CAS that lead to different treatment approaches (2). There are the motor control models and the psycholinguistic theories (3) that try to define the disorder. The ASHA committee (4) defines CAS as "A neurological childhood (pediatric) speech sound disorder in which the precision and consistency of movements underlying speech are impaired in the absence of neuromuscular deficits (e.g., abnormal reflexes, abnormal tone)". CAS may occur as a result of a known neurological impairment, in association with complex neurobehavioral disorders of known or unknown origin, or as an idiopathic neurogenic speech sound disorder. The core impairment in planning and/or programming spatiotemporal parameters of movement sequences results in errors in speech sound production and prosody.

One of the diagnostic markers for CAS examines the ability to imitate movements of the three basic systems of speech: articulators (oral imitation), breathing (blowing out a candle, blowing bubbles) and vocal cords (sound production of any kind). The ability to imitate speech means that there is an ability to imitate combined movements of each of these systems. Speech is both the combined and timed work of these three systems. If there is a problem in imitating movements of one of these systems in the absence of muscle tone deficits, lack of muscle power or anatomic disorder, than the speech problem is probably due to CAS.

One of the deficits in CAS is the lack of intonation. The child has difficulties in delivering a non-verbal message through his speech. Verbal language without intonation becomes poor and robotic. The loss of intonation has been well demonstrated among people after a head injury (5). Without intonation, the non-verbal message is unclear just as reading would be if it was done without punctuation marks. Teaching intonation to a child who doesn't understand how to produce the sound is not an easy task. Very few articles have been written on this subject. Exceptions are Helfrich-Miller (6) who demonstrated the Melodic Intonation Therapy Method which used melody patterns in order to organize speech patterns and Boutsen and Christman (7) who described the prosody issues in apraxia of speech.

Prosody is the patterns of stress and intonation in a language. The term generally covers intonation, rhythm, and focus in speech (8). Acoustically, prosody describes changes in the syllable length, loudness, pitch (frequency of a sound), and certain details of the formant structure of speech sounds. From the speech articulator's perspective, prosody is a result of changes in the velocity and range of motion in articulators like the jaw and tongue, along with change in the air pressure in the trachea and a change in the tension of the laryngeal muscles. Phonologically, prosody is described by tone, intonation, rhythm, and lexical stress (9).

The VML method is a set of Manual techniques, motor learning principles and multi-disciplinary therapeutic guidelines that is aimed at treating apraxia of speech. The method was developed via field work with children diagnosed with CAS. Based on theory and previous research, the practical techniques framework, and evaluation, analysis and treatment forms were created. The method is being taught in Hebrew and English. The VML method includes hundreds of different techniques to treat CAS.

In this case study the influence of several manual techniques on prosody was examined. One of the techniques is the Distal Dynamic Stabilization Technique (DDST). The basic principle of the DDST is to stabilize dynamically the distal end of the moving system in order to perform movement in the proximal end. The specific DDST in this case study relates to dynamic stabilization of the jaw movement in order to elicit movement around the vocal cords in order to influence intonation. For further information about the DDST see appendix 1. Other techniques were breathing control via diaphragmatic breathing and candle blowing control.

The main purpose of this study was to test the impact of DDST and breathing control techniques on prosody parameters. More specifically, the goals of the intervention were to decrease the loudness of the child's voice, to achieve expressive differentiation between high and low pitch and to reduce word duration.

A CASE STUDY

The subject was a 14 years old teenager, diagnosed with severe general motor apraxia and severe Apraxia of speech. A few years after this intervention took place the subject was diagnosed with OCD (obsessive compulsive disorder). He attended a small special class in a regular school together with 10 other children diagnosed with learning disabilities.

At birth the subect received high Apgar scores of 9 and 10 and there were no reported complications. He was very quiet as a baby and didn't babble during his first year of life. His motor development was unusual; at the age of a year and two months he stood up for the first time, sat down and then crawled. He was very clumsy as a child. He couldn't pronounce phonemes through imitation or spontaneously. The physician who saw him at the age of two years said that the child wasn't mentally retarded since he had "smart eyes" and that he wasn't autistic either. As a child he used to cry a lot and would occasionally bang his head on the floor. His behavior and lack of speech caused his parents to send him to special kindergartens where the educational team didn't know exactly what to do with him. At the age of four, a speech language pathologist (SLP) was the first to diagnose him with Severe Apraxia of speech.

I started working with him using the VML method when he was 6 years old. At that age he still couldn't pronounce phonemes, syllables or words through imitation or spontaneously, he couldn't walk up stairs without support and would walk down stairs in a step to step manner (STS) with poor control. He couldn't stand on one leg or jump. However he could read. In the entrance to the kitchen in his home was a big board on which he posted written words in short sentences such as "I want to eat". He taught himself to read through working on the computer. His reading ability was the proof of his academic potential. He was in a special kindergarten just before entering the first grade and was supposed to go to a special-education school.

We worked primarily on speech for the first 6 months and then integrated gross motor skills into the program. He acquired all the syllables in Hebrew after six months and started forming words and using them. Thanks to that he entered a regular school the year after.

In the following nine years he acquired motor-speech abilities and could use his speech pragmatically though his pronunciation wasn't clear. The main problem with his speech was the prosody of speech. The child couldn't control the loudness of his speech nor did he have versatility of tones in his speech. These prosody problems prevented him from delivering non semantic messages via speech which is a very important element in pragmatic verbal interactions. Four years of treatment on prosody in different ways such as changing head position, practicing asking questions, playing the piano, singing and working on voice control didn't bring a change in intonation.

The DDST idea came to my mind and we decided to give it a chance while performing the therapy in a research paradigm.

Procedure

The child had a 30 minute professional VML treatment session once a week and 6 more similar sessions a week conducted by his mother. The mother was watching the professional session and performed the same during the week under the guidance of the VML therapist. Each session included four exercises: 1) Blowing on a candle without extinguishing the flame 15-20 times 2) Imitating words of two open syllables faster then usually with a focus on reducing the fragment of time it takes to pronounce the vowel in the syllable 3) DDST was used to teach high and low pitch differentiation 4) Imitating words while lying on the back and breathing diaphragmatically. For protocols of the intervention see appendix 1. The program was conducted for four weeks. Tests were taken at the beginning of the first session of the program and at the end of the last session.

Measurements

The child performed two tests: 1) producing the highest pitch using /I/ sound without and with DDST, 2) Imitation of 18 words at a regular pace. The child's voice was recorded using a microphone attached to professional headphones. The voice recording took place in the child's room in the pre and post intervention testing. The microphone was placed as near as possible to the child's mouth in order to prevent inaccuracy of sound recordings and to prevent inconsistency in voice recordings. We used the same headphones for both measurements. We used "speech analyzer version 1.5" software (10) for voice analysis.

The dependent variables that were examined are: 1) words length, 2) Maximum loudness of words, 3) Maximum frequency of words, 4) Maximum frequency of pitch with and without DDST, 5) Minimum frequency of pitch with and without DDST, 6) Maximum loudness of pitch with and without DDST, 7) length of pitch with and without DDST.

Variables one and seven were measured in seconds. Variables 2 and 6 were measured as the percentage of loudness relative to a level provided by the software. Variables 3-5 were measured in Hertz units.

Statistical analysis

Paired T tests were used to examine the statistical significance of the difference between the word lengths, loudness and frequencies before and after the intervention. In regards to the pitch, as only the best measures out of 10 attempts was recorded for each condition (i.e., before, after, with, without), no significance test was used. However, there was a substantial difference in few of the pitch variables.

FINDINGS

Tables 1 & 2 provides the results of the experiment. Word length decreased significantly (p<0.001). The average words length at the beginning of the experiment was 0.7 seconds while after the experiment it decreased to 0.52 seconds. The maximum loudness of the words also decreased significantly from 27.37% on average at the beginning of the experiment to 20.29% (p<0.001). The maximum frequency of the words also decreased significantly from 198.88 HZ on average at the beginning of the experiment to 158.62 HZ (P<0.0001) at the end.

The pitch tests were examined for tendency. Maximum pitch frequency tends to increase with the DDST in comparison to no DDST condition. No tendency for change was observed between beginning and end of intervention as for results of Minimum frequency of pitch with and without DDST. The length of pitch tends to be higher at the end of the intervention in comparison to the beginning. Maximum pitch loudness tends to be higher for the DDST condition in comparison to no DDST condition.

Table 1. Pitch results summary

	with support	without support	Time
max' pitch frequency (HZ)	280	243	Beginning
	276	232	End
Min' pitch frequency (HZ)	186	176	Beginning
	192	172	End
length of pitch (seconds)	0.68	0.61	Beginning
	2.24	1.15	End
max' pitch loudness (% of max	56.8	33.8	Beginning
	21.9	12.2	End

Table 2. Words results summary

	before		after				
Var	avg	std	avg	std	t test	df	Sig'
word loudness	27.37059	6.152211	20.29412	5.726088	3.719139	16	<0.0001
word frequency	198.8824	10.50525	158.6235	7.208114	12.43725	16	<0.0001
word length	0.709829	0.16586	0.526741	0.133803	5.30602	16	<0.0001

DISCUSSION

The use of DDST support shows tendency for changes in maximum pitch frequency and in maximum pitch loudness. Usually, we can find proximal dynamic stabilization for an angular movement in the body's joints. For example, the shoulder muscles give proximal stabilization to the elbow movements; the muscles that surround the elbow stabilize the elbow joint in order to allow movement around the wrist joint etc. In this case; a distal dynamic stabilization was given through DDST technique since it encouraged proximal muscles to work. Using the distal dynamic stabilization technique was crucial in this case as there was no other apparent way to approach these deep muscles. There may be two possible explanations for the tendency using the distal dynamic stabilization mechanism. The first explanation is that the vocal cord muscles and the jaw retraction muscles work as a group in this specific task. In order to perform the task all the muscles that belong to the group must work together otherwise the task can't be performed. This group of muscles might have neuronal connections (similar to agonist-antagonist neuronal connections) thus, activating part of the group with intention to activate the other parts as well, might cause a neurological overflow from one part to the other.

The other explanation is simpler. A co-contraction of the jaw openers and the Masseter muscles creates a distal stabilization that performs a close kinematic chain. Stabilization of the distal part of the chain enables movement in the proximal part of the chain, just as when performing push up exercises the distal part (i.e., the wrists) are stabilized while the proximal parts (i.e., the elbow and shoulder joints) are moving.

The decrease in loudness between the baseline and end can be explained by the improved control in breathing in general and exhalation in particular. The control of breathing enables the child to exhale with more control while talking thus more accurately monitoring the air pressure in the vocal cords area. Increased loudness usually increases pitch frequency because of the increased air pressure beneath the vocal cords. An ability to decrease the air pressure beneath the vocal cords (decreased loudness) while increasing pitch frequency (rather then decreasing) shows movement discrimination.

The DDST was developed in order to increase tone. This explains the child's inability to decrease tone beyond the baseline measurements. The improved control over breathing were due to the candle blowing and diaphragmatic exercises while practicing speed pronunciation intensively. It brought a significant change in the words length. The change wasn't only numeric but was expressed functionally as the child became more understandable in interactions with unfamiliar people.

The results are even more impressive when taking into consideration the child's age, history of previous failures and the relatively little amount of practice (15 minutes a day for a month). Since this is only a case study and no statistical analysis was made for the pitch variables we should be very careful in generalizing the study findings. There might have been other factors that influenced the results such as maturation or intensity of practice (rather than the technique itself). The techniques should be employed in other treatment programs in bigger study designs in order to determine its efficacy on other children or adults. The influence of the techniques on prosody should be examined functionally in an objective study.

ACKNOWLEDGMENTS

Many thanks to the child and his family for participation and commitment. Without the support and active participation of the family we wouldn't have been able to perform the study.

APPENDIX 1

Protocols of intervention

1. Blowing on a candle without extinguishing the flame – the therapist explains the exercise to the child. The child sits on a chair and the therapist faces him. The therapist lights the candle and puts it 40-50 cm in front of the child's face. The child is instructed to blow on the candle without extinguishing the flame. If he succeeds the therapist will put the candle closer and the child tries again. If he succeeds again then the candle is put closer to the child at approximately 15 cm. the child will blow 15-20 times in each session.
2. Imitating words of two open syllables faster then usual with special consideration of reducing the fragment of time it takes to pronounce the vowel in the syllable. The child is introduced to the same list of 20 words each session.
3. Distal Dynamic Stabilization Technique (DDST) was used to teach high and low pitch differentiation. The child is asked to say the sound /I/ in a regular tone and in a low tone without support and in a high tone with and without DDST. DDST technique is performed by putting the first fingers (left and right) under the chin while pressing caudally. Simultaneously the two indexes are placed above the zygomatic arc. The child is asked to open his mouth. When he presses his jaw down the therapist asks him to say /I/ in a high pitch. It can be performed also with the support of only the first fingers. The exercise is done 10-15 times each session.
4. Imitating list of 20 words while lying on the back and breathing diaphragmatically

REFERENCES

[1]   Denes PB, Pinson EP. The speech chain. New York: WH Freeman,1993.

[2]   Ziegler W. Psycholinguistic and motor theories of apraxia of speech. Semin Speech Lang 2002;23:231-44.

[3]   Ken RD. Research on speech motor control and its disorders: A review and prospective. J Commun Disord 2000;33(5):391-428.

[4]   Asha.org/policy [Internet]. Childhood apraxia of speech [Position Statement]. Accessed 2013 Aug 01. URL: http://www.asha.org/docs/html/PS2007-00277.html.

[5]   Toshniwal SS, Joshi NA. Residual speech impairment in patients with traumatic brain injury. Indian J Neurotrauma 2010;7(1):61-6.

[6]   Helfrich-Miller KR. A clinical perspective: melodic intonation therapy for developmental apraxia. Clin Commun Disord1994;4(3):175-82.

[7]   Boutsen, FR. Christman SS. Prosody in apraxia of peech. Semin Speech Lang 2002;23:245-56.

[8]   Rom A, Segal M, Tchur B. [Child, what does he say?] Tel Aviv: Mofet Institute. 2003. [Hebrew].

[9]   http://en.wikipedia.org [Internet]. Prosody. Accessed 2013 Aug 01. URL: http://en.wikipedia.org/ wiki/Prosody_%28linguistics%29

[10]   http://www.sil.org [Internet]. Speech Tools. Accessed 2013 Aug 01. URL: http://www.sil.org/ computing/speechtools/SATdownloads2.htm

In: Disability and Chronic Disease   ISBN: 978-1-62948-288-0
Editors: J. Merrick, S. Aspler and M. Morad   © 2014 Nova Science Publishers, Inc.

Chapter 7

ALERTNESS OBSERVATIONS IN CHILDREN WITH PROFOUND INTELLECTUAL AND MULTIPLE DISABILITIES

Vera Munde, MScPhD[*] and Carla Vlaskamp, PhD

Department of Special Education, University of Groningen, Groningen, the Netherlands

Assessment of cognitive, motor, sensory and communicative functions in children with profound intellectual and multiple disabilities (PIMD) is still in its infancy and there is a lack of standardised instruments (checklists and observation scales have so far been used). The level of alertness in the child has been one very specific factor in assessment that is related to the complexity and severity of the disability, but observers/assessors have not been sure when it is the 'best moment' to start assessment and unaware of which conditions can help provoke and maintain optimal alertness levels for assessment. Alertness, however, is not only a means to optimize the assessment process; it can also be the objective of the assessment process itself. An observation list was developed to assess the level of alertness in children with PIMD. In this paper, a description of the content of the list is presented. For this list, inter observer and intra observer reliability were determined by comparing scores of three groups of observers: teachers, an external observers who had received additional information about the clients and an external observer who did not know the clients at all. Results of the reliability scores for 78 situations exceed the previously formulated criterion of 80%. The observation list seems to be a functional and sensitive instrument that gives direct support staff the opportunity to discern individual differences in alert moments and the impact of different stimuli on alertness. This information can be of use in clinical practice.

INTRODUCTION

A key objective of assessment is to determine the progress a child is making developmentally. There is, however, a category of children for whom progress or development in the generally

[*] Correspondence: Vera Munde, University of Groningen, Department of Special Education, Grote Rozenstraat 38, 9712 TJ Groningen, The Netherlands. E-mail: V.S.Munde@rug.nl.

accepted sense is lacking. Children with profound intellectual and multiple disabilities (PIMD) certainly do progress as they get older, but not always towards goals that are generally seen as crucial or important in our society. Some children with PIMD even have such profound cerebral lesions that based on neurological evidence no functional adaptation is said to be possible (1). On the other hand, most parents and direct support persons (DSPs) believe firmly in the abilities of children with PIMD, even when these seem to run counter to clinical or educational assessment (2).

In this paper, the characteristics of children with PIMD will be described. The importance of alertness in assessment, both as a mean and as an objective, is then explained. The implications of such a complex pattern of disabilities for assessment of alertness will be considered. We will then describe the content and use of an observation list that was developed in order to establish the optimal period or periods during the day to offer a stimulus and to establish the pattern of alertness and the contextual influences on this pattern. Results of the inter observer reliability and intra observer reliability of this list are given, and its practical use is illustrated by an example. Though the list seems sufficiently useful and reliable, its actual use may still be problematic.

CHILDREN WITH PROFOUND INTELLECTUAL DISABILITY

A profound intellectual disability is almost always the consequence of neurological impairments arising from trauma or genetic influences (3) with implications for overall functioning. Central nervous system (CNS) damage results in profound intellectual, severe or profound motor disorders (e.g., spastic quadriplegia) and sensory disorders. Characteristically, children with PIMD will be at the preverbal stage of communication, though some will have limited spoken or signed expressive language, and limited communicative comprehension. Understanding of causality and space will be limited, and adaptive, self-help abilities will be at such a level that the support they require will be pervasive. Other consequences of such CNS damage are that most children with PIMD are wheelchair users, frequently have limited use of hands and arms and have difficulties in maintaining postural balance. Both gross motor and fine motor functions are usually profoundly disturbed. Sensory impairments are common, and recent studies showed that at least 85% of people with profound intellectual disabilities experience visual impairments (4, 5). In most cases these are caused by damage to the visual cortex in the occipital lobe (cortical blindness) (4, 5). Between 25% and 33% of children with profound intellectual disabilities have auditory impairments, but it is suspected that a substantial number of cases may have remained unidentified (4). In addition, dysfunctions of taste and smell are relatively common (6), but usually ignored. The tactile and coetaneous senses that include the receptors of touch, pressure, temperature and pain are frequently thought to be impaired to some degree as well (7, 8). In addition to the intellectual, motor and sensory disabilities just noted, further concomitant impairments should also be mentioned as they, too, have significant implications for assessment. Extensive 'additional' impairments include: seizure disorders, chronic pulmonary infections, and skeletal deformations (4, 5, 9, 10). As each child with PIMD represents a unique configuration of abilities and constraints to functioning, children with PIMD form a heterogeneous group in terms of central nervous system integrity, physical growth, development and behavioral repertoires (11). Notwithstanding this huge diversity, children with PIMD are comparable in the degree of profound intellectual and severe or profound motor disabilities, and may be considered to constitute the most disabled group of people in the populations of individuals with intellectual disabilities. They form a very vulnerable group with heavy or total dependence on personal assistance for their physical care, education, stimulation and recreation.

ASSESSMENT

The assessment of children with PIMD presents special challenges. Even though a child with PIMD cannot be understood as a simple combination of assessment results of different impairments, it is still necessary to know what his or her disabilities and potential entail in order to understand how these may affect the overall functioning of the child (2). But to assess intellectual, motor or sensory functioning means that we encounter a wide range of barriers to the conventional types of assessment that are feasible with more able individuals. Partly because of the multiplicity of the disabilities and the fact that each child with PIMD represents a unique configuration of abilities and constraints to functioning, but also because there are not many specific instruments available (2).

As there are as yet insufficient research data relating to the way these profoundly disabled children develop (or can develop), it is indeed not an easy task to design and develop reliable and valid instruments. The lack of valid and reliable instruments for determining a children's abilities on the various development domains are likely to have contributed to the development of situation-based observation lists and the use of observations in every-day life situations. In such cases, validity and reliability are often considered to be limited. It is therefore necessary to formulate observation regulations and certain targeted areas for observation prior to the start of the observation. The reliability of the observations is determined not only by setting requirements to inter and intra assessment reliability. The inclusion or exclusion of environmental factors may play a role concerning factors such as the extent of reliability of the direct staff, the occurrence of audible noises in the background during observation, the presence of other persons and the position and posture of the child under observation (12).

Moreover, children with PIMD may have specific, idiosyncratic thresholds for stimuli, with children reacting in a hypersensitive way and subsequently trying to ignore certain stimuli or parts of stimuli. Others may need very strong stimuli before they can actually respond. Selecting the focus and maintaining attention to sensory stimuli can be hampered. In addition, understanding behavioural responses is difficult because of the complexity of the behaviour of children with PIMD. The same expression, sound or movement may have different meanings in different situations (13). Therefore, ascribing meaning to any behaviour is at least partly the assessor's interpretation, which is a potential threat to reliability. To overcome this threat, some researchers use physiological reactions (e.g., muscle tone) or measurements of brain activity to study the reactions of children with PIMD to sensory stimuli (14). However, these types of instruments are difficult to use in practice as they may be intrusive. Furthermore, one might question how practical such methods are, as specialized equipment and technicians are necessary to measure the children's physiological reactions and, even more importantly, the results do not elucidate the meaning for the children themselves of the behaviour that is registered.

ALERTNESS

As stated in the previous paragraph, we encounter a wide range of barriers to the conventional types of assessment that are feasible with more able individuals lacking complex disabilities. One of the barriers that we may experience is timing. In children with PIMD, the focus on the environment is irregularly and rapidly changing (15). Additionally, these short moments are often difficult to detect because of individual differences in expressing 'being focused on the environment'. Based on these difficulties, we face returning questions when assessing children of the target group: what may be the best moment to assess the cognitive, motor and sensory abilities of a child with PIMD? How can we determine such a 'best moment' and what may be the duration of such a moment? Only if we know that the stimuli that are presented in the assessment can enter the consciousness of the child, we can expect the assessment to be unbiased (16). Consequently, it is very important to take these 'best moments' into account during the assessment, even though they only endure shortly.

Looking at the 'best moments' more closely in the literature, we encounter various terms and descriptions (17). Authors introduce terms such as 'behavior state', 'alertness', 'involvement' and 'on-task behavior'. Thereby, mainly two types of descriptions can be found. One group of the given terms is linked to an internal state of the individual that becomes manifest and visible in the individual's behavior. In contrast, other authors shift the focus from the individual only to the individual in his or her environmental context. Authors emphasize interaction and engagement with the environment which can be observed on different levels. The highest level then equals the 'best moments'. Despite this differentiation, all descriptions consider the 'best moment' for individuals with PIMD to be observable in the individual's behavior.

Since the term 'alertness' is the most used in behavioral observations with individuals of the target group, we will use this term in the continuation of this paper.

OBSERVING ALERTNESS

Since alertness is not only considered a precondition, but an objective of assessment at the same time, a number of instruments to observe alertness in individuals with PIMD are presented in the literature (17). All instruments are based on observations to detect the subtle alertness expressions of individuals with PIMD. Since the meaning of one signal may differ for different situations, DSPs need to register the behavior of their client and interpret the signal based on their knowledge about the client and the situation at the same time. Individual differences in alertness expressions as well as contextual factors can, thereby, have an impact on the interpretations (18). Because the subjectivity of interpretations is a potential threat to validity and reliability (2), physiological measures might be considered as an alternative. However, these do not reveal detailed information about the complex behavior of individuals of the target group and, still, observations are the most obvious method to determine alertness in individuals of the target group (15, 19).

The instruments described in the literature differ in the number of alertness levels (17). Thereby, the observation system of Guess and his colleagues (20) can be described as a standard scale. Nine alertness levels are differentiated: Asleep-Inactive, Asleep-Active, Drowsy, Daze, Awake Inactive-Alert, Awake Active-Alert, Awake-Active/Stereotypy, Crying/Agitated and Seizures. In other studies, authors modified the scale and used a different number of levels. The number of levels for the analyses was always reduced to a maximum of six (e.g., 15). Determining the number of observation levels, several authors discuss the position of self-injuring behavior. Whereas Woodyatt et al. (21) expect this behavior to occur in all states, Siegel-Causey and Bashinski (22) classify self-injurious behavior as a form of communication, not as an alertness level.

Scoring is another aspect of alertness observation in individuals with PIMD that is discussed in the studies mentioned above. Two problems have been described in literature: the frequency with which observations are measured, and whether or not to include the context in the observations. As for the frequency, authors mention that in order to register the quick changes and reveal a maximum of information, short scoring intervals or continuous scoring seems necessary (15). For continuous observations, hand-held registration systems can be used, allowing a new score after minimally three seconds (23, 24). However, since continuous scoring is time-consuming and registration systems are expensive, most studies use interval scoring with 10 seconds intervals (25, 26). For scoring in real time, these intervals of observations are alternated with 10-seconds intervals for the scoring of the behavior (25, 27). To prevent information loss, other authors first videotaped the situations. Then, in a second step, they looked at the tapes for intervals of 10 seconds and stop the videotapes for the scoring (20, 23). The size and impact of loss of information when interval scores are used instead of continuous scores, is, as yet, not clear. Even more important in clinical practice is the fact, that continuous scoring is almost impossible to realize. Observations are very time-consuming (28) and continuous scoring is found to be difficult to integrate in daily routines.

The second problem is related to the context. Contextual information will influence the observational judgments. Although the context does not seem to have an influence on the judgment per se, expectations and experiences about the way of influence can make the observers' judgment more extreme (18). Thus, when the client is not expected to appreciate the situation, DSPs tend to interpret the expressions more negatively. Additionally, scoring of the context itself is another challenge. In real time observations, registration of behavior and context at the same time is only possible by employing two observers. For observations with one observer, videotapes can solve the problem of information loss. Observers can, then, register behavior during the first time they look at the videotapes and note contextual factors at a second time (20, 25). However, realizing observations in such a way is again difficult to realize in clinical practice.

Taking both problems into account, it is clear that to be able to attune to the clients 'best moment', practice needs an instrument that is on the one hand easy to use and not too time consuming, but on the other hand reliable.

ALERTNESS OBSERVATION LIST

In an analogous manner as an assessor can optimally conduct the assessment when the child is alert, DSPs can best start an activity when the child with PIMD is susceptible for the stimulus (29). In general, DSPs offer stimuli to promote learning and development of their clients. However, timing and the choice of the stimulus are returning issues in the care for children of the target group.

Based on the need of DSPs to determine the 'best moment' to start an activity, Vlaskamp, Fonteine and Tadema (30) developed the Alertness Observation List (AOL). This list was developed for use by DSP's and is aiming to formulate an individual alertness profile in five steps.

As a first step, and before actually starting the observations, DSPs need to decide whether the agreed day for observation is a representative day for the child with PIMD - or not. Only if the child is 'feeling good' (e.g., did not have any seizures prior to the observation) and did not receive any unusual medication, observations may reveal representative picture of alertness. When the first step reveals that the selected day is an 'ordinary' day for the client who is to be observed, the agreed observation takes place. In this second step, alertness levels are noted every 15 minutes to determine the best moment in terms of alertness during the day. This first and second step are executed for three days, not necessarily three days in a row, but at least within a fortnight. In the two following steps [3 and 4], the relation between an activity and alertness is determined. Based on the previous observations, the best moment in terms of alertness during the day is determined. At that selected 'best moment', the DSP offers a stimulus to the child with PIMD.

We therefore distinguish between three sorts of stimuli: visual, auditory and tactile, but combinations are also possible. When offering the stimulus, DSPs have to take into account the following. Only if the stimulus is considered to have an impact on the alertness of this child with PIMD, we can expect to see changes. Consequently, the choice of a stimulus has to be made based on the child's preferences and reactions. Additionally, DSPs are advised to take the time when offering the stimulus. Since children with PIMD often process information in a different way, it is especially important that DSPs act in their clients' speed. Furthermore, an explicit description of the presented stimulus on the scoring form is necessary. Based on observations before, during and after offering a stimulus, changes due to the stimulus can be recognized. Thereby, scoring frequency increases. Whereas alertness levels are noted every five minutes in step 3, scores have to be noted every 20 seconds in step 4. Finally, all observations are summarized in an individual alertness profile (step 5). During all observations, alertness is assumed to occur on four different levels: alert, drowsy, asleep and agitated. For the scoring, every alertness level is associated with a color: green, orange and red, respectively. To include the frequently occurring self-injuring behavior of children with PIMD, blue was added as a forth color. In the alertness profile, individual behaviors and reactions that are associated with the four alertness levels are described.

Before introducing the Alertness Observation List to clinical practice, the psychometric quality was investigated. The instrument was used in a children's special educational centre, with a focus on establishing the reliability. We were able to determine only sufficient reliability (kappa = .60) in five cases (31). We therefore decided to try to calculate the reliability for a larger sample. A Dutch school for special education volunteered to use the list. Four classes were chosen at random and all 23 children of the four classes were included in the study. The observation list was completed for the children and observations of the fourth form were videotaped. Because a number of videotapes were of low quality, they had to be excluded. A pool of 120 situations remained. Out of the pool, we chose 39 situations to calculate the inter observer reliability. For another 39 situations, we determined the intra observer reliability. Therefore, three groups of observers were involved in the study: the teachers, an external observer who received additional information about the children and an external observer who was not familiar with the children at all. Reliability was calculated by employing the overall agreement formula: agreement/disagreement+agreement)*100. A criterion of 80% was applied (15).

Based on the scores of the fourth form, the reliability of the observation list was estimated. Calculations resulted in an inter observer reliability of 81% (Mdn = 81,44; M = 81,46; SD = 13,88). The intra observer reliability was 87% (Mdn = 86,79; M = 85,23; SD = 11,75). The detailed results are given in table 1 and 2.

Table 1. Results for the inter observer reliability

	T and E+*	T and E-	E+ and E-	
	83,33	50,00	83,33	
	75,00	75,00	80,00	
	87,50	70,83	86,67	
	75,17	79,17	75,86	
	80,00	83,33	93,33	
	100,00	91,67	100,00	
	75,00	100,00	50,00	
	62,50	100,00	64,86	
	100,00	87,50	81,82	
	87,50	91,67	94,74	
	62,50	79,16	64,44	
	100,00	66,67	100,00	
	87,50	75,00	76,00	**TOTAL**
M	*82,77*	*80,77*	*80,85*	**81,46**
Mdn	*83,33*	*79,17*	*81,82*	**81,44**
SD	*12,80*	*13,98*	*14,86*	**13,88**

* The letters refer to the different (groups of) observers. Teachers are named with 'T', the external observer who received additional information about the children is named with 'E+' and the external observer who did not know the children at all is named with 'E-'.

Because the results exceed the formulated criterion, we conclude that the Alertness Observation List reveals reliable information to determine alertness in children with PIMD. But next to this general result, the data show additional information. A striking fact is the differences in reliability scores for the different groups of observers. Calculations of the inter observer reliability revealed higher percentages for the observers who had more information about the children, but intra observer reliability was higher for the observer who did not know the children at all.

Table 2. Results for the intra observer reliability.

T *	E+	E-	
70,83	95,83	91,07	
70,83	66,67	96,77	
91,67	76,67	63,64	
100,00	93,10	72,88	
79,17	93,55	95,16	
83,33	100,00	82,98	
70,83	88,89	100,00	
70,83	61,11	90,48	
100,00	87,10	91,53	
70,83	78,95	86,05	
100,00	86,36	97,73	
91,67	100,00	86,84	
83,33	85,00	72,22	**TOTAL**
M	*83,33*	*85,63*	*86,72*	*85,23*
Mdn	*83,33*	*87,10*	*90,48*	*86,97*
SD	*12,15*	*12,02*	*11,09*	*11,75*

* The letters refer to the different (groups of) observers. Teachers are named with 'T', the external observer who received additional information about the children is named with 'E+' and the external observer who did not know the children at all is named with 'E-'.

These differences in results may be explained as follows. Firstly, as research shows, proxies tend to be influenced in their judgment by their knowledge and daily experiences (32). When they are in doubt about the correct interpretation of the child's behavior, they may decide differently based on a recent experience with their client. In contrast, external observers, missing this type of additional information, only judge the visible behavior. This, in consequence, leads to more consistent scores. Secondly, observations of children who remain in the same alertness state for a prolonged period of time have been scored with a higher reliability. Total agreement was reached when the observed children were clearly focused on their environment for the entire session. Most children, however, show frequent changes in alertness levels. Thereby, changes between alert and drowsy states aggravate alertness observations in particular, because expressions of these alertness levels are difficult to differentiate for some children with PIMD. We may conclude that a large number of quick changes in alertness level complicates the realization of reliable observations for DPSs, as suggested previously others (15, 23). Thirdly, low reliability scores can be linked to the heterogeneity of the target group. Thereby, the ability of an individual to show a clear focus of the eyes and control over his or her own movement are the main influencing factors. It is far more difficult to give a reliable score about the level of alertness of individuals with visual impairments, as these individuals will not always show their focus on the environment by fixation with the eyes. Additionally, severe spasticity and difficulties to direct the movements to the presented stimuli may be interpreted as low alertness or incapacity to control the body movements.

The results of our study underline the complexity of alertness observations in individuals with PIMD. To clarify the issues discussed here above, the alertness observations of a girl called Emily will be described in the following section. First, we will introduce Emily as well as the questions DSPs have concerning Emily's alertness. Then, the results of the Alertness Observation List for Emily will be presented. Finally, observations results will be linked back to the DSPs' questions concerning the alertness of Emily.

CASE STORY: EMILY

Emily is a 10-year old girl with profound intellectual and multiple disabilities. She attends a special educational center from the age of three. Emily has a friendly and outgoing nature, but since quite some time, Emily has periods in which she is rather withdrawn. Too, during these withdrawn periods, Emily has crying fits, apparently without clear cause. These periods have increased in number and duration in the last six months. DSPs feel ambiguous about the most adequate reaction towards this behavior. On the one hand, they think that it is better to 'leave her be' when she apparently feels uncomfortable; on the other hand, they would like to keep offering a balanced educational program that supports and stimulates Emily's development. A central issue in this balanced educational program is the optimal moment for stimulation.

Name: *Emily*

Active, focused on the environment (green)	Concrete examples of behavior:
Emily is mainly active and focused on her environment in the morning. Because of low vision, she shows activity by listening and touching. Her strongest reactions are on tactile stimuli. *Emily is mainly focused on DSPs. When you stay close to her and do not interrupt the tactile contact with her, she can keep her focus for about 1 to 5 minutes on an activity.*	*Emily turns her face to the sound, her eyes are open, she is smiling permanently. She produces sounds when you touch her. At the same time, she tries to touch you back. Emily clamps objects and touches them.*
Inactive, withdrawn (orange)	**Concrete examples of behavior:**
Emily is mainly inactive and withdrawn after mealtimes or after other activities, such as physiotherapy. This condition can then last for longer periods.	*Emily is focused on her hands, she fiddles and plucks. She picks her cloth,(using her thumb and index finger), sucks her thumb, makes humming noises and rubs her eyes.*
Sleeping, drowsy (red)	**Concrete examples of behavior:**
Emily does not fall asleep during the day. You can only see periods of drowsiness, especially following therapy sessions or group activities	*Emily sits very quietly, her eyes close and open slowly and repeatedly.*
Agitated, discontented (blue)	**Concrete examples of behavior:**
Emily sometimes cries out loud when everything overstrains her. Crying fits mainly occur in the afternoon.	*Emily cries with long exhalation, but without tears. When you do not give her your attention immediately, she begins to bit on the heel of her hand.*

Figure 1. Form D – the 'traffic light'.

To determine such an optimal moment, the Alertness Observation List has been completed. Form A was filled in twice: a day before the observations and just before the observations. This form showed that Emily is not ill, nor was she unusually passive or active, that she wasn't in an unusual environment, that there was no change in medication and that she did not have unusual epileptic activities prior to the observations. With form B, DSPs search for alertness patterns that Emily shows normally. The DSPs observe Emily during three entire days. From the observations, it becomes clear that Emily's best time of day is the morning, and she is most alert between 9 and 10 o'clock. Except for lunch, Emily is in the orange and red level for the remains of the day. With form C, a DSP offers Emily a preferred activity, and assesses Emily's level of alertness every five minutes during 10 minutes. Before and after the activity, the DSP scores for another 15 minutes, giving a score every five minutes. The observations show that after about 5 minutes of the activity, Emily's alertness decreases from green to orange levels. Observing Emily's reaction to an activity every 20 seconds during 5 minutes (with form D) shows quick changes from to being active and focused on the environment to being inactive and withdrawn during the 5 minutes of offering an activity. Additionally, observations with both form shows that Emily becomes drowsy after the activity. The information that resulted from the observations of the Alertness Observation List was summarized in a 'traffic light' for Emily (see figure 1).

Based on the 'traffic light', DSPs made a number of decisions about Emily's program. All activities were now planned in the morning and activities were presented for a short period (about 5 minutes). Moments of rest were planned between two activities (again of about 5 minutes). During the afternoon, DSPs created periods of sufficient rest for Emily. Therapy sessions were planned in the afternoon, and such sessions were followed by a period of rest. In a next step, DSPs can evaluate Emily's reactions on her new schedule and may want to try to prolong the duration of Emily's alert periods.

DISCUSSION

The results of our study and the given example show that the Alertness Observation List is a reliable instrument, and may serve as a starting point in a further understanding of alertness, like: does starting an activity when the child is in an alert state lead to more preferable reactions than using an activity to make the child alert? Or: which aspect of the activity evokes changes in alertness levels; do children with PIMD react because of the stimulus itself, because of the interaction with the DSP or because of another, unknown factor? In several studies, a number of factors that were expected to have an impact on alertness were included in the observations themselves (25, 33, 34). These can be summarized in aspects of the interaction, the activity and the setting. Whereas interaction is described as a general precondition to increase alertness, frequency, type and content of the activity can have an individually different impact (33). Settings with a limited number of stimuli have been found to lead to higher alertness levels in general (35, 36). Even if all studies including ours have been realized for a relatively small number of participants and large individual differences in this target group, they still are important for a better understanding of the meaning of contextual influence on individual alertness levels.

The use of the Alertness Observation List in clinical practice is a challenge for DSP. They act as proxies, and literature yields conflicting results concerning the value of using a proxy-approach. Several researchers have attempted to evaluate consumer-proxy agreement by comparing proxy responses about people who can respond for themselves with self-reports from the same people. In some of these studies concerning aspects of quality of life, the answers given strongly disagreed with one another (37,38); others found greater concordance (39,40). Though the use of proxies may negatively influence validity, the fact remains that children with PIMD are unable to speak for themselves directly. Indirectly, the use of the Alertness Observation List enables children with PIMD to speak out: when the results of the Alertness Observation List are valid, and children are offered appropriate stimuli at an appropriate time, the child with PIMD will show the validity to us by being alert.

ACKNOWLEDGEMENTS

We would like to thank the children and teachers who agreed to participate in this study. Special thanks are owed to the observers for their time and effort.

REFERENCES

[1]   Robertson IH, Murre JMJ. Rehabilitation of brain damage: Brain plasticity and principles of guided recovery. Psychol Bull 1999;125: 544-75.

[2]   Vlaskamp C. Assessing people with profound intellectual and multiple disabilities. In: Hogg J, Langa A, eds. Assessing adults with intellectual disability: A service provider's guide. Oxford: Blackwell Publishers; 2005.

[3]   Arvio M, Sillanpää M. Prevalence, etiology and comorbidity of severe and profound intellectual disability in Finland. J Intellect Disabil Res 2003;47:108-112.

[4]   Evenhuis H M, Theunissen M, Denkers I, Verschuure H, Kemme H. Prevalence of visual and hearing impairment in a Dutch institutionalized population with intellectual disability. J Intellect Disabil Res 2001;45:457-64.

[5]   Van Splunder J, Stilma JS, Bernsen RMD, Evenhuis HM. Prevalence of visual impairment in adults with intellectual disabilities in the Netherlands: cross-sectional study. Eye 2006;20:1004-10.

[6]   Bromley SM. Smell and taste disorders: A primary care approach. Am Fam Physician 2000;61:427-36.

[7]   Dunn W. The sensorimotor systems: A framework for assessment and intervention. In: Orelove FP, Sobsey D. Educating children with multiple disabilities: A transdisciplinary approach, 2nd ed. Baltimore, MD: Paul H Brookes, 1991:33-78.

[8]   Oberlander TF, Gilbert CA, Chambers CT, O'Donnell ME, Craig KD. Biobehavioral responses to acute pain in adolescents with a significant neurologic impairment. Clin J Pain 1999;15:201-9.

[9]   Hogg J. The administration of psychotropic and anticonvulsant drugs to children with profound intellectual disability and multiple impairments. J Intellect Disabil Res 1992;36:473-88.

[10]   Janicki MP, Dalton AJ. Sensory impairments among older adults with intellectual disability. J Intellect Dev Disabil 1998;23:3-11.

[11]   Zijlstra HP, Vlaskamp C. The Impact of Medical Conditions on the Support of Children with Profound Intellectual and Multiple Disabilities. J Appl Res Intellect Disabil 2005;18:151-61.

[12]   Lohrmann-O'Rourke S, Browder DM. Empirically based methods to assess the preferences of individuals with severe disabilities. Am J Ment Retard 1998;103:146-61.

[13]   Grove N, Bunning K, Porter J, Olsson C. See what I mean: Interpreting the meaning of communication by people with severe and profound intellectual disabilities. J Appl Res in Intellect Disabil 1999; 12:190-203.

[14]   Chaney RH, Givens CA, Aoki MF, Gombiner ML. Pupillary Responses in Recognizing Awareness in Persons with Profound Mental-Retardation. Percept Mot Skills 1989;69:523-8.

[15]   Mudford OC, Hogg J, Roberts J. Interobserver agreement and disagreement in continuous recording exemplified by measurement of behavior state. Am J Ment Retard 1997;102:54-66.

[16] Nelson C, Van Dijk J, McDonnell AP, Thompson K. A framework for understanding young children with severe multiple disabilities: The van Dijk approach to assessment. Res Pract Persons Severe Disabil 2002;27:97-111.

[17] Munde VS, Vlaskamp C, Ruijssenaars AJJM, Nakken H. Alertness in individuals with profound intellectual and multiple disabilities: a literature review. Res Dev Disabil 2009;30:462-80.

[18] Hogg J, Reeves D, Roberts J, Mudford OC. Consistency, context and confidence in judgements of affective communication in adults with profound intellectual and multiple disabilities. J Intellect Disabil Res 2001;45:18-29.

[19] Vlaskamp C, Cuppen-Fonteine H. Reliability of assessing the sensory perception of children with profound intellectual and multiple disabilities: A case study. Child Care Health Dev 2007;33:547-51.

[20] Guess D, Roberts S, Siegel-Causey E, Ault M, Guy B, Thompson B. Analysis of Behavior State Conditions and Associated Environmental Variables among Students with Profound Handicaps. Am J Ment Retard 1993;97:634-53.

[21] Woodyatt G, Marinac J, Darnell R, Sigafoos J, Halle J. Behaviour State Analysis in Rett Syndrome: Continuous data reliability measurement. Int J Disabil Dev Educ 2004;51:383-400.

[22] Siegel-Causey E, Bashinski SM. Enhancing initial communication and responsiveness of learners with multiple disabilities: A tri-focus framework for partners. Focus Autism Other Dev Disabil 1997;12: 105-20.

[23] Guess D, Roberts S, Rues J. Longitudinal analysis of state patterns and related variables among infants and children with significant disabilities. Res Pract Persons Severe Disabil 2002;27:112-24.

[24] Mellstrom BP, Saunders MD, Saunders RR, Olswang LB. Interaction of Behavioral State and Microswitch Use in Individuals With Profound Multiple Impairments. J Dev Phys Disabil 2005;17:35-53.

[25] Arthur M. Patterns amongst behavior states, sociocommunicative, and activity variables in educational programs for students with profound and multiple disabilities. J Dev Phys Disabil 2004;16: 125-49.

[26] Lancioni GE, O'Reilly MF, Mantini M. Activity arrangements with or without mobility and performance of persons with profound multiple disabilities over long sessions. Ir J Psychol 1999;20:124-35.

[27] Parsons MB, Rollyson JH, Reid DH. Improving day-treatment services for adults with severe disabilities: A norm-referenced application of outcome management. J Appl Behav Anal 2004;37: 365-77.

[28] Petry K, Maes B. Identifying expressions of pleasure and displeasure by persons with profound and multiple disabilities. J Intellect Dev Disabil 2006;31:28-38.

[29] Arthur-Kelly M, Bochner S, Center Y, Mok M. Socio-communicative perspectives on research and evidence-based practice in the education of students with profound and multiple disabilities. J Dev Phys Disabil 2007;19:161-76.

[30] Vlaskamp C, Fonteine H, Tadema A. Manual of the list 'Alertness in children with profound intellectual and multiple disabilities'. [Handleiding bij de lijst 'Alertheid van kinderen met zeer ernstige verstandelijke en meervoudige beperkingen]. Groningen: Stichting Kinderstudies; 2005. [Dutch]

[31] Petitiaux WSD, Elsinga GM, Cuppen-Fonteine H, Vlaskamp C. Alertheid van kinderen met ernstige verstandelijke en meervoudige beperkingen: een casestudy. [Alertness in children with profound intellectual and multiple disabilities: a case study]. NTZ 2006;32: 241-54. [Dutch]

[32] Swennenhuis P, Vermeer A, Rispens J, Teunissen J, Wensing M. Quality of the care process for children with intellectual disabilities: A Delphi study. Eur J Spec Needs Educ 2004;19:241-53.

[33] Guess D, Roberts S, Guy B. Implications of behavior state for the assessment and education of students with profound disabilities. In: Repp AC & Horner RH, editors. Functional analysis of problem behavior − from effective assessment to effective support. Belmont: Wadsworth, 1999:338-94.

[34] Vlaskamp C, De Geeter KI, Huijsmans LM, Smit IH. Passive activities: The effectiveness of multisensory environments on the level of activity of individuals with profound multiple disabilities. J Appl Res Intellect Disabil 2003;16:135-43.

[35] Belfiore PJ, Browder DM, Mace FC. Effects of community and center-based settings on the alertness of persons with profound mental retardation. J Appl Behav Anal 1993;26:401-2.

[36] Green CW, Gardner SM, Canipe VS, Reid DH. Analyzing alertness among people with profound multiple disabilites: Implications for provision of training. J Appl Behav Anal 1994;27:519-31.

[37] Cummins RA. Proxy responding for subjective well-being: A review. In: Glidden LM, Glidden LM, eds. International review of research in mental retardation, Vol. 25. San Diego, CA: Acad Press, 2002:183-207.

[38] Stancliffe RJ. Proxy respondents and quality of life. Eval Program Plan 2000;23:89-93.

[39] McVilly KR, Burton-Smith RM, Davidson JA. Concurrence between subject and proxy ratings of quality of life for people with and without intellectual disabilities. J Intellect Dev Disabil 2000;25:19-39.

[40] Stancliffe RJ. Proxy respondents and the reliability of the Quality of Life Questionnaire Empowerment factor. J Intellect Disabil Res 1999; 43:185-93.

In: Disability and Chronic Disease   ISBN: 978-1-62948-288-0
Editors: J. Merrick, S. Aspler and M. Morad   © 2014 Nova Science Publishers, Inc.

Chapter 8

MODELING WATER THERAPY FOR CHILDREN WITH COGNITIVE IMPAIRMENTS

Alessandro Pollini, PhD[*]

BSD Design, Consulting and Research, Italy

User research in the health care domain is valuable per se as a way to gather more and more structured information about the settings, the actors, the impairments and the therapeutic practices. User research methods are then particularly valuable if used within a design process with the goal of eliciting user knowledge and requirements in delicate settings such as the water therapy for children with cognitive impairments. This work examines the current existing practices in order to gain a firm understanding of the involved users, i.e., the therapists and the children; the features of the therapeutic setting and the support tools. The investigation prepared the knowledge base that have been elaborated into user requirements for the design of therapeutic technologies for water therapy. The activity analysis informed the interaction design and the development of the enabling software architecture. User and activity modelling have been conducted following combined interaction design and ethnographic methods. The outcomes of the research have provided guidance and support for the design, development and field evaluation of the therapeutic technologies developed.

INTRODUCTION

Therapeutic technologies have been explored for physical activation (1), aesthetic resonance (2) and cognitive and psychological treatment (3, 4). Many national or EU funded research projects deal with disabilities and special needs with a specific focus on play and therapy, but none of the currently existing projects deals with designing therapeutic technology for the aquatic environment. In fact the application of interactive and embedded technologies as support for the practices of rehabilitation in water for disabled children is still an emerging field that has to be explored.

---

[*] Correspondence: Alessandro Pollini, PhD, BSD design, Via Boezio 14, 00192, Rome, Italy. E-mail: alessandro.pollini@bsdesign.eu.

In a domain in which the needs of the users, whether they are the therapists or the patients, are heterogeneous and the context dynamically modifies itself, the introduction of interactive technologies represents a challenge and an opportunity for the research and for the evolution of the rehabilitation practices. In particular, the design of interactive and embedded technologies in the rehabilitative context presupposes and contributes to a specific reflection regarding the environment, the objectives and the instruments utilized in the rehabilitation interventions.

The interventions in water are in fact characterized by manifold factors, such as the psycho-dynamic characteristics of the water, the particular profiles of the recipients of the treatment, the needs and the abilities of the disabled children and the richness and the potentialities of the aids used in the practices.

The activities in water for the disabled are currently characterized by non-structured games in which the children can explore the aquatic environment and learn to move, float and swim. The activities in water are particularly well adapted to disabled children, since the water is a facilitating element; the ideal context for going beyond ones own limits, whether they be physical or psychological. In the water psychomotor therapists, teachers and educators work with children with motor disabilities and mental retardation, with the aim of intervening on the relational, sensorial and functional aspects and on the particular needs of the disabled child (7).

The therapeutic practice in water has as its objective the consolidation of the available cognitive and motor abilities and the stimulation of the global development of the child. This is achieved through functional activities that support the experiences of coordination in space and time, equilibrium, postural adjustment and dynamic/general coordination (7).

Another very important aspect of the therapeutic interventions in water is the work that is done on muscular tone. This permits the child to balance their physical instability and also to influence the difficulties they experience with managing their attentive and cognitive capacities. With this therapy the water element is utilized to progressively permit the child to feel comfortable and to express their individuality. Thus in the water the dynamics of relation, equilibrium, movement in the space and in the dynamics of perception change (8). Global interventions such as those that take place in the water then support the development of the child's central nervous system, favouring a balanced development of the mind and body.

The main objectives of the therapeutic intervention in the water can be summarized into specific and global skills related to movement, manipulation, social coordination and physical dialogue.

As regard these objectives, the intervention begins with the acquisition of basic skills, e.g., learning elementary and purposeful actions, in order to subsequently reach complex skills, such as integrated sets of actions, following rules and sequencing and coordinating actions. Each objective can thus be specified according to issues related to different degrees of complexity (from very basic to complex skills).

The intervention can be supported by the use of instruments specifically designed for water therapy. Through the movement and the physical manipulation of objects, children with varying degrees of ability (multiple disabilities, physical-motor deficits and mental retardations) can progressively achieve a greater knowledge of their own bodies and of their own capacity for action.

In this paper we describe the water therapy as it is currently carried out trying to focus on those aspects that could be used to leverage the design of interactive system. In particular the fieldwork and activity modeling described in this paper guided the design of the software architecture for ubiquitous computing technology developed within the EU funded PalCom project (9). Key requirements coming from the users' profile and from the therapeutic practice have therefore been elicited in order to ground the future design of interactive and embedded therapeutic technologies.

FIELDWORK

Fieldwork has been carried out with the aim of directly exploring the field of therapeutic intervention in water. The fieldwork has been conducted in two settings for psychomotor therapy in water, the Disabled Children Parents Association, Siena and the D. Chiossone Institute in Genova. In the former context, trainers specifically trained for working with children with special needs mainly conduct the activities in the water. The activities are not structured and, while personalized to each patient, are not formally assessed. The latter is a rehabilitation center where the therapy in the water has been carried out in a more formal way by therapists specifically trained for treating cognitive and physical disabilities in the water. Therapists and trainers in both the settings followed a mixed functional-relational approach mainly based on playful activities and direct contact with the children.

The fieldwork provided us with a meaningful collaboration with trainers and therapists; with their valuable suggestions and comments they gave us a sense of the activities taking place and the challenges they pose. The participation of the actors resulted in a number of activities both during the fieldwork and the experimental phases of the process. Thus a variety of methods and techniques have been adopted ranging from ethnographic methods - such as field observation and interviews - to design methods - such as user workshops and creative brainstorming.

The ethnographic activities attempted to observe and reveal relevant issues related to the environment (the features of the water, the physical structure of the swimming pool), the actors (therapists, disabled children, parents), the tools (objects, toys and water noodles) and, above all, the activities (the procedures, the different phases, the practices). The outcomes of this activity resulted in a number of key observations that informed the whole design process. The development of activity scenarios summarized many of the outcomes described in the following sections.

In the following sections the descriptions of the tools, actors and environment, the procedures and activity models and the summary discussion refer primarily to the research activity conducted at the D Chiossone Institute, where the therapy in the water is part of a clinical rehabilitative plan, the activities are structured within a multifaceted rehabilitation plan and specific and coordinated objectives are pursued.

CONTEXT

The context in which the activity takes place is essentially an immersive physical and emotional environment that is experienced with the whole body. The setting is the public or private swimming pools where non-specific or dedicated pools are used as therapeutic settings for people with special needs.

Special pools dedicated to disabled people generally differ from the others by the higher water temperature (around 30-32°C) and the presence of equipment to aid disabled people with entering and exiting the water. These pools may also be of different dimensions and depth and may be characterized with respect to the activity taking place within them. There may be lanes in order to favour the swimming or the walking of the disabled or all water surfaces may be available for social and symbolic games.

The water temperature is one characteristic that makes a noticeable difference in the treatment. The appropriate temperature has valuable effects on muscular tone and prepares to sustain demanding tasks and physical efforts. In fact, as described at the beginning of this paper, entering the water means living the holistic experience of perceiving the whole body under different physical laws (e.g., buoyancy). This provides new and different capacities for action, especially for those who have severe physical and motor impairments. These people can particularly enjoy the perception of an uncommon autonomy and ability to move. Being in the water also alters the perspective on the surrounding environment. Depending on the position (if you lie or if you stand), you may change between different point of views on objects and persons.

The water environment is also immersive for what regards the lights - because of the reflections and transparencies - and the sounds - because of the echoes and the amplification of voices and noises due also to the presence of other people (parents, trainers, and people in other pools).

It is very difficult to communicate exclusively by voice, and that's why the interaction is also a more physical dialogue, based more on facial expressions, gestures and physical facts rather than words. In the water you may also feel the waves created by movement. The sensorial experience is thus predominant; sight, hearing, touch and whole body experiences are the key senses the therapists' play on throughout the therapy.

ACTORS

The main actors of this therapeutic setting are the children with special needs. Other actors involved are the therapists and caregivers, who take part in the activities, and the parents, who are usually present at the intervention, accompanying their children to the pool and helping them to enter and exit the water.

In this paragraph the needs of the main actors are described in order to provide insight on the nature of the disabilities treated and on the current therapeutic activities being used. Such information can hardly be expected from children with mental delays or cognitive impairments. The profiles briefly described below stem from interviews with caregivers and parents and from the available literature.

Children with very diverse profiles actually benefit from therapeutic play in the water. The users we have observed can be summarized in three main groups: children with cognitive and socio-relational disabilities, such as autism, children with physical impairments like cerebral palsy and those with a mental retardation such as Down syndrome.

Autistic spectrum disorders and other affective and socio-relational disturbances

In general terms, the main disabilities that are characteristic of people with autism are impaired social interaction and social communication and having a limited range of imaginative activities. People with autism also typically show little reciprocal use of eye-contact, and have a tendency toward repetitive behaviour patterns and resistance to any change in routine. Some children with autism do not interact with other children on their own initiative, and although some of them can play interactive games with others if they are told to, they will need to be instructed and supported during the game, otherwise they very quickly return to their own solitary 'obsessive activities'. Children with other affective and socio-relational disturbances will also have these kinds of impairments, even if in different degrees.

Physical and motor disabilities and cerebral palsy

These children have limitation or an impossibility of movement, restrictions in force, abnormal postures, the presence of neurological movement disorders such as dystonia, tremor, ataxia, etc. Children with mild or severe motor impairments particularly benefit from treatment in the water. Children with CP can be severely impaired in playing by their motor disability, but also by speech and communication disabilities, and sensory impairments (visual and/or hearing). These children can differ a lot from each other because the degrees to which they experience disabilities vary, resulting in a large number of different levels of functioning.

Mental retardation/ intellectual disabilities/learning disabilities

Children with mental retardation also referred to as intellectual disabilities or learning disabilities (for example children with Down's syndrome), have a reduced capacity for attention and might not understand the meaning of the proposed activity. They might not understand the meaning of language and many of them have speech limitations too.

It is also important to focus on age ranges to be able to make sense of the practice. Current therapeutic play activities are mainly for children in the age range of 3-6 years, who would like to do things with others and experiment with movements and actions; and children in the age range of 7-13 years, who would also like to perform activities on their own, such as trying, inventing, building, even when nobody else is available to assist them. Note that the chronological age is not suitable to be applied to these target users without an understanding of their developmental level.

The therapists and trainers are the other main actors of this setting. They essentially have the role of facilitating the playful physical, social and emotional experience. They have to mediate the social relationships, the experience in the water and offer a reassuring presence to the child. They are the scaffolds that allow the child to express and freely explore the space of the pool. The therapists have to facilitate the activity, and not impose rules or, on the opposite extreme, abandon the child without a guide. Even when the child would like to explore by herself the therapist should also be present and support her independent action.

The intervention is considered successful when the therapist interprets the meanings of the behaviors of the child. Having an intimate knowledge of the child is central to achieving this interpretation.

TOOLS

The therapists use two different kinds of tools during the current practice in the swimming pool. There are not therapy specific tools and the professionals have to define their own set of tools to rely upon. Being responsible for the care of the child, they pay attention to the materials, to how they react to the water and the potential dangers they may bring. After this careful analysis they choose the common noodles and tubes for swimming pool and water resistant toys that can be particularly pleasing for children.

The noodles are usually used as aids for buoyancy and as a means for engaging in symbolic play, e.g., the tube frequently becomes the horse that brings the child to the end of the lane.

The other kinds of tools are generally common toys that are water resistant and can be used in the water. They are special materials and toys available in the market and not specifically designed for the water environment or for therapeutic activity.

Those toys are generally made of coloured plastics and preferably have dynamic parts. An example is the polyp that floats and adapts to the surface of the water. The presence of these kinds of objects is also emphasized by the use of a torch for discovery games based on light.

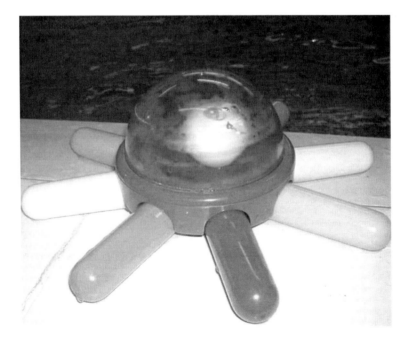

Figure 1. The polyp.

The most popular objects are those that produce some kind of effect and make use the dynamic property of the water (see the examples in figure 1, 2, 3). They capture the interest of the children and have been used for symbolic play or for play that involves physical causality. Those objects are also used for many of the game activities described in the next paragraph (e.g., give and take, push and pull, reaching with the extremities). Examples of these toys are the mill and the boats in the figures below.

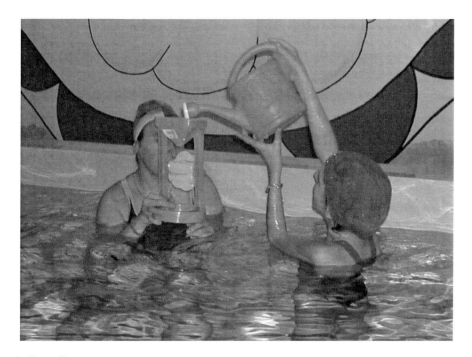

Figure 2. The mill.

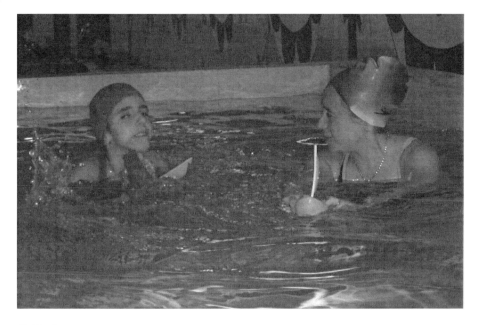

Figure 3. The boats.

It must then be noted that no interactive or digital tools have been used in the current practices examined.

ACTIVITY MODELLING

The children enter the therapeutic treatment in the water by way of a coordinated process characterized by:

- The initial assessment focused on the profile of the patient, their history of previous therapeutic treatments, the observation of the mother-child relationship and the assessment through profile specific Scales, e.g., the Learning Accomplishment Profile (LAP), for learning disabilities, or the Renè-Zilkin Scale, for evaluated sight impairments.
- The design of the therapeutic plan. The primary indication is to start from the needs of the child, which makes the identification of the rehabilitative project and, later on, the single rehabilitation sessions with the child possible. The rehabilitative project is defined by the group of therapists that usually treat the child (speech therapist, psychologist, psychomotor therapist and physician) and it consists of coordinated activities in different areas such as the visual stimulation, basal sensorial stimulation, physiotherapy, pet therapy and, among the others, the therapy in the water. In all of the treatments the objectives are defined by the relationship established between the adult and the disabled child within a rehabilitative context that makes use of play activities.
- Throughout the treatment periodic assessments take place. They are based on protocols defined ad hoc with respect to the therapeutic plan. In fact specific protocols for the therapy in the water are not currently used in the practices we have observed. The therapy in the water is mainly assessed by the therapist's individual qualitative assessment, which is based on the global wellness of the child and how the acquired behaviours can be transferred to other settings (i.e., self confidence and self awareness). In this respect, the water context makes exception with respect to other common therapeutic settings. In particular, it is hard to evaluate whether some changes or improvements are due to the role of the specific therapy in the water, to the global treatment of the child (physiotherapy, pet therapy, etc.) or to the growth of the child.

To my knowledge there are not, in fact, scales to measure and assess the activities in the water. The qualitative criterion adopted is the overall improvement of the child. In particular, as other research suggests (10), the therapist might observe if the behavior changes:

- from involuntary to voluntary
- from accidental to intended
- from indifference to interest
- from random to purposeful
-

- from exploratory to preconceived
- from isolated to integrated

These headings may summarize the overall picture of development for each individual (10). Other criteria for assessing the outcomes of the intervention in the water are the improvements in the social interactions with peers, family members and operators and the increase in vocalizations or in the physical dialogue through the contact with the caregiver.

One of the outcomes of the fieldwork and activity analysis is the activity model, in which the different phases of the practice have been described in detail. We have addressed the whole practice starting from the Planning, entering the Activity and proceeding with the Evaluation phase. The Activity has been better analyzed and modelled with respect to the other two phases of the practice, which are less structured and comprehensive.

PLANNING

When the therapist plans the therapeutic activity she primarily needs to focus on the therapeutic objectives established together with the other therapists in the integrated rehabilitation plan. She then rehearses the overall picture of the child, focusing on the history of the treatment, the child's previous behavioural answers, their needs and interests. In order to arrange the plan for the session the therapist obviously relies on previously performed successful activities, her personal set of best practices. By identifying play scenarios, along with objects and rules, it becomes possible to create a unique intervention, based on a careful analysis of the child's capabilities and their limits, as well as their preferences and attitudes.

The diverse abilities and personalities of the children have to be specifically taken into account. To avoid imposing their desires on the child, the therapist has to construct the therapeutic situation in a way that it is significant and motivating for that child. Forcing the child into rigid and repetitive activities is the least effective way of engaging the children. On the other hand, neither is it positive to hyper stimulating the child with many different initiatives. They have to be able to understand the requests and to choose the strategies that are most suitable to them in order to carry out the task.

Another element to consider in this phase is the proposed place for all of the activity. The presentation of games and toys and the structure of the activity must also be organized within the swimming pool environment. These choices must match with the purpose of the therapy and the child's individuality. The therapist needs to set up all of the available tools, which must already be configured but should also allow for customization and adaptation. The availability of ready at hand resources contributes to the prevention of distraction and loss of attention and allows the therapist to keep exclusive focus on the patient. Key requirements of the planning are summarized below:

- Focus on user needs
- Focus on acquired objectives
- Creative and novel proposals
- Re-use of successful solutions
- Minding the history of the therapy
- Purposeful set-up of the resources

ACTIVITY

The play activities must be started, maintained or changed in accordance with the child and their specific way of dealing with the problems and the provocations that the environment and the actors provide her. The play situation is not based on and characterized by the functional limitations and the pathology; rather, it is highly individualized according to these factors, and is based on an extensive knowledge of the child, their preferences, skills and frustrations. In this way the therapist may obtain the connection indispensable to establishing a play relationship with the child. The selected play activity also involves objects that have a role with respect to the exercise and to the relationship. The tools are used to stimulate imagination and curiosity, and involve the child in social and collaborative game dynamics. The activity is highly distinguished by the opportunity to provide the child with free movement in a very pleasing environment. The movement in the water is determined in relation to the treatment, e.g., treating children with attention deficit hyperactivity disorder requires a restrained space of action that does not favor free exploration and initiative taking.

In the following figure a specific model of the activity has been elaborated and evaluated on the basis of the ethnographic analysis and the participation of the therapist in the research process. The model is inspired by and adapted from the Body schemas Intelligent Learning approach (11) that consist of three phases:

- Exploration: Situating the problem and free exploration
- Dissociation: Proposal of different behavioural patterns
- Stabilization: Repetition on interiorization of body schemas

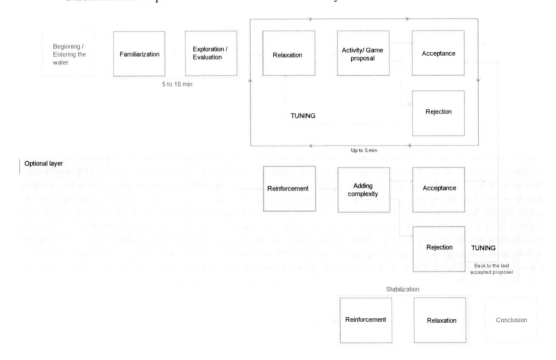

Figure 4. The Activity model.

The activity is detailed in the model by a sequence of actions each represented in the squared box. The model shows the relations among the events occurring throughout the therapeutic session. The sequence of actions is described to a large extent as follows.

With the entrance to the pool and the first contact with the water the child begins to familiarize themselves with the novel and uncommon environment of the swimming pool. They must deal with the novelty of meeting the therapist and the extensive experience of entering the water.

This phase is very relevant at the beginning of the therapy. Especially for very young children everything constitutes a novelty, both the unusual bodily experience of the water and the therapeutic play. As they continue with the sessions the children takes less and less time to adapt and to take part in the play activity.

The therapist must then explore the potentials of the intervention, what can be done and what is feasible. They have to evaluate the health conditions of the child, if they are tired or ill. It is also important to contextualize the activity within the events of the week and the daily experiences.

At the beginning of the treatment the exploration takes place almost exclusively on the child, on her abilities and her interests. Then the therapist may also use toys and objects to understand how the child feels, e.g., asking the child to discover objects, to reach and move them.

After these initial phases the therapist tries to relax the child and create the right atmosphere. They can remind the child of the last pleasing experience they have undergone together within the therapy, or they can work on the pleasing effect of the water to start the game activity with a feeling of wellness.

The game proposal is not conceived as a persistent demand that the therapist ought to make. The proposal has to be tailored to user needs and the therapist doesn't have to unreasonably insist in order to avoid the opposite effect, i.e., a rejection. The therapist involves the child in playful situations always asking the child for an answer, whether it be the acceptance or the rejection of the game. The child has to adhere to and, in some way, declare her interest in the game. This is necessary for the activity to achieve its goals.

The therapist has to tune the game activity with respect to the child's, often only behavioural, response. They have to reconfigure the tools as well by using them in a newly created way. This is an emergent behaviour throughout the interventions. The therapists need to tailor the stimuli and the feedback with respect to the needs of the children, and also using rigid objects and toys not specifically designed for therapeutic use.

When the game proposal is rejected the therapist has to set all of the tools aside and try to re-establish stability. Time needs to be given (usually 2-3 min) where the therapist steps back and permits the child some breathing space in the session, which is referred to as the "stillness zone" (12). This could indicate a preference for the next phase, for example if the child is bored with the choice they rejected it could be a defined pause to reflect upon what had been happening; or it could be an indication of exhaustion and a desire to stop the session.

In these few minutes the therapist may try again following another strategy. After an eventual rejection the therapist ought to go back to a positive situation in order to re-establish a positive attitude. Then the therapist retries the stimulus previously rejected or tries a novel initiative.

Optionally, the therapist may want to add complexity to the activity by adding elements to the game or modifying the activity by using only one object and varying some conditions. It can be proposed within a change in the game or a change of the physical dynamic.

In any case the child doesn't have to lose interest in the object/ game. If this risk is present, it is always better to remove the elements of complexity previously added and go back to the game that was originally established. In this particularly delicate domain the therapist has to be sensitive and able to capture interest and anticipate disinterest.

When the child accepts and participates in the game, the experience of novel capabilities happens with an understanding and awareness of novel spatial, physical and functional relationships. The therapist also aims to reinforce the positive results by repetition and slight variation in the play dynamics.

Towards the end of the session the therapist tries to stabilize the child by providing them with relaxing and pleasing activities. They remove all of the stimuli utilized and set all the objects apart in order to make the environment simpler and plainer. In this phase the objective is mainly to support the propioceptive experience of the children and to favor the contact with themselves. They exit the pool with a sensation of wellness and a rewarding memory of the experience. It is, in fact, very important to create bridges among the sessions in the pool due to the need for making the unique environment of the water more and more familiar. This phase usually takes from 5 to 10 min.

EVALUATION

After the activity is completed, the therapist makes a qualitative assessment of the session by considering the particular type of interaction established with the child. The evaluation phase usually takes place in a different environment with respect to the pool. The therapist has gone to the rehabilitation center or home and a certain time has passed.

This phase is not structured according to any procedure. The therapist chooses the suitable ways to organize her notes and comments about the child and the therapy.

The therapists are mainly interested in evaluating the intervention with relation to the therapeutic objectives they have defined in the plan, if and how sub-goals, intermediate and functional goals have been achieved. Another focus of the evaluation is on the child herself and on her attitudes and experience. The play activity is analyzed within the context of the relationship established between the child and the therapist. An exercise may be reproduced during different sessions or with different children, but the relationship within which the exercise and the environments are proposed is unique and built around the therapy. The therapists analyze the roles that have been carried out and how the interaction has evolved.

They also evaluate the methods used during the session and if they were appropriate for attaining the objectives. The therapist indeed chooses tools and games throughout the planning that are then experimented with in the real context of use. She doesn't know a priori if the planned resources would be effective and appropriate. The assessment of each intervention constitutes a piece of knowledge that the therapist has to formalize in order to collect and make these contents shareable. She usually takes a notebook to write down the assessment of each intervention in the water. Key requirements of the evaluation are summarized below:

- Feasibility of the pursued objectives
- Appropriateness of the adopted resources
- Adding notes

PACE OF THE ACTIVITY AND NEEDS OF THE ACTORS

Entering into a more detailed description of the activity (b), in the following section we discuss the key characteristics of the activity that have triggered the design process: the pace of the activity and the needs of the actors.

Each session in the water lasts 50 minutes with a few minutes provided to enter the water and exit the pool. The general structure of the session is based on the periods of activation/ excitement of the child. In fact, the therapist does recognize the fatigue of the child and the appropriateness of the stimulation, and eventually may choose to relax the child.

We describe a general model for the arousal/ relaxation dynamics that take place into the therapeutic activity by considering the outstanding function of the water and the events hereby described. The therapist allows a recreational pause (10 min ca.) between the two most demanding phases of physical and mental activation/ stimulation (20 min each ca.)

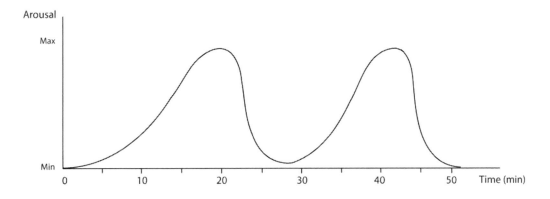

Figure 5. Arousal Model.

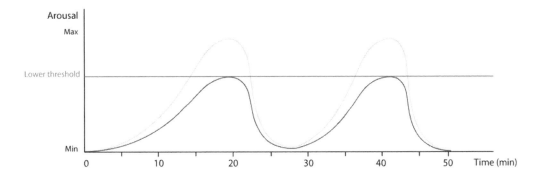

Figure 6. Arousal model representing the case of hyperactive children.

This graph can serve to model the general behaviour of the therapists and children throughout each session. Of course it may be slightly adapted according to the different patients. For example, in the case of hyperactive children the maximum level of stimulation would be lower than other patients and wouldn't go beyond a certain threshold (see figure 6). In the case of children with severe physical-motor impairments, the activity will probably follow a different path, with a higher periodicity of high arousal and rest (Figure 7).

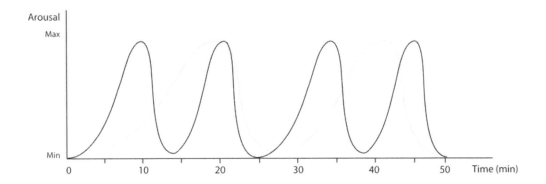

Figure 7. Arousal model representing the case of severe physical-motor impaired children.

A specific pace then characterizes the therapeutic activity in the water. The pace of each session is based mainly on the attention span and on the engagement of the child. The therapy has to remain a pleasing activity that captures and motivate the child to perform demanding tasks while engaging in playful activities.

Generally, children with cognitive deficit and delays are not able to remain focused for more than an average of 5 minutes. Even when involved in purely physical tasks, this special need has to be taken into account. In the figure below we tried to represent the pace of the activity with the same template used in the arousal model. Within the two periods of activation/ stimulation of the child, the activity can't be represented by a linear curve that increases homogenously. The pace of the activity is characterized by 5 minutes intervals during which each proposed game dynamic is maintained and pursued. After no longer than 5 minutes the therapist has to change the stimulus and vary the activity in order to avoid a loss of attention and motivation.

The pace of the activity can be represented with a sinusoid where the games are interrupted by very short intervals during which the child is free to take initiative and thus recover from the efforts made.

During the period of recreation the pace of the activity becomes linear to the lowest level. The overall therapeutic session is thus constituted by up to 10 short game dynamics. It may of course vary depending on the conditions of the children and on how the intervention proceeds.

The models proposed in this paragraph permit a greater comprehension of the current practices and provide a generalization of the knowledge gained from the fieldwork. In this perspective our aim is to pass from the description of single cases to general models through which each intervention can be explained and described.

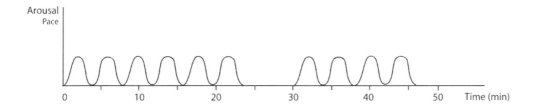

Figure 8. Activity Pace.

The game dynamic proposed by the therapists stems from the main objectives of the therapy that can be grouped into areas like Movement, Manipulation, Coordination and Physical Dialogue. Examples of short game dynamics are basic tasks such as following the objects, pushing / pulling, give and take, positioning and orientating objects in the pool, and more complex and structured games where multiple tasks are integrated in meaningful ways. Very often these games are part of playful activities of mutual exchange and reciprocal action. Key requirements of the activity are summarized below:

- Readily available resources
- Exploration
- Tuning/adaptation
- Pace
- Increasing complexity
- Emergent use of resources due to changing conditions

CONCLUSION

From our field and participatory work we have determined key issues referred the environmental conditions and the users' needs. As described throughout this paper, the properties of the water enable new opportunities for rehabilitation. The reassuring and calming qualities of the water, as well as the facilitation of body movement that it provides create a pleasant setting in which cognitive tasks can be easily combined with physical ones. The swimming pool represents an environment where different actors own specific spaces and the water play a central role in the activity. The therapists, who are possibly in or near the pool need to re-configure complex assemblies depending on which child they are working with and which support for planned and ad-hoc changes of complex configurations is needed.

The outcomes from the activity and the user modelling were used to explore interactive, embedded and distributed technology. Within the health care domain the field of therapeutic technology for the water therapy was selected as considered very promising for challenging the development of the software architecture for future ubiquitous computing technology (9).

In fact, as described above, the therapeutic practice in water poses challenges due to the changing conditions of the users and especially to the dynamic nature of the context. Furthermore, from a technological point of view the water challenged the development of embedded, interactive and distributed technologies. Water impacts floating objects by enforcing incessant dynamicity and is particularly challenging to the development of the communication module and the discovery protocol. This issue was of interest since the major focus of ubiquitous computing is on embedded, distributed and networked technology.

The ethnographic data described in this paper aimed at revealing key aspects of user practices that have been reviewed and analyzed within the technological research and design (13-15). These data have been assessed through different user workshops: i.e., discussions, focus groups and brainstorming sessions in which, in turn, the professionals have actively participated as an integrated part of the design team.

The data elaborated in this way have been used for organizing the software evaluation in the following phases of the process. In particular the software architecture for these technologies have been evaluated through performance testing (16-18). This method was based on a user-oriented perspective and we assumed human practice in the therapeutic setting, described in this paper, as baseline for the experiments. The measurements, i.e., time responses, delays or frequency of errors, have been observed with respect to the requirements coming from the activity analysis. For what regards timeliness, the major requirements from the therapeutic activity in the water are the duration of the whole session (45 minutes), the pace of the interaction (cycles of 3 to 5 minutes games to the utmost) intervened by the restless time pauses (2-3 minutes). These are the main criteria that allowed us to define the baseline for the performance testing' experiments.

The outcomes of the fieldwork and activity analysis were also elaborated from a more qualitative perspective. In fact the key issues outlined at the end of each session have been re-formulated with the active participation of the users. They can be summarized as follows:

- Looking for creative solutions: The therapists usually deal with dynamic settings and changing conditions. This implies the ability to manage and rearrange the available resources in purposeful and creative ways.
- Dynamic configuration of the tools: In dealing with continuously changing conditions and rehabilitation demands, the therapists should always find new solutions for adapting their tools and the environment to the patients and for maintaining their attention throughout the session. Consequently a core characteristic is that the tools have to be easily re-configurable and adaptable to this evolving situation.
- Resource availability and opportunities for action: The therapist needs to feel in control of the available resources and how they might be adopted, changed and exploited. As in many workplaces, since their attention is exclusively directed to the patients, the resources the therapists use have to be ready at hand and immediately understandable.
- Exploration and performance: This practice facilitates and encourages exploratory experimentation by users. Tools have to be used, customized and altered according to established degrees of freedom and constraints.

These data have been then elaborated into Activity Scenarios in order to define, as thoroughly as possible, what is relevant and appropriate in this specific domain of use, the therapeutic practice in the water. The Activity Scenarios have been developed to interpret the user and activity requirements determined through the fieldwork, and to describe the daily practice of water therapy in a rich, narrative form. These were also tools that provided guidance for and that informed the whole design process. In this way the user and activity modelling allowed us to elicit the requirements for the design of therapeutic technologies and the evaluation of the enabling middleware architecture.

ACKNOWLEDGEMENTS

My gratitude goes to Professor Patrizia Marti, who was responsible of the research team and supervisor of this research at the University of Siena, and my colleagues, Dr. Alessia Rullo and Dr. Erik Gronvall, who directly contributed to this work.

I especially thank the therapists at the Functional Rehabilitation Unit, Le Scotte Hospital, Siena, and the director Maria Grazia Burroni; the trainers, therapists and friends of the Parental Disabled Children Association, Siena, especially Laura Cardosi; and the therapists Alessio Persico and Alessandra Picasso at the D. Chiossone Institute, Genova, for their kind collaboration and enthusiasm during the different design activities. This study was supported by PalCom, an integrated project in EU 6th Framework Program undert he proactive initiative' The Disappearing Computer in Future and Emerging Technologies' (FET), part of the Information Society Technologies.

REFERENCES

[1]   Lund HH, Jessen C. Playware: intelligent technology for children's play. Odense: Maersk Inst, Univ Southern Denmark, Tech Rep, 2005.

[2]   Brooks A, Hasselblad S. CAREHERE. Creating aesthetically resonant environments for the handicapped, elderly and rehabilitation: Sweden. In: Sharkey P, McCrindle R, Brown D, eds. 5th Int conf disabil virtual reality assoc tech, 2004:191-8.

[3]   Spagnolli A, Gamberini L, Cottone P, Mantovani G. Ergonomics of virtual environments for clinical applications. In: Riva G, Botella C, Lgeron P, Optale G, eds. Cybertherapy: internet and virtual reality as assessment and rehabilitation tools for clinical psychology and neuroscience. Amsterdam, IOS Press, 2004:217-30.

[4]   Sharry J, McDermott M, Condron J. Relax to win: treating children with anxiety problems with a biofeedback video game. J Irish Assoc Couns Psychother2003;2:22-5.

[5]   MEDIATE Project – Accessed 2013Jul 26. URL: http://www.port.ac.uk/research/mediate/

[6]   ELDERGAMES Project - Accessed 2013Jul 26. URL: http://www.eldergames.org/

[7]   Belloni L. Psicomotricità in acqua. Percorso educativo e terapeutico. Trento: Erickson, 2007.

[8]   Lapierre A. Dalla psicomotricità relazionale all'analisi corporea della relazione. Roma: Armando, 2001.

[9]   PalCom Project - Accessed 2013Jul 26. URL: http://www.ist-palcom.org

[10] Ellis P, Van Leeuwen L. Living sound: human interaction and children with autism. Paper presented ISME Comm Music Spec Educ, Music Ther Music Med, Regina, Canada, July 2000.

[11] Vayer P. Per ritrovarsi nella complessità dei fenomeni umani. In: Perfetti C, Pieroni A, eds. La logica dell'esercizio. Idelson Liviana, 1992.

[12] Brooks T, Petersson E. Stillness design attributes in non-formal rehabilitation. CADE2007 - Computers in Art Design and Education. Perth: Curtin Univ Technol, 2007:36-44.

[13] Grönvall E, Marti P, Pollini A, Rullo A. Active surfaces: a novel concept for end user composition, NordiCHI, Oslo, Norway, 2006 Oct 14-18.

[14]   Pollini A, Grönvall E. Constructing assemblies for purposeful interactions. In: Proceed Mobile Interaction Real World Workshop, MUIA06 at Mobile HCI, 8th Int Conf Hum Comput Interaction Mobile Devices Serv, Espoo, Finland, 2006 Sept 12..

[15]   Pollini A, Experimenting with an ubiquitous computing open architecture. Dissertation. Firenze: Electr Engineering Dept, Univ Florence, 2008.

[16]   O'Brien L, Bass L, Merson P. Quality attributes and service-oriented architectures. Technical Note. Software CMU/SEI-2005-TN-014.Accessed 2013 Aug 01. URL: http://www.sei.cmu.edu/pub/documents/05.reports/pdf/05tn014.pdf

[17]   Bass LJ, John BE. Supporting usability through software architecture. IEEE Computer 2001;34(10):113-5.

[18]   Bass LJ, John BE, Kates J. Achieving usability through software architecture. Carnegie Mellon Univ, Software Engineering Inst, Tech Rep CMU/SEI-2001-TR-005, 2001.

In: Disability and Chronic Disease
Editors: J. Merrick, S. Aspler and M. Morad

ISBN: 978-1-62948-288-0
© 2014 Nova Science Publishers, Inc.

Chapter 9

NEUROPSYCHOLOGY FINDINGS AND PHARMACOLOGICAL TREATMENT OF ATTENTION DEFICIT HYPERACTIVITY DISORDER

Donald E Greydanus, MD, DrHC (ATHENS)[*,1],
Gabriel Kaplan, MD[2,3] *and Kevin M Antshel, PhD*[4]
[1]Department of Pediatric and Adolescent Medicine,
Western Michigan University School of Medicine, Kalamazoo, Michigan, US
[2]Rutgers New Jersey Medical School, Newark, New Jersey, US
[3]Behavioral Health Services, Bergen Regional Medical Center, Paramus, New Jersey, US
[4]Department of Psychiatry and Behavioral Sciences, SUNY – Upstate Medial University,
Syracuse, New York, US

Attention deficit hyperactivity disorder (ADHD) is noted in 3-9% of children and adolescents by American research, three times more common in males than females; it is found in 3%-5% of adults with equal male to female ratios if the diagnostic criteria are based on the DSM. The neuropsychiatric etiology of ADHD was suspected from early on so that significant research was aimed at elucidating its neuropsychological deficits. Impairments in attention, impulse control, and motor activity -the condition's core deficits- are well documented in neuropsychological studies. So are the beneficial effects of medication for ADHD which have been unambiguously supported by hundreds of studies in the expert academic literature. While stimulants are the most effective therapeutic agents, non stimulants also play an important role. Theoretical constructs linking molecular neurotransmitter actions to neuroanatomical macro structures and cognitive and behavioral findings have found solid empirical confirmations. Although medication related cognitive improvements appear to be supported only in short term studies, it is recommended that ADHD be actively treated, as patients with this condition can show serious long term disabilities that go beyond academic failure, and overall clinical improvements are strong and the agents prescribed relatively safe.

---

* Correspondence: Donald E Greydanus, MD, Dr. HC (ATHENS), Professor and Chair, Department of Pediatric and Adolescent Medicine, Western Michigan University School of Medicine, 1000 Oakland Drive, D48G, Kalamazoo, MI 49008-1284, United States. E-mail: Donald.greydanus@med.wmich.edu.

INTRODUCTION

Few conditions in the mental health field have shown a closer link to neuropsychological constructs than the Attentional Disorders. From the word "attention", prominently listed in the current Diagnostic Statistical Manual of Mental Disorders (DSM-5) (1) nomenclature of "Attention Deficit Hyperactivity Disorder (ADHD)" and recent sophisticated neurotransmitter findings, to previous descriptions such as "minimal brain dysfunction", the disorder has been associated with neuropsychiatric substrates throughout its history (2).

ADHD is noted in 3% to 9% of children and adolescents by American research, three times more commonly in males than females; it is found in 3%-5% of adults with equal male to female ratios if the diagnostic criteria are based on the DSM(3). Clinicians in European countries tend to use criteria based on the International Classification of Diseases in which the condition is called "attention-deficit/hyperkinetic disorder", and estimate a much lower prevalence for ADD/ADHD(4). However, various studies from different countries based on similar diagnostic criteria confirm the widespread prevalence of ADHD (5, 6). In 2006, 5 million individuals in the United States were prescribed psychostimulant medications, the most commonly recommended ADHD agents, 3.5 million between ages 3 to 19 years, and 1.5 million between ages 20 and 64 years (3).

COREFEATURES

The DSM-IV-TR presents a detailed list of symptoms and criteria for arriving at a diagnosis. Core features include attention dysfunction along with variable degrees of hyperactivity and impulsivity that interfere with day to day functioning (1, 7). This disorder is a lifelong condition with persistence from childhood and adolescence into adulthood in approximately up to 66% of those diagnosed with ADHD in childhood (2). Sometimes, ADHD is not diagnosed until adolescence or adulthood. Inattention in childhood may evolve into difficulty sustaining attention, paralyzing procrastination, and severe disorganization skills in teens or adults. The impulsivity of childhood may persist manifesting in adults as severe impatience characterized by frequent losing one's temper, quitting or losing jobs, or ending relationships. The classical hyperactivity of childhood is observed less commonly in the older populations and may evolve into an inner restlessness, excessive talking, and/or self-selection of jobs that mask ADHD symptomatology (8).

ADHD is considered a neurobehavioral disorder with abnormalities in various neurotransmitter systems, mainly dopaminergic and noradrenergic (9-11). Neuroimaging (i.e., PET scans) and genetic studies further suggest that dopamine transporter dysfunction (6) appears to be implicated in the pathophysiology of ADHD. Heritability is about 75% with at least seven genes involved in ADHD: DRD4, DRD5, DAT, DBH, 5-HTT, HTR1B, and SNAP25 (12).

Current research is attempting to identify different types of attentional dysfunction based on what areas of the brain are involved and then using specific medication to correct or moderate the identified defects; these areas include the cortex (prefrontal and parietal), brain stem (reticular formation), thalamus, basal ganglia, cingulate gyrus, and limbic structures (amygdala-hippocampus) (13). It is hoped that this brain mapping may allow more specific ADHD medications in the future.

CURRENT PSYCHOPHARMACOLOGIC PRACTICES

There are over 70 years of research noting that medication can ameliorate ADHD symptoms in children, adolescents, and adults (9). Drugs used for treatment include US Food and Drug Administration (FDA) approved stimulant and non stimulant agents as well as other various non - FDA approved agents.

FDA APPROVED AGENTS

A-stimulant agents

Hundreds of research studies on patients with ADHD have established the beneficial effects of stimulant medications in all ages: children, adolescents, and adults (3, 14-17). Approximately 75% or more of those with ADHD achieve some benefit (9) and the utilization of medication has become a standard part of management for these patients by many clinicians. A comprehensive study was sponsored by the National Institute of Mental Health (NIHM) in the United States; this research was named the NIMH Collaborative Multisite Multimodal Treatment Study of Children with Attention-Deficit/Hyperactivity Disorder, Combined type (or the MTA study) (18, 19). The MTA study posed 3 questions. How do long-term medication and behavioral treatments compare with one another? Are there additional benefits when they are used together? What is the effectiveness of systematic, carefully delivered treatments versus routine community care? In this study, 579 children with ADHD Combined Type, aged 7 to 9.9 years at study entry, were randomly assigned to 14 months of treatment with: rigorous medication management; intensive behavioral treatment; the 2 combined; or standard community care (delivered by community providers who in two thirds of the cases treated patients with medications). Seventy-four percent of the MTA Study subjects in the medication management group received methylphenidate immediate release (MPH IR) 3 times per day with an average dose of approximately 31 mg/d, which was well tolerated overall. Because of ethical concerns about the duration of the trial, a placebo or sham treatment control group was not included; the community care group served as the comparator arm. Although all groups showed considerable reductions in symptoms with time, there were significant differences between the 4groups. For core ADHD symptoms, children in the combined treatment and medication management groups showed significantly greater improvement than those given intensive behavioral treatment and community care. However, the combined treatment offered no significantly greater benefits than medication management alone for core ADHD symptoms. The MTA results validated the clinical experience that children who largely adhere to a well-titrated regimen of stimulants continue to benefit significantly for at least 14 months.

Methylphenidate preparations

MPH, the stimulant most commonly prescribed for patients with ADHD since its production started in 1957, is a sympathomimetic agent with mild central nervous system (CNS) stimulant properties. Preparations are available forracemicdl-MPH as well as the single d-MPH isomer. Its beneficial effect on attention span dysfunction results from blocking the presynaptic dopamine transporter in the CNS striatal and prefrontal areas, leading to rise in extracellular dopamine (20). It also causes a blockade of the CNS norepinephrine transporter in the norepinephrine system. Stimulant medication therapeutic actions include reduced motor restlessness (i.e., less gross/fine motor movement), reduced impulsivity, reduced hyperarousal, enhanced concentration and less aggressive and/or antisocial behavior. There is no correlation between weight of the patient and optimal MPH dose, and plasma levels of MPH are not useful. A number of tools, some of which are listed in table 1, are used to assess treatment effectiveness and include patient/family interviews, parent ratings, school grades or reports, and others. These instruments are helpful to monitor the efficacy of any type of ADHD therapy.

Table 1. Most commonly used ADHD rating scales

NAME	MAIN FEATURES
Conners Scales	Available in Parent, Teacher, Adolescent Versions Long, Short, and Abbreviated (10 item) Forms www.mhs.com
ADHD Rating Scale-IV	Based on the DSM-IV 18 symptoms, School and Home versions available. www.guilford.com
Brown ADD Scales	Available in Parent, Teacher, and Adolescent self report versions. Assess executive functions psychcorp.pearsonassessments.com
SKAMP	Brief 10 item version for Teacher or Observer www.adhd.net
CBCL	Not ADHD specific but one of the oldest and most studied tool. Multiple informant versions www.aseba.org

Various IR or short acting preparations of MPH had been popular until recently, when a number of longer-acting products were developed. All these agents are listed in table 2. There is only one "head to head" study comparing agents (21), so the absence of comparison data at this time makes the selection of the most appropriate agent truly a veritable blend of art and science (9). The process of identifying the best agent for specific patients is addressed later in this chapter. Reasons for failure of MPH to be effective are listed in table 3 and its side effects in table 4.

Amphetamine preparations

The description of beneficial effects of amphetamine (AMP) on hyperactivity and inattention date back to 1937(22). The amphetamines are non-catecholamine, sympathomimetic amines that act as CNS stimulants. Their putative mechanism of action involves reuptake blockade of neurotransmitters (dopamine and norepinephrine) into presynaptic neurons, as well as an increased release of those neurotransmitters into the synaptic cleft (20). Amphetamines are available as dextroamphetamine sulfate (the dextro isomer of d,l amphetamine sulfate) or as mixed amphetamine salts (dextroamphetamine plus levoamphetamine) as well as lysdexamfetamine, a prodrug formulation of d-amphetamine. The potential adverse effects of amphetamines are the same as of MPH (see table 4). Available amphetamine products are listed in table 5.

Table 2. Methylphenidate Preparations

| Brand name (in USA) | Dosage form | Dosing regimen | | Maximum per day | Duration of effect in hours |
		Start	Titrate weekly		
Active ingredient: d,l,methylphenidate					
Ritalin; Generic form available	Scored tablets: 5,10,20 mg	5 mg 2-3 times/day; 1 dose before breakfast, 1 before lunch	5-10 mg; Give a third dose in the afternoon if needed	Not to exceed 20 mg/dose; 60 mg/day	3-4
Methylin	Scored tablets: 5,10,20 mg; chewable tablets: 2.5,5,10 mg; oral solution: 5mg/ml, 10 mg/10 ml	5 mg 2-3 times/day; 1 dose before breakfast, 1 before lunch	5-10 mg; Give a third dose in the afternoon if needed	Not to exceed 20 mg/dose; 60 mg/day	4-8
Ritalin SR	Sustained release tablets: 20 mg	20 mg before breakfast	20 mg; Give a second dose in afternoon if needed; for desired dose and duration, short acting form may be used	60 mg	6-8
Metadate ER	Extended release tablets: 10, 20 mg	10 mg before breakfast	10 mg; Give a second dose in afternoon if needed	60 mg	4-8
Methylin ER	Extended release tablets: 10, 20 mg	10 mg before breakfast	10 mg; Give a second dose in afternoon if needed	60 mg	4-8
Metadate CD	Extended release capsules: 10, 20, 30 mg. Can be sprinkled	20 mg before breakfast	20 mg; Give a second dose in the afternoon if needed	60 mg	4-8
Ritalin LA	Long acting capsules: 10,20,30,40 mg; can be sprinkled	10 mg before breakfast	5-10 mg; Use short acting form (Ritalin) to titrate if needed	60 mg	4-8
Concerta	Capsules: 18,27,36,54 mg; do not split or chew or crush	18 mg before breakfast	18 mg	72 mg	8-12
Daytrana	Transdermal patch: 10,15,20,30 mg	10 mg patch applied 2 hour before desired effect; remove 9 hours later	10 mg	30 mg	12
Active ingredient: d, methylphenidate					
Focalin	Scored tablets: 2.5, 5, 10 mg	2.5 mg 1 to 2 times a day	2.5 mg; Give a third dose in afternoon if needed.	30 mg	4-5
Focalin XR	Extended release capsules: 5, 10 mg; can be sprinkled	5 mg before breakfast	5 mg; Give a second dose in afternoon if needed; for desired dose and duration short acting form (Focalin) may be used	30 mg	8-12

Table 3. Reasons for failure of Methylphenidate

- Inaccurate diagnosis
- Comorbid disorders that overshadow the ADHD
- Medication doses that are too high or not high enough
- Medication is diverted to others in or outside the family
- Intolerable medication side effects
- Medication is used as a drug of abuse for its euphoric effects
- Patient and/or family not accepting of medication
- Patient does not respond to MPH but does to other stimulants or alternative medications
- Patient does not respond to medications of any kind

Source: Modified with permission from: Greydanus DE, Pratt HD et al: Psychopharmacology of ADHD in adolescents. *Adolesc Med* 2002;13:604.

Table 4. Potential Side Effects of Stimulant Drugs

Headache*
Nausea/vomiting*
Anorexia*
Insomnia (delayed onset of sleep)
Weight loss*
Moodiness (irritability)
Tachycardia
Palpitations
Sudden cardiac death
Increase in blood pressure
"Unmasking" of Tourette Syndrome
Rebound phenomenon
Reduced seizure threshold
Irritability/ restlessness
Emotional lability
Appearance of psychosis or psychotic features
Growth retardation (at higher doses, over longer times,
 in those with short stature or slow axial growth)
Skin rash (rare)
*Commonly seen side effects

Source: Modified with permission from: Greydanus DE, Pratt HD et al:
Psychopharmacology of ADHD in adolescents. *Adolesc Med* 2002;13:607.

Table 5. AMP preparations

NAME/FORMULATION DOSE DURATION	DOSE FORMS	STARTING DOSE	MAXIMUM (May increase as per MD judgment)
SHORT ACTING			
Adderall	5, 7.5, 10, 12.5, 15,	3-5y: 2.5 mg q.d	40mg.
(Mixed AMP salts)	20, 30 mg tab	>6y: 5 mg q.d.	
Dexedrine	5 mg cap	3-5y: 2.5 mg q.d	40mg.
(d-AMP)		>6y: 5 mg q.d.	
LONG ACTING			
Dexedrine Spansule	5, 10, 15 mg cap	>6y: 5-10mg q.d.	40mg.
Adderall XR	5, 10, 15, 20, 25,	>6y: 10 mg q.d.	30mg;
(Mixed AMP salts XR)	30 mg cap		contents can be sprinkled
PRODRUG			
Vyvanse	20, 30, 40, 50, 60,	>6y: 20mg q.d.	70 mg
(LDX)	70 mg cap		contents can be dissolved

Contraindications for stimulant use

Unless stated otherwise, it is assumed that any medication will have as a contraindication sensitivity to that medication or any of its ingredients. Patients with significant levels of anxiety, inner tension, or psychomotor agitation should generally not be on psychostimulants. Other contraindications include glaucoma, psychosis, and hyperthyroidism. Due to significant comorbidity with substance abuse disorders, the field has taken a fresh look at the traditional contraindication of drug and alcohol dependence although it is still present on the labels (9). Because of potential cardiovascular side effects, stimulants should not be used in patients with uncontrolled hypertension, symptomatic cardiovascular disorder (i.e., angina, heart failure), serious structural cardiac abnormalities, cardiomyopathy, and serious heart rhythm abnormalities.

The use of stimulants in the presence of motor tic disorder or Tourette's syndrome is relatively contraindicated along with a history of epilepsy. Stimulants should not be combined with monoamine oxidase inhibitors since this combination can lead to a hypertensive crisis. Therefore, two weeks should be allowed between prescribing a stimulant and discontinuing a monoamine oxidase inhibitor. Mixing a stimulant with a tricyclic antidepressant may lead to sudden death from cardiac arrhythmias in rare cases. MPH can interfere with the metabolism of some anticonvulsant drugs, such as phenytoin and phenobarbital.

Side effects of stimulants

Adverse effects of stimulants, some of which are transient, can be reduced if the patient starts with a low dose and slowly increases the dosage to maximize benefit. Nausea or emesis that may occur with stimulants often improves if the medication is taken with meals. Dizziness occurs in some patients and is worse with short-acting stimulants versus long-acting types. If dizziness occurs, dehydration or blood pressure changes may be responsible and need to be treated as necessary. Headaches may develop while taking stimulants and this may be related to peak plasma levels or related to drug withdrawal. A change to a different formulation may provide symptomatic relief. The use of stimulant medication does not appear to increase the risk of substance abuse, although it is important to be cognizant of potential stimulant diversion and prescribe longer acting formulations that are less preferred in patients with drug dependence histories (23).

The phenomenon of stimulant related delayed growth remains controversial and seems to be, in part, related to appetite suppression with decreased caloric intake (24). It appears to be a transient effect, and most children eventually seem to attain expected adult height. However, youth on stimulants who are not growing properly need careful supervision. If the appetite is blunted while on stimulants, a number of measures can be taken, including taking food when the stimulant wears off (as in the evening), using high-caloric foods or nutritional supplements, taking the patient off stimulants when not in school (such as during vacation or on weekends), and trying other non stimulant ADHD medications (9).

Tolerance may develop in some patients receiving high stimulant doses. Management involves tapering off the stimulant and trying a different ADHD medication. Rebound can develop in which increased ADHD symptoms (i.e., irritability, sadness, and excitability) develop as the stimulant effect wears off. This can be managed by giving a smaller immediate-release dose in the afternoon or changing to a sustained release product. Stimulants may interfere with sleep and this side effect tends to diminish with time. In addition to stimulant side effect, the patient with sleep disturbances should be carefully evaluated for other causes of sleep disturbances(25).Administering the last dose of the day earlier, eliminating or reducing the last dose of the day, or the use of a long-acting preparation are some of the strategies that may help with sleep problems. Pharmacological options for sleep problems in children are limited. Drugs such as tricyclic antidepressants, alpha2 agonists [i.e., clonidine, guanfacine], trazodone, and melatonin have been used. However, potential complications of combination of these drugs with stimulants must be carefully considered, in particular regarding antidepressants. Recent data suggests that combinations with melatonin (26) and guanfacine XR (27) are safe.

ADHD is found in 50% to 75% of patients with Tourette Syndrome (TS) and TS may become apparent in some children or adolescents after starting stimulant drugs. Research does not suggest that stimulant medications cause TS and the presence of tics is a relative, not absolute contraindication to stimulant medication. Patients with both ADHD and TS may be given both stimulant medications (if effective) and anti-tic medication (such as risperidone, haloperidol, or pimozide). If the tics are worsened by the stimulant drugs, other ADHD medications may be tried that do not typically worsen tics such as guanfacine and atomoxetine.

Because of reports of serious cardiovascular adverse events in recent years, the FDA has required that a strong warning be placed on the label of stimulant drugs. Before starting a patient of any age on a stimulant drug a careful cardiovascular screening is recommended with the goal of identifying those at risk for serious underlying cardiovascular disease and adverse events related to stimulant use (28).

How to monitor patients on stimulants

In cases of long term use of stimulants, periodic complete blood count (with differential and platelet count) is recommended. Height and weight should be monitored routinely in pediatric patients, and any significant slowing should prompt further evaluation and possible discontinuation of the stimulant medication. Blood pressure and pulse should be checked as both values can increase with stimulant treatment. The use of rating scales is recommended to aide in the periodic assessment of therapy efficacy.

B-NON STIMULANT AGENTS

Atomoxetine

Atomoxetine is a selective inhibitor of norepinephrine reuptake. Its actions include the blockade of the presynaptic norepinephrine and dopamine transporter in the prefrontal cortex (29). The efficacy of atomoxetine has been documented in many short and long term studies in children and adults (30). Full therapeutic effect can take up to 4 weeks to develop. It can be used in those not wishing to take a stimulant, where stimulant or other medications are ineffective, or in patients with anxiety symptoms. Table 6 shows the main features of the preparation. The duration of atomoxetine effect is 18-24 hours.

Table 6. FDA approved non stimulant preparations main features

NAME/FORMULATION	DOSE FORMS	STARTING DOSE	REMARKS
Strattera (Atomoxetine)	10, 18, 25, 40, 60, 80, 100 mg cap	<70 kg: 0.5mg/kg/day. Increase up to 1.2mg/kg/day not faster than every three days. Can be given in 2 divided doses.	Maxdaily dose=100mg or less than1.4mg/kg. Higher doses have not shown greater efficacy. In CYP 2D6 poor metabolizers or with 2D6 potent inhibitors, titrate dose after 4 weeks of initial dose if symptoms fail to improve
Intuniv (Guanfacine extended release)	1, 2, 3, 4 mg	1mg at bedtime, then increase by 1mg per week up to 4 weeks.	Max daily dose=4mg. However, if tolerated, doses up to 0.12mg/kg may provide additional benefit. Do not crush or chew. Upon d/c, ↓ dose by 1mg every 3-7 days to prevent withdrawal.
Kapvay (Clonidine extended release)	0.1 & 0.2mg	0.1mg at bedtime, may increase by 0.1mg daily at weekly intervals	Max daily dose = 0.4mg. Do not crush or chew. Upon d/c, ↓ by 0.1mg every 3-7 days to prevent withdrawal.

Table 7 lists potential adverse effects. Atomoxetine has been associated with an increased risk of mydriasis, and should not be used in patients with narrow angle glaucoma. Due to reporting of several cases of severe liver injury, the manufacturer's package insert was modified in December 2004 to recommend baseline liver function tests with periodic monitoring. Patients should be monitored for an increased risk of suicidality due to reports of increased risk of suicidal ideation and behavior as atomoxetine carries an FDA black box warning similar to that for antidepressants. Drug-drug interactions can occur with inhibitors of the cytochrome P450, 2D6 isoenzyme, including selective serotonin reuptake inhibitors.

Guanfacine XR

Guanfacine is a selective alpha 2A adrenoreceptor agonist. An extended branded release formulation (GXR), was approved by the FDA in 2009 for the treatment of ADHD in children ages 6-17 years. It appears that guanfacine strengthens pre frontal cortex (PFC) regulation of attention and behavior by directly stimulating postsynaptic alpha 2A adrenocreceptors in that region. Controlled short term studies as well as open label studies of up to 24 months duration concluded that GXR was effective and safe as monotherapy. These studies also found that GXR improves both hyperactive as well as inattentive symptoms (31).

The side effect profile is considered mild with a preponderance of sedation which attenuates with continued use. Because guanfacine is a hypotensive agent, researchers followed its cardiovascular effects in detail in both the controlled and open label studies and results were similar across subject populations. Mild decreases in blood pressure and heart rate were noted which tended to normalize with continued treatment. In clinical settings, it would be prudent to obtain baseline and follow up readings of blood pressure and pulse. Research did not show weight loss or delayed growth and some patients experienced the opposite. Commonly reported side effects include abdominal pain, dizziness, dry mouth, and constipation. GXR does not carry a black box warning. It is contraindicated in patients showing sensitivity to guanfacine. Discontinuation should take place over time because while this was not observed with GXR, there are reports that immediate release a2 agents can cause rebound hypertension. It is recommended that dosing be titrated upwards slowly and based on a mg/kg method. Improvement can be seen in some cases at the second week of treatment (9).

Clonidine XR (Kapvay)

Clonidine is another á 2 agonist that was approved as an extended release formulation in October 2010 for the treatment of ADHD in those aged 6-17 years. This agent, like guanfacine, was originally approved for the treatment of hypertension and has been used off-label for ADHD for many years. Dosage is initiated at 0.1mg daily at bedtime and can be titrated up to a maximum of 0.4mg daily (two divided doses) at weekly intervals. Side effects most commonly reported include sedation, fatigue, irritability, nightmares, constipation, and dry mouth. Due to the potential for bradycardia/hypotension, patient's heart rate and blood pressure should be monitored at baseline, after dosage increases and periodically thereafter. Due to the risk for rebound hypertension, abrupt withdrawal should be avoided (no more than 0.1mg decrease every 3-7 days).

Non **FDA** approved agents

Over the years, clinicians have searched for alternatives to the traditional stimulant treatments. A few agents that were found to be effective to some degree have not been approved by the FDA. Due to their effects on central neurotransmission, antidepressant agents were among the first options researched. For instance, multiple controlled and open label studies showed that imipramine and desipramine are effective for ADHD symptoms.

However, they appear to improve behavioral problems more than cognitive deficits. Despite their efficacy, they are rarely used today due to concerns regarding cardiovascular toxicity (9). Bupropion considered to be a safer antidepressant from the cardiovascular perspective, has shown efficacy in controlled ADHD studies as well (32) and can be considered a second line agent. It works by inhibiting dopamine and norepinephrine reuptake into the presynaptic neuron. At higher doses, bupropion is associated with an increased seizure risk. In contrast to the tricyclics and bupropion, the SSRI antidepressants have not shown efficacy in ADHD. Modafinil, a wake-promoting agent with actions similar to amphetamine and methylphenidate, showed efficacy in ADHD (33). Nonetheless, the FDA rejected its approval because of concerns regarding Stevens Johnson syndrome, reason for which it is not often recommended. Clonidine is a presynaptic, central-acting alpha2-adrenergic agonist that is used by some clinicians to manage ADHD symptoms, though it may take 4 to 6 weeks to achieve full benefit and is less effective than stimulants (34, 35). Abrupt discontinuations can result in severe rebound hypertension, cerebrovascular accidents and sudden death. Blood pressure should be monitored for hypotension and rebound hypertension. Clonidine is used as an alternative or adjunctive medication to MPH. It is often given with MPH to treat the insomnia related to MPH.

LINKING PSYCHOPHARMACOLOGIC NEUROPHYSIOLOGY AND PATHOPHYSIOLOGY

A brief outline of current thinking regarding the pathophysiology of ADHD is helpful in understanding the potential remedial role that pharmacological agents play. The cognitive and behavioral impairments experienced by ADHD patients can be viewed from a unifying neuropsychological perspective as representing deficits in executive functions (EF). These functions encompass higher order cognitive tasks such as organizing, prioritizing, focusing, sustaining effort, managing frustration, utilizing working memory, monitoring and self regulating, as well as certain aspects of behavior and emotion (36). The literature shows that the neuronal substrate for these functions is located in the PFC and its connections to other cortical and subcortical structures and that anatomical as well as neurochemical integrity are instrumental for healthy EF. For instance, dopamine (DA) and noradrenaline (NA) are essential to PFC function and a growing body of evidence suggests that normal PFC activity is attained when NA/DA availability reaches an optimal level. Either too much or too little catecholaminergic presence can result in PFC dysfunction (37). DA and NA appear to exert different actions at the cortical level. While NA strengthens network connections, sometimes referred to as increasing "signal", DA seems to weaken unnecessary connections or decrease "noise". Not surprisingly, all the agents with demonstrated efficacy in improving ADHD symptoms are believed to improve catecholaminergic transmission. As mentioned, stimulants increase synaptic cleft DA and NA by inhibiting their intracellular reuptake; atomoxetine blocks the NA transporter resulting in higher synaptic levels of both NA and DA; and guanfacine selectively blocks post synaptic alpha 2a receptors thus mimicking increased levels of NA (37).

NEUROPSYCHOLOGICAL OUTCOMES

Because stimulant medications exert a primary effect on the DA system by preventing catecholamine reuptake it is not surprising that the most heavily researched neurological regions in ADHD are those that have inputs and outputs which affect the DA system. These regions are the PFC, basal ganglia, and cerebellum. This is logical given that these same areas are also involved in executive functioning, a core cognitive vulnerability in individuals with ADHD.

The PFC and basal ganglia are the primary targets of two ascending dopamine pathways, the neocortical and nigrostriatal pathways (38). The cerebellum, especially the posterior-inferior lobules of the cerebellarvermis, is also a target of DA projection from the ventral tegmental area (39). There are also reciprocal connections between the PFC, basal ganglia, and cerebellum via the pons, dentate nucleus and thalamus (40). The cerebellar vermis also has projections to the ventral tegmental area and locus ceruleus, affecting the turnover of DA and NA in the basal ganglia (41). In sum, there is much connectivity between these regions, permitting feed-forward and feedback loops.

Stimulant medications reduce unwanted ADHD symptoms (hyperactivity) and increase desired symptoms (attention), in both individuals with ADHD as well as those without ADHD (42, 43). Investigators found that non ADHD children who received MPH showed improved response inhibition and memory, and healthy adults who were administered stimulants displayed improved attention, vigilance, and working memory (44). Thus, a positive response to a stimulant medication is not diagnostic of ADHD. These cognitive benefits appear to be mediated not only by DA stimulation but also by NA release (45).

A great deal of research has been centered on studying the cognitive effects of stimulants which has focused more on short-term treatment effects rather than long term effects. The methodologies utilized varied greatly in the doses prescribed, length of treatment, presence of comorbidity, and outcome measures. MPH and AMP salts are thought to increase availability of DA in the striatum. Research shows that increasing striatal DA availability increases the salience of task-relevant stimuli (46), decreases impulsivity (47) and decreases the variability of response patterns (48). Stimulant medications, however, do not appear to reliably improve task motivation (49). A recent exhaustive review of the cognitive effects of MPH in children found that it reliably improved saccadic eye movement, planning/cognitive flexibility, attention/vigilance, and inhibitory control (44). On the other hand, in adults, studies evaluating stimulant effects of cognition in ADHD patients showed consistent effects only in improving attention and less reliable findings in other domains of executive function. (50)

Regarding effects on behavior, stimulant medications have been demonstrated to reduce disruptiveness (51, 52) and negative verbalizations (53) as well as increase compliance to rules / expectations (54, 55). Motor planning, motor coordination, and motor sequencing have all been demonstrated to be improved with stimulant medications (56-58). Physical aggression, however, does not appear to be as easily decreased by stimulant medications (59).

Atomoxetine and guanfacine both reduce core ADHD symptoms, although their effect size is lower than that of MPH and AMP (9). In contrast to stimulants, atomoxetine and guanfacine have received less neuropsychological research foci. Of the existing data, atomoxetine has been demonstrated to decrease impulsivity on a laboratory measure of inhibition (60), increase visuospatial working memory (61), and improve the memory and learning domains of the NEPSY children's battery (62). Guanfacine was associated with significant decreases in both commission and omission errors on the CPT (63) as well as improved planning and spatial working memory (64).

While there is a large body of literature documenting medication cognitive improvements, clinicians do not measure these routinely in order to determine therapeutic effectiveness and treatment progress. In part, this is due to the absence of user friendly instruments to assess cognitive domains in ADHD beyond inattention. In fact, the most widely utilized rating scales for ADHD (Table 1) preponderantly document behavioral manifestations of inattentiveness.

Despite improvements found in attention, task attractiveness, impulse control, response control, and multiple other domains, research has not been able to demonstrate that medication has an impact on long-term academic achievement (50, 65, 66). This lack of evidence has been puzzling to clinicians and researchers alike. If ADHD subjects experience acute medication improvements on a number of skills that are necessary for learning, why has this not resulted in verifiable enhancement of academic long term outcomes? The literature explains this contradiction in part by pointing out to methodological research issues. For instance, studies have varied greatly in their use of pharmaceutical formulations, dosage ranges -some perhaps suboptimal-, and times of medication administration. It is also possible that duration of treatment was not sufficient enough to demonstrate change or that patients did not adhere to treatment as prescribed. These issues may have interfered with the power to demonstrate effectiveness for an outcome measure that is very complex and multi determined to begin with. Recent studies continue to show uneven results; for instance even in the context of treatment considered optimal (67), while stimulants significantly improved cognition in ADHD children, they did not normalize it. On the other hand, in a large group of urban elementary and middle school students diagnosed with ADHD, stimulant adherence, although found to be low among was associated with a marginal improvement in GPA (68). A 2013 thought provoking paper suggests that while stimulants have demonstrated effects on aspects of cognition they may also increase the interfering effect of environmental distractions that therefore may prevent academic gains (69). Ultimately, it is also possible that for long term academic achievement to occur, medication alone may be insufficient and much more comprehensive wraparound modalities may be necessary.

AGENT SELECTION

The selection of a specific starting agent is not guided by its neuropsychological effects because as noted above, all agents improve core ADHD deficits alike. The decision of which agent to use is based on the assessment of individual patient needs and the pharmacodynamic/pharmacokinetic properties of a particular medication, as follows (9). Before beginning pharmacotherapy, it is important to record baseline measures to help determine the safety and feasibility of treatment. More specifically, information should be obtained from a recent physical examination that includes blood pressure, heart rate, and growth rate. Also, parents and teachers can complete pretreatment symptom rating scales or if this is not possible, a clinical estimation of baseline severity can be made. It is essential to discuss target symptoms to determine improvement, and carefully review possible adverse effects with the patient and family. Despite guidance from specialty medical associations, the multiplicity of agents available and the variety of patient clinical presentations call for a true blending of art and science in order to tailor the choice of medication to individual patient circumstances. It is normally recommended that treatment be started with an FDA approved agent but should it be a stimulant or a non stimulant? Unless specific contraindications exist, stimulants are the favored first choice because of their high degree of efficacy for core ADHD symptoms, rapid onset of action, ease of use, and generally benign side effect profile. Non stimulants could be used first if there is patient/caretaker preference, patient/caretaker substance abuse (due to diversion or abuse concerns), comorbidity, prior stimulant failure, or recent intolerance to stimulant side effects.

Longer acting preparations are the best first option for children and adults, for several reasons. First, once daily administration affords the patient full day symptom coverage in school, afterschool activities, homework, and evening family time. In addition, by virtue of the ease of following a once/day regimen, these agents may improve adherence. Unquestionably, they eliminate the need to involve school nurses, and they potentially are less likely to be abused. In general, the longest acting preparation that induces no side effects or side effects that are deemed acceptable to the patient is the one preferred. On the other hand, children under 6 are usually started on short acting preparations because they are more sensitive to dose dependent adverse effects and long acting agents are not available in low enough strengths. However, once a safe dose of an IR formulation has been established, conversion to a longer acting agent maybe considered.

While AMP was the first described agent to treat ADHD, concerns about its illicit use led the way for MPH to become more frequently prescribed. Nonetheless, in the past few years, AMP has regained considerable popularity. There have been several studies comparing AMP with MPH formulations that show differences in effectiveness and side effect profiles but these differences are not clinically meaningful enough to dictate choice of one type over another. It is important to understand that both types of stimulants have demonstrated high efficacy. When one fails, the other kind could be recommended next in order to increase overall treatment effectiveness to 80%. Usually, clinicians tend to become comfortable with one stimulant type they start patients with and use the other if the first trial fails. For example, a clinician may recommend Concerta but switch to Vyvanse if there are problems or vice versa. In special circumstances, such as children who cannot swallow pills, physicians may recommend one of the various preparations described in Tables 2 and 5 that do not require ingesting an intact pill.

For treatment of naive patients, the rule of thumb is to start with the lowest possible stimulant dose and to monitor side effects and efficacy every few days. If parent/teacher rating scales show inadequate improvement and there are few significant side effects, it is reasonable to increase to the next dose level. This strategy can continue until either the desired effect is reached or intolerable side effects appear. In general, doses can be titrated upwards until improvements in rating scale scores of 40-50% are obtained.

In cases where the patient is not improving and has side effects, the first step is to discontinue the initial stimulant and switch to the other type, or switch to a non-stimulant. There are no evidence based data that preferentially support continuation with either strategy after a first treatment fails. If the main issue is intolerance to stimulant side effects, then switching to a non stimulant is preferred. There is evidence that adding a non stimulant to stimulant therapy potentiates the effectiveness of the overall regimen; thus, combination therapy is another accepted strategy. However, if there is no improvement after two ADHD treatments, a diagnostic reassessment is necessary. For instance, is there comorbidity with affective disorder, anxiety disorder, or substance abuse? Can adherence be clearly ascertained? Are there psychosocial stressors that require resolution?

Only a small minority of patients will not respond to FDA approved treatments, either as monotherapy or in combination. Therefore, if there is little or no improvement, a diagnostic reassessment is mandatory. In the absence of diagnostic issues, non FDA approved treatments can be entertained. On the other hand, these have yielded lower effect sizes than approved agents. A trial of behavior therapy for which there are evidenced based data of effectiveness should also be presented to the family. If medication is preferred by caretakers, a trial of bupropion, modafinil, or tricyclics can be entertained as long as appropriate informed consent is obtained.

The need for continued treatment should be reevaluated periodically, as some patients may no longer require pharmacotherapy. In order to avoid disruptions in school function, treatment should generally be maintained through the academic year. On the other hand, it is important to have school input when assessing the need for continued care. Thus, a reasonable strategy is to taper first and finally discontinue treatment near the end of the year. For adolescents, it is important to maintain treatment until final examinations are taken. By the end of the year, teacher input is still available but final grades are not jeopardized as there is time to reinstitute treatment if the patient relapses off medication. Regarding medication use during the summer, for non stimulants, unless the goal is to reassess need for ongoing care, it is not advisable to stop treatment because it may take several weeks to return to therapeutic success. Weekend holidays are impractical for the same reason. With respect to stimulants, if a patient becomes symptomatic without them, routine discontinuation on weekends is not recommended. However, in cases in which there is notable growth delay, drug holidays have been recommended as a strategy to allow for "catch up" growth. Routine summer discontinuations are no longer recommended since symptom relapse often occurs in the absence of medication. On the other hand, if growth delay is a concern or the patient prefers stopping, summer discontinuation should be considered.

CONCLUSION

The neuropsychiatric etiology of ADHD was suspected from early on so that significant research was aimed at elucidating its neuropsychological deficits. Impairments in attention, impulse control, and motor activity -the condition's core deficits- are well documented in neuropsychological studies. So are the beneficial effects of medication for ADHD which have been unambiguously supported by hundreds of studies in the expert academic literature. While stimulants are the most effective therapeutic agents, non stimulants also play an important role. As described above, theoretical constructs linking molecular neurotransmitter actions to neuroanatomical macro structures and cognitive and behavioral findings, have found solid empirical confirmations. However, medication related improvements appear to support only short term gains (50) and just while patients remain under carefully monitored treatment conditions (70). Plausible reasons exist for the apparent lack of scientific proof in documenting long term academic gains and further research is needed in this respect.

Nonetheless, because of the strong beneficial effects in alleviating current symptomatology and the relative safety of the agents used, the clinical psychiatric community strongly recommends that ADHD be appropriately treated, as patients with this condition show very serious long term disabilities that go beyond academic failure (71).

REFERENCES

[1]   American Psychiatric Association. Diagnostic and statistical manual of mental disorders,5th ed,. Washington, DC: American Psychiatric Association, 2013:59-61.

[2]   Barkley R. The nature of ADHD in attention-deficit hyperactivity disorder, third edition: A handbook for diagnosis and treatment. New York: Russell A Guildford, 2006.

[3]   Greydanus DE, Pratt HD, Patel DR: Attention deficit hyperactivity disorder across the lifespan. Disease-a-Month 2007;53(2):65-132.

[4]   Faraone SV, Sergeant J, Gillberg C, Biederman J. The worldwide prevalence of ADHD: is it an American condition? World Psychiatry 2003;2:104-13.

[5]   Katragadda S, Schubiner H. ADHD in children, adolescents, and adults. Prim Care Clin Office Pract 2007;34(4):111.

[6]   Biederman J, Farone SV. Attention-deficit/hyperactivity disorder. Lancet 2005;366;237-48.

[7]   Barkley RA: Attention-deficit/hyperactivity disorder. Sci Am 1998;3:66–71.

[8]   Adler L, Cohen J. Diagnosis and evaluation of adults with attention-deficit/ hyperactivity disorder. Psychiatr Clin North Am 2004;27:187-201.

[9]   Kaplan G, Newcorn JH, Ivanov IS. Pharmacologic management of ADHD in children and adolescents. Int J Child Adolesc Health 2010; 3(2):143-61.

[10]   Biederman J. Attention-deficit/hyperactivity disorder: A selective overview. Biol Psychiatry 2005;57:1215-20.

[11]   Greydanus DE, Pratt HD. Attention deficit/hyperactivity disorder in adolescents. In: Greydanus DE, Patel DR, Pratt HD,eds. Essential adolescent medicine. New York: McGraw-Hill, 2006:751-68.

[12]   Faraone SV, Khan SA. Candidate gene studies of attention-deficit/hyperactivity disorder. J Clin Psychiatry 2006;67(Suppl 8):13-20.

[13]   Wilens T. Personal Communication, 2007.

[14]   Clarke SD. ADHD in adolescence. J Adolesc Health 2000;27:77–78.

[15]   Pliszka SR, Crismon ML, Hughes CW, et al. The Texas Children's Medication Algorithm Project: Revision of the algorithm for pharmacology of attenton-deficit/hyperactivity disorder. J Am Acad Child Adolesc Psychiatry 2006;45(6):642-57.

[16]   Schubiner H, Robin AL, Young J. Attention-deficit/hyperactivity disorder in adolescent males. Adolesc Med 2003;14:663–76.

[17]   Staufer WB, GreydanusDE. Attention-deficit/hyperactivity disorder psychopharmacology for college students. Pediatr Clin North Am 2005;52:71-84.

[18]   Jensen PS, Hinshaw SP, Swanson JM, Greenhill LL, Conners CK, et al. Findings from the NIMH Multimodal Treatment Study of ADHD (MTA): Implications and applications for primary care providers. J Dev Behav Pediatr 2001;22:60–73.

[19]   National Institute of Mental Health (NIMH): Attention Deficit Hyperactivity Disorder. NIMH, NIH Publication No. 01-4589, 2001. Available at: http://www.nimh.nih.gov/publicat/helpchild.cfm.

[20]   Solanto MV, Arnsten AFT, Castellanos FX.The neuroscience of stimulant drug action in ADHD. In: Solanto MV, Arnsten AFT, Castellanos FX, eds. Stimulant drugs and ADHD. London: OxfordUniversity Press, 2001:355-79.

[21]   Muniz R, et al. Efficacy and safety of extended-release dexmethylphenidate compared with d,l-methylphenidate and placebo in the treatment of children with attention- deficit/hyperactivity disorder: a 12-hour laboratory classroom study. J Child Adolesc Psychopharmacol 2008;18(3):248-56.

[22]   Bradley C. The behavior of children receiving Benzedrine. Am J Psychiatry 1937;94:577-85.

[23]   Ivanov I, Pearson A, Kaplan G, Newcorn J. Treatment of adolescent ADHD and comorbid substance abuse. Int J Child Adolesc Health 2010; 3(2):33-40.

[24]   Swanson JM and MTA Cooperative Group. National Institute of Mental

[25]   Health Multimodal Treatment Study of ADHD Follow-up: Changes in effectiveness and growth after the end of treatment. Pediatrics 2004;113:762–9.

[26]   Chhangani BS. Sleep disorders in children and adolescents. In: Greydanus DE, Patel DR, Reddy VN, Feinberg AN, Omar HA, eds. Handbook of clinical pediatrics: An update for the ambulatory pediatrician. Singapore: World Scientific, 2010:87-115.

[27]   Weiss MD, Wasdell MB, Bomben MM, Rea KJ, Freeman RD. Sleep hygiene and melatonin treatment for children and adolescents with ADHD and initial insomnia. J Am Acad Child Adolesc Psychiatry 2006;45(5):512-9.

[28]   Spencer TJ, Greenbaum M, Ginsberg LD, Murphy WR. Safety and effectiveness of coadministration of guanfacine extended release and psychostimulants in children and adolescents with attention-deficit/hyperactivity disorder. J Child Adolesc Psychopharmacol 2009;19(5):501-10.

[29]   Vitiello B, Towbin K. Stimulant treatment of ADHD and risk of sudden death in children. Am J Psychiatr 2009;166(9):955-7.

[30]   Atomoxetine: Strattera revisited. MedMed Lett 2004;46:65.

[31]   Faraone SV, Glatt SJ. A comparison of the efficacy of medications for adult attention-deficit/hyperactivity disorder using meta-analysis of effect sizes.J Clin Psychiatry 2010;71(6):754-63.

[32]   Biederman J, Melmed RD, Patel A, McBurnett K, Donahue J, Lyne A. Long-term, open-label extension study of guanfacine extended release in children and adolescents with ADHD. CNS Spectr 2008;13(12):1047-55.

[33]   Paykina N and Greenhill L. Attention deficit hyperactivity disorder. In: Findling RL, ed. Clinical manual of child and adolescent psychopharmacology. Washington, DC: APP, 2008:33-87.

[34]   Biederman J, Spencer TJ. Psychopharmacological interventions. Child Adolesc Psychiatr Clin North Am 2008;17(2):439-58.

[35]   Greydanus DE, Sloane MA, Rappley MD. Psychopharmacology of ADHD in adolescents. Adolesc Med 2002;13:599–624.

[36]   Greydanus DE, Pratt HD, Sloane MA, et al. Attention-deficit/hyperactivity disorder in children and adolescents: Interventions for a complex costly clinical conundrum. Pediatr Clin North Am 2003;50:1049–92.

[37]   Barkley RA. Behavioral inhibition, sustained attention, and executive functions: Constructing a unifying theory of ADHD. Psychol Bull 1997;121(1):65-94.

[38]   Arnsten AF. Toward a new understanding of attention-deficit hyperactivity disorder pathophysiology: an important role for prefrontal cortex dysfunction. CNS Drugs 2009;23(Suppl 1):33-41.

[39]   Swanson J, Volkow N. Pharmacokinetic and pharmacodynamic properties of methylphenidate in humans. In: Solanto MV, Arnsten AFT, Castellanos FX, eds. Stimulant drugs and ADHD: Basic and clinical neuroscience. Oxford: Oxford University Press, 2001:259-82.

[40]   Ikai Y, Takada M, Mizuno N. Single neurons in the ventral tegmental area that project to both the cerebral and cerebellar cortical areas by way of axon collaterals. Neuroscience 1994;61:925-34.

[41]   Middleton FA, Strick PL. Basal ganglia and cerebellar loops: motor and cognitive circuits. Brain Res Brain Res Rev 2000;31:236-50.

[42]   Snider RS, Maiti A, Snider SR. Cerebellar pathways to ventral midbrain and nigra. Exp Neurol 1976;53:714-28.

[43]   Berridge CW, Devilbiss DM, Andrzejewski ME, et al. Methylphenidate preferentially increases catecholamine neurotransmission within the prefrontal cortex at low doses that enhance cognitive function. Biol Psychiatry 2006;60(10):1111-20.

[44]   Rapoport JL, Inoff-Germain G. Responses to methylphenidate in attention-deficit/hyperactivity disorder and normal children: update 2002. J Atten Disord 2002;6(Suppl 1):S57-60.

[45]   Pietrzak R, et al. Cognitive effects of immediate-release methylphenidate in children with attention-deficit/hyperactivity disorder. Neurosci Biobehav Rev 2006;30:1225–45.

[46]   Arnsten AF, Dudley AG. Methylphenidate improves prefrontal cortical cognitive function through alpha2 adrenoceptor and dopamine D1 receptor actions: Relevance to therapeutic effects in attention deficit hyperactivity disorder. Behav Brain Funct 2005;1(1):2.

[47]   Volkow ND, Wang GJ, Fowler JS, Telang F, Maynard L, Logan J. Evidence that methylphenidate enhances the saliency of a mathematical task by increasing dopamine in the human brain. Am J Psychiatry 2004;161:1173–80.

[48]   Scheres A, Oosterlaan J, Swanson J, Morein-Zamir S, Meiran N, Schut H. The effect of methylphenidate on three forms of response inhibition in boys with AD/HD. J Abnorm Child Psychol 2003;31:105–20.

[49]   Pliszka SR, Liotti M, Bailey BY, Perez R, Glahn D, Semrud-Clikeman M. Electrophysiological effects of stimulant treatment on inhibitory control in children with attention-deficit/hyperactivity disorder. J Child Adolesc Psychopharmacol2007;17:356–66.

[50]   Groom MJ, Scerif G, Liddle PF, Batty MJ, Liddle EB, Roberts KL. Effects of motivation and medication on electrophysiological markers of response inhibition in children with attention-deficit/hyperactivity disorder. Biol Psychiatry 2010;67(7):624-31.

[51]   Advokat C. What are the cognitive effects of stimulant medications? Emphasis on adults with attention-deficit/hyperactivity disorder (ADHD). Neurosci Biobehav Rev 2010;34:1256-66.

[52]   Bukstein OG, Kolko DJ. Effects of methylphenidate on aggressive urban children with attention deficit hyperactivity disorder. J Clin Child Psychol 1998;27(3):340-51.

[53]   Reitman D, Hupp SD, O'Callaghan PM, Gulley V, Northup J. The influence of a token economy and methylphenidate on attentive and disruptive behavior during sports with ADHD-diagnosed children. Behav Modif 2001;25(2):305-23.

[54]   Pelham WE, Gnagy EM, Greiner AR, Hoza B, Hinshaw SP, Swanson JM. Behavioral versus behavioral and pharmacological treatment in ADHD children attending a summer treatment program. J Abnorm Child Psychol 2000;28(6):507-25.

[55]   Evans SW, Pelham WE, Smith BH, Bukstein O, Gnagy EM, Greiner AR. Dose-response effects of methyphenidate on ecologically valid measures of academic performance and classroom behavior in adolescents with ADHD. Exp Clin Psychopharmacol 2001;9(2):163-75.

[56]   Pelham WE, Gnagy EM, Burrows-Maclean L, Williams A, Fabiano GA, Morrisey SM. Once-a-day Concerta methylphenidate versus three-times-daily methylphenidate in laboratory and natural settings. Pediatrics 2001;107(6): E105.

[57]   O'Driscoll GA, Dépatie L, Holahan AL, Savion-Lemieux T, Barr RG, Jolicoeur C. Executive functions and methylphenidate response in subtypes of attention-deficit/hyperactivity disorder. Biol Psychiatry 2005;57(11):1452-60.

[58]   Rubia K, Noorloos J, Smith A, Gunning B, Sergeant J. Motor timing deficits in community and clinical boys with hyperactive behavior: the effects of methylphenidate on motor timing. J Abnorm Child Psychol 2003;31(3):301-13.

[59]   Sheppard DM, Bradshaw JL, Georgiou N, Bradshaw JA, Lee P. Movement sequencing in children with Tourette's syndrome and attention deficithyperactivity disorder. Mov Disord 2000;15(6):1184-93.

[60]   Matier K, Halperin JM, Sharma V, Newcorn JH, Sathaye N. Methylphenidate response in aggressive and nonaggressive ADHD children: distinctions onlaboratory measures of symptoms. J Am Acad Child Adolesc Psyciatry1992;31(2):219-25.

[61]   Chamberlain SR, Del Campo N, Dowson J, Müller U, Clark L, Robbins TW, Sahakian BJ. Atomoxetine improved response inhibition in adults with attention-deficit/hyperactivity disorder. Biol Psychiatry 2007; 62(9):977-84.

[62]   de Jong CG, Van De Voorde S, Roeyers H, Raymaekers R, Allen AJ, Knijff S. Differential effects of atomoxetine on executive functioning and lexical decision in attention-deficit/hyperactivity disorder and reading disorder. J Child Adolesc Psychopharmacol 2009;19(6):699-707.

[63]   Maziade M, Rouleau N, Lee B, Rogers A, Davis L, Dickson R.A tomoxetine and neuropsychological function in children with attention-deficit/hyperactivity disorder: results of a pilot study. J Child Adolesc Psychopharmacol 2009;19(6):709-18.

[64]   Chappell PB, Riddle MA, Scahill L, Lynch KA, Schultz R, Arnsten A. Guanfacine treatment of comorbid attention-deficit hyperactivity disorder and Tourette's syndrome: preliminary clinical experience. J Am Acad Child Adolesc Psychiatry 1995;34(9):1140-6.

[65]   Jäkälä P, Riekkinen M, Sirviö J, Koivisto E, Kejonen K, Vanhanen M. Guanfacine,but not clonidine, improves choice reaction time performance in young healthy volunteers. Neuropsychopharmacology 1999;21(4):495-502.

[66]   Raggi VL, Chronis AM. Interventions to address the academic impairment of children and adolescents with ADHD. Clin Child Fam Psychol Rev 2006;9:85-111.

[67]   Schachar R, Jadad AR, Gauld M, Boyle M, Booker L, Snider A, et al. Attention-deficit / hyperactivity disorder: Critical appraisal of extended treatment studies. Can J Psychiatr 2002;47:337-48.

[68]   Gualtieri T, Johnson L. Medications do not necessarily normalize cognition in ADHD patients J Attend Dis 2008;11(4):459-69.

[69]   Marcus SC, Durkin M. Stimulant adherence and academic performance in urban youth with attention-deficit/hyperactivity disorder. J Am Acad Child Adolesc Psychiatry. 2011;50(5):480-9

[70]   AdvokatC, Scheithauer M Attention deficit hyperactivity disorder (ADHD) stimulant medications as cognitive enhancers. Front Neurosci. 2013 29;7:82

[71]   Molina BS, et al. The MTA at 8 years: prospective follow-up of children treated for combined-type ADHD in a multisite study. J Am Acad Child Adolesc Psychiatry 2009;48(5):484-500.

[72]   Barkley R. Appendix A. International Consensus Statement on ADHD in attention-deficit hyperactivity disorder, third edition. In: A Russell, ed. A handbook for diagnosis and treatment. New York: Guildford, 2006.

In: Disability and Chronic Disease   ISBN: 978-1-62948-288-0
Editors: J. Merrick, S. Aspler and M. Morad   © 2014 Nova Science Publishers, Inc.

Chapter 10

WOMEN CARING FOR ADULTS WITH INTELLECTUAL DISABILITIES

*Michelle Rowbotham, BA (Hons), Monica Cuskelly, PhD** and Annemaree Carroll, PhD*

School of Education, University of Queensland, Brisbane, Australia

Most adults with intellectual disabilities are cared for across their life-spans by their families. The processes that link long-term care-giving to the psychological functioning of family care-givers is unclear, as most research is cross-sectional, preventing the study of how care-giving demands, satisfactions, and coping strategy usage impact upon care-giver well-being. In this chapter we examine the course of coping and the relationships of caregiving stressors and satisfaction for carers of adults with an intellectual disability. Four female carers were interviewed for five consecutive months, and questionnaire and interview data collected, to examine whether their appraisals of these variables changed over time. Results: Data revealed direct relationships between care-giving difficulties and satisfactions, as well as evidence that for some individuals there was development of competence in meeting the demands of care-giving as carers aged whereas for others, the demands of care-giving depleted their resources. Conclusion: These results suggest that cross-sectional studies may provide an incomplete picture and may overlook the cumulative impact of stressors, as well as the role of satisfactions and resources, upon care-givers' well-being.

INTRODUCTION

Various research studies attest to the stressfulness of long-term care-giving (1, 2). This concern is of particular relevance to the families of adults with intellectual disabilities, who typically provide care to the individual with intellectual disability for either the entire lifespan of the adult or for the entire lifespan of the care-giver (3). One of the most common observations in the literature on stress and coping is the need for more longitudinal research,

---

* Correspondence: Monica Cuskelly, School of Education, University of Queensland, Queensland 4072, Australia. E-mail: m.cuskelly@uq.edu.au.

in order that the relationships between various stressors and the ways people cope with the demands associated with them can be identified and tracked over time (4, 5). This paper reports on a short-term longitudinal examination of stress and coping in female carers of an adult with intellectual disabilities.

Theories explaining the impact of long-term, unrelieved demands on care-givers suggest that the psychological well-being of carers is eroded as a consequence of the unrelenting exposure to stressors (i.e., the wear and tear hypothesis) (6) or that the experience builds resilience within carers, because exposure to constant stressors facilitates the development of skills for their management (i.e., the adaptation hypothesis) (7). Current Australian research (8) has concluded that most carers of people with disabilities report higher rates of poor physical and mental health than the general population, as predicted by the wear and tear hypothesis (6). However, the oldest group in their study were an exception to this, according with past US research where older mothers who were full-time carers of their daughters and sons with intellectual disabilities rated their physical health as better than that of women without care-giving responsibilities (9). These women also experienced more life satisfaction than women caring for elderly relatives and considered that they had no greater care-giver burden than younger mothers caring for their children with intellectual impairments (9). Commensurate with the adaptation hypothesis, these contrary findings have been explained in terms of care-givers' extensive experience in managing stressors (10).

CARE-GIVER STRESS

Pearlin's stress process model (11) is an example of an adaptation theory. In this model, stress is conceptualised as the end-product of interactions between chronic role strains (or daily hassles) and negative life events (e.g., death). These interactions are complex, because while life events usually occur at clearly identified points in time, role strains often emerge less clearly. While most carers buffer the negative impact of stressors through the use of moderators, such as social support and coping strategies, of particular concern are situations where care-givers have been exposed to continual, high-level role strains, such as caring for a person with pervasive daily support needs, in addition to accumulated residual stress from negative life events. Interactions between these role strains and life events can result in stress proliferation, which may lead to poor psychological well-being. Women carers providing care to family members in addition to their adult child or sibling with an intellectual disability constitute a group potentially at risk of stress proliferation because of the various role demands they encounter (12); for example, those combining full-time employment and parental/child-care roles (13).

One of the most frequently reported types of care-giving demand faced by female carers is the management of episodes of challenging behaviour (14). Mothers of adults engaging in violent behaviours reported higher levels of care-giving burden; particularly those who care for adults exhibiting self-injurious behaviours or stereotypies (15, 16). These findings show that carers' role responsibilities are complex: not only are they required to meet the demands associated with the additional support needs of their adult child or relative with an intellectual disability, but also those associated with their other roles.

COPING WITH ROLE DEMANDS

The cognitive model of stress and coping (17) remains one of the most influential theories of coping with stress. This model posits that situations which tax or exceed carers' coping resources have the potential to either harm or threaten goal attainment, or represent challenges to be overcome, depending upon how they are cognitively appraised. Individuals' appraisals of situations, in turn, influence their decision to implement emotion-focussed (i.e., regulate affect) or problem-focussed (i.e., courses of action taken to address the issue) coping strategies, although these strategies are not mutually exclusive and can be used interchangeably at any given stage of the coping process (4). In instances where coping attempts have failed, Folkman and Moskowitz (4) argue that individuals will turn to meaning-based coping (e.g., positive reappraisal), which triggers the positive emotional states essential to motivating individuals to continue attempting to resolve the distressing situation. The co-existence of positive emotion in the face of extreme stress is well documented (4, 18). According to the dynamic model of affect (19), carers experiencing psychological stress within the clinical range would be expected to simultaneously experience high levels of positive affect, hypothesised to counter the negative impact of these stressors. This seeming paradox explains the decisions of care-givers to continue in their difficult role.

Research has shown that problem-focussed coping is more likely to lead to better outcomes than is the adoption of emotion-focussed coping for carers of adults with intellectual disabilities (16, 18, 20). However, it is not known whether female carers of adults with intellectual disabilities use meaning-focussed strategies, such as positive reappraisal, in highly stressful care-giving situations.

CARE-GIVING SATISFACTION

Grant and his colleagues have observed that, even when faced with multiple demands from a variety of roles, most care-givers continue to derive satisfactions from their care-giving role, which is instrumental in the continuity of care to their family member, even in instances where they must deal with onerous, long-term demands (21, 22). Grant (21) attributes these satisfactions to three sources: the carer and care-recipient relationship (e.g., carer feelings of pleasure at seeing the care recipient well-turned out), the carer's self-esteem (e.g., the development of assertiveness following difficult interactions with service providers), and meeting the needs of the person cared-for (e.g., success in organizing access to an appropriate training program).

OUR STUDY

Accordingly, this research investigated the experiences of four female carers over a five-month period. The aim of this research is to provide a more complete, and consequently more complex, description of the experiences of carers and to explore some of the differences in these experiences that are obscured when using group data. First, the actual care-giving demands faced by these women and how stressful they perceived these demands to be each month was identified, to investigate whether carers managing high levels of role demands also exhibited symptoms consistent with stress proliferation. Secondly, we investigated the types of strategies used by carers over the 5-month interview period to cope with a stressful care-giving incident nominated at the outset of the study and whether these were the same or different over the 5-monthly intervals. We also examined whether carers used problem-, emotion-, or meaning-focussed strategies to manage highly stressful demands. Thirdly, the amount of satisfaction experienced by care-givers was measured, to determine if it fluctuated in response to care-giving demands. Finally, the relationship between positive affect and psychological stress was examined, to determine whether highly stressed carers also reported high levels of positive affect.

Four women who had participated in a study of stress and coping (23) agreed to participate in a further four interviews concerning how they coped with care-giving stress: three were mothers and one was a sister carer. Three carers were interviewed in their homes while the fourth carer was interviewed via phone, as she lived several hundred kilometres from the university. Two carers were aged 45-55 years, one was aged 55-65 years and the other was aged 65-75 years. Two were full-time carers and the other two participants worked on a full-time basis, their work schedules planned around the work and leisure activities of the person for whom they cared as far as was practicable. Two of the carers were married and two were divorced.

All of the adults cared for lived in the family home. Two of the adult children were male. Demographic details pertaining to the carer and the adult cared-for, including details on behavioural difficulties of the adults with intellectual disabilities are contained in Table 1. Pseudonyms are used throughout the paper.

Table 1. Demographic details for the carers and adults with intellectual disabilities

Carer		Adult Cared-for							
Adjustment Category	Age Range	Work Status	Marital Status	Relationship to Adult Cared-for	Age or Adult	Personal Adjustment Standard Score	Category	Social Adjustment Standard Score	Category
1. Phillipa Roberston	45-55	Full-time carer	Married	Mother of Bruce	24	100	Average	95	Average
2. Pamela O'Rourke	65-75	Full-time carer	Divorced	Sister of Clara	54	106	Average	83	Below Average
3. Camilla Williams	45-55	Full-time employee	Married	Mother of Scott	25	122	Superior	95	Average
4. Jackie Di Mattia	55-65	Part-time employee	Divorced	Mother of Stella	34	89	Below Average	91	Average

[a] M = 100; SD = 15

Measures in initial interview

This semi-structured interview comprised 29 questions concerning carer and adult child demographics (including employment and health histories), types of stressors encountered by carers and sources of care-giving and emotional support. Carers were encouraged to answer questions in as much detail as they wished to provide. At the conclusion of the interview, carers were asked to nominate a stressful care-giving incident that had occurred in the last seven days (i.e., Time 1 Incident – see Table 3) and to rate this incident on a Likert scale (anchored by 0=Not Stressful and 10=Extremely Stressful). When completing the Ways of Coping Questionnaire (WOCS), carers were asked to recall this stressful incident as vividly as possible and then to nominate all of the strategies listed on the WOCS they had used to cope with the ensuing stress, as well as the intensity with which they used these strategies. A copy of the interview schedule is available from the second author upon request.

Follow-up Interviews

These interviews comprised 13 questions concerning additional care-giving stressors that had occurred since the first interview and ratings of their stressfulness on a Likert scale (anchored by 0=Not Stressful and 10=Extremely Stressful). These are reported in Table 3, along with the level of stress attributed to that particular stressor in subsequent interviews. Finally, participants rated the current stressfulness of the Time 1 incident, and nominated the strategies they were currently using to cope with any continued stress, and the intensity with which they used these strategies.

Instruments

Some additional standardized questionnaires were included as part of the data gathering, to compliment the interview data and to illuminate some of the findings (23). Table 2 provides a detailed description of these measures.

Table 2. Description of measures

	Focus	Range and meaning of scores	Cronbach's alpha[a]
Bradburn Affect Scale (BAS) Bradburn, N. M. (1969). *The structure of psychological well-being.* Chicago, IL: Aldine.	10 items describing positive (5 items; e.g., 'Pleased about having accomplished something') and negative (5 items; e.g., 'Very lonely or remote from other people') experiences.	After reversing the negatively worded items, positive experiences are calculated as the sum of positive experiences and the absence of negative experiences. Possible scores range from zero to ten with high scores indicating positive affect.	.78[a]
Carers' Assessment of Difficulties Index (CASI) Nolan, M., Grant, G., & Keady, J. (1988). Carers' Assessment of Satisfactions Index. In M. Nolan, G. Grant & J. Keady (Eds.), *Assessing the needs of family carers* (pp. 29-30). Sheffield, UK: The University of Sheffield.	30 items concerning common care-giving difficulties experienced by care-givers.	Total obtained score represents different levels of stress in the following way: 0-30=Low 31-60=Moderate 61-90=High.	.95

Table 2. (Continued)

	Focus	Range and meaning of scores	Cronbach's alpha[a]
Carers' Assessment of Satisfactions Index (CASI) Nolan, M., Grant, G., & Keady, J. (1988). Carers' Assessment of Satisfactions Index. In M. Nolan, G. Grant & J. Keady (Eds.), *Assessing the needs of family carers* (pp. 31-32). Sheffield, UK: The University of Sheffield.	30 items concerning common satisfactions experienced by care-givers.	Total obtained score represents different levels of care-giver satisfaction: 0-30=Low Satisfaction 31-60=Moderate Satisfaction 61-90=High Satisfaction.	.96
Family Inventory of Life Events (FILE) McCubbin, H. I., Patterson, J. M., & Wilson, L. R. (1983). *Family Inventory of Life Events*. Madison, WI: University of Wisconsin-Madison.	71 items cataloguing changes that may occur in the life of a family or its individual members.	Respondents are asked to indicate which of these events occurred in their family during the last 12 months. Scores range from 0 to 950+ with high scores indicating the occurrence of a large number of potentially stressful life events.	Not applicable
The General Health Questionnaire-28 (GHQ-28) Goldberg, D. (1981). *The General Health Questionnaire-28*. London: nferNelson.	28 items concerning carer psychological well-being. Four sub-scales: Somatic Symptoms; Anxiety and Insomnia; Social Dysfunction; Severe Depression.	Likert rating of items: 0, 1, 2 & 3, collapsed into GHQ scores, where items rated 0 or 1 are scored 0 and items rated 2 or 3 are scored 1 (Goldberg, 1981). Scores of 6 or higher suggest distress.	Total GHQ-28 .88 Somatic Symptoms .77 Anxiety and Insomnia .77 Social Dysfunction .75 Severe Depression .75
Hassles and Uplifts Scale DeLongis, A., Folkman, S., & Lazarus, R. S. (1988). Hassles and Uplifts Scale. *Journal of Personality and Social Psychology, 54*(3), 486-495.	53 items measuring both hassles and uplifts experienced across 53 aspects of family life.	Likert rating of items: 0=None or Not applicable; 1=Somewhat; 2=Quite a bit; 3=A great deal. Scores on both elements range from 0 to 159, with high scores indicating high Hassles or high Uplifts	Hassles .68 Uplifts .95
Ways of CopingQuestionnaire (WOCS) Folkman, S., & Lazarus, R. S. (1988). *Ways of Coping Questionnaire*. Redwood City, CA: Mind Garden.	66 coping strategies in checklist format. Respondents think of a specific stressful incident that occurred in the last seven days, indicate which strategies they used and rate the frequency with which they used each strategy.	Items are clustered into eight different ways of coping: Confrontive; Distancing; Self-controlling[b]; Seeking Social Support; Accepting Responsibility[b]; Escape-Avoidance[b]; Planful Problem Solving; and Positive Reappraisal.	Confrontive .81 Distancing .68 Seeking Social Support .80 Problem Solving .79 Positive Reappraisal .76

[a] Cronbach's alpha refers to the data for the cross-sectional study from which these participants were drawn

[b] Cronbach's alphas were below .65 and so were not used in this study.

Procedure

The study was formally approved by the Social and Behavioural and Social Sciences Ethics Review committee at The University of Queensland. Participants for the original study were recruited through 12 organizations who agreed to forward recruitment letters to carers. It is not possible to determine how many carers received letters of invitation to participate in the study. Upon contact from a carer indicating willingness to participate in the study, information about both the cross-sectional and longitudinal aspects of the study was provided. Thirty-one participants agreed to contribute to the cross sectional study and four to participate in the longitudinal study.

The interview and questionnaire data collected from the four participants were compiled into summaries for each of the families, the aim of which was to identify specific areas of similarity and difference in their experiences (e.g., areas of high stress or high satisfaction), and these summaries are contained in the following section. Longitudinal data collection also enabled the comparison of how certain variables changed over time (e.g., changes in carer's ratings of the stressfulness of events and coping strategy usage).

PARTICIPANTS

Phillipa Robertson and her son, Bruce

Phillipa and Bill Robertson have been married for over 30 years. They have two daughters, Margaret and Paula, aged 18 and 24 at the time of the study and one son, Bruce, who is in his early twenties and has Down syndrome. Margaret is studying at a tertiary institution and still lives at home. Paula lives with several friends far from the family home. Bill currently works full-time and has been involved in numerous industries. Phillipa also worked until Bruce's birth.

Bruce has always lived at home with his parents. He is unable to speak and engages in stereotypic behaviour that is self-injurious; thus, he requires constant supervision to ensure that he is not harming himself. Bruce has also been diagnosed with Pica, a potentially life-threatening condition where non-nutritive substances are ingested. On most nights, Bruce will wake several times, requiring Phillipa to rise, turn him in bed and calm him. She often feels exhausted yet, irrespective of the demands of Bruce's care on a given day, she then has to meet the responsibilities of running the household and caring for Margaret.

Phillipa reported that Bruce often ingests substances such as nails and cleaning products when her attention is directed elsewhere; for example, when she is answering the telephone. She then has to discern what it is that Bruce has swallowed, and if it is a chemical or sharp object, she must take him to the local hospital to have it removed, and on some occasions, leave Bruce at the hospital so that his health status can be monitored. Phillipa described her monitoring of Bruce as a constant strain: she is always worried that one day, he may ingest something that will kill him.

Phillipa reported that, aside from Bill, local respite and activity workers are her greatest source of support. This is because they understand and cater for Bruce's need for pervasive support and Phillipa's need for respite from care-giving. These staff members are very responsive to Bruce's interests in the types of support provided. For example, they know that Bruce loves sport and so organise a variety of different sporting activities for him to participate in throughout the year. According to Phillipa, they also readily solicit Phillipa and Bill's views about what is or is not helpful and take the necessary steps to amend Bruce's programme, wherever possible.

Pamela O'Rourke and her sister, Clara

Pamela O'Rourke is in her seventies. She took over caring for her sister, Clara, who is in her early 50s and has Down syndrome, when her mother became too frail to do so. Pamela assumed Clara's care for two reasons; so that her mother would not worry about Clara and because she wanted to ensure that Clara was well cared-for. Pamela describes herself as a strong and determined person; she has several sons and daughters whom she raised without their father. She prefers not to access other sources of social support out of concern that when she is coping alone, if such support falls through, she will be left much more vulnerable.

Clara periodically engages in prolonged episodes of perseveration which are extremely stressful to Pamela. These episodes typically consist of Clara repeating a particular behaviour over and over again, sometimes for weeks at a time. On account of these episodes, Pamela considers Clara's care to be extremely demanding. She also feels no-one else has the patience and devotion to care for Clara as she does. However, Pamela now faces a dilemma: as she ages, her own physical health is deteriorating. The thought of placing Clara in an institution causes Pamela much mental distress; however, she is reluctant to discuss her concerns with others, for fear that they may consider her unable to cope and consequently rescind her role as Clara's primary care-giver.

Camilla Williams and her son, Scott

Camilla and John Williams have three children: Barbara, Helen and Scott, aged 31, 28 and 25 respectively at the time of the study. Barbara and Helen now live away from home: both are married with young families of their own. Camilla and John both work in highly-demanding management positions that require them to work in excess of 40 hours per week. John is also often required to attend interstate and international meetings as part of his job, leaving Camilla alone to manage family matters, in addition to her work commitments. This is particularly demanding on Camilla even though her family is extremely close-knit and provides her with immense satisfaction. However, supporting Helen and Barbara and their spouses, as well as helping to care for her grandchildren, is extremely stressful, because it requires a significant time commitment on her behalf.

Scott's intellectual disability occurred as a result of an illness he suffered when he was a young child, which led to extensive brain damage. Scott's recovery was long and intensive, and at one point it was possible that he may not have survived. Both parents reported that this placed the family under extreme emotional pressure for a long period of time. Scott still needs ongoing support as the nature of his brain injury has resulted in pervasive decrements in his functioning. For example, Scott can become fatigued at irregular intervals, due to the erratic operation of his endocrine system. Because of this, it is difficult to secure any employment for him, despite his desire to have a job. Although this is frustrating to Camilla and John, they understand that employers need reliable staff capable of meeting the demands of the job. They report that an inability to find long-term employment for Scott adds to their stress; at the very time Scott should be leading an independent life, he remains in their care with few ongoing community contacts.

Jackie Di Mattia and her daughter, Stella

Jackie Di Mattia lives with her daughter, Stella, who is in her mid-20s and has a dual diagnosis of intellectual disability and autism spectrum disorder. Jackie is divorced from Stella's father and works part-time. Jackie's son, Rhys, is in his mid-30s and works as a health-care professional in another state, so their only sources of contact are regular phone conversations and holiday visits. Jackie reported that she receives very little support from her own siblings and none from her ex-husband's family. Stella goes to a variety of day respite activities. From time to time, Stella also stays with Mary Briggs, a respite-care worker who cares for Stella every second weekend. Jackie reports that Stella enjoys her time with Mary immensely.

Stella has also been diagnosed with Pica and frequently ingests dangerous items, such as coins, tacks, screws and sometimes faeces. Jackie reported that Stella also engaged in perseverative behaviours and gave an example of how Stella can repeat the same sentence, at intervals of approximately five minutes, for four consecutive days. Jackie also stated that when she is unable to understand what Stella is trying to communicate to her, Stella will become physically violent towards her and sometimes, Stella has broken furnishings and other household items.

Jackie explained that work provides her with many benefits, such as opportunities to practise her profession and interact with others in the community. However, the lack of flexible respite care remains a source of stress. An example she gave of these stresses concerned restrictions on the number of hours she is permitted to work before her respite care hours are reduced. Another of her concerns is the lack of empathy on the part of employers and certain respite providers in relation to the complexities of Stella's care. For example, there are times when Jackie has to take Stella to the hospital, when she has swallowed a dangerous substance. As they live alone, she cannot delegate this task, and if this happens to fall on one of the mornings she is working, she is late for work. However, her employers are not very tolerant of such emergencies, even though Jackie works back to make up the time she has lost while seeking help for Stella.

FINDINGS

Table 3 contains a list of all of the stressful care-giving incidents nominated by carers from Times 1 to 5, including ratings of how stressful these same incidents were for them at each subsequent interview. Scores on the measures of care-giving difficulties and satisfactions, psychological stress and positive affect for each carer are provided in Table 4. The change in scores and their relationships to each other are illustrated in Figure 1.

Table 3. Ratings of time 1 incident and additional stressful care-giving events for times 2-5

CARER 1: Phillipa Robertson	TIME 1	TIME 2	TIME 3	TIME 4	TIME 5	CARER 2: Pamela O'Rourke	TIME 1	TIME 2	TIME 3	TIME 4	TIME 5
Time 1 Incident: Personnel changes in respite care team. Coping strategy: Distancing	10	0	0	0	0	*Time 1 Incident:* Episodes of late-night challenging behaviour. Coping strategy: Confrontive	10	10	0	2	2
Time 2 Incidents: Pica		7	7	8	10	*Time 2 Incidents:* Poor personal hygiene		10	10	10	10
Pica		7	8	8	10	Pacing angrily around house		10	10	10	10
Uncontrollable binge eating		7	10	6	10	Refusal to leave bedroom		10	6	10	10
Playing with cleanser		8	10	5	10	Hoarding mail in bedroom		10	3	10	10
Time 3 Incidents: Pica			10	9	10	*Time 3 Incidents:* No additional incidents					
Smashing eggs on floor			10	10	10						
Time 4 Incident: Walking around house at night				10	9	*Time 4 incidents:* Going into carer's bedroom without permission				10	10
						Dialling "Census" numbers on phone				10	10
Time 5 Incident: Getting out of bed several times per night					6	*Time 5 Incidents*:* Dialling "000" + visit from Police					10
						Mixing up paid and unpaid accounts					10

CARER 3: Camilla Williams	TIME 1	TIME 2	TIME 3	TIME 4	TIME 5	CARER 4: Jackie Di Mattia	TIME 1	TIME 2	TIME 3	TIME 4	TIME 5
Time 1 Incident: Arranging for medical treatment with new doctors. Coping strategy: Problem-Solving	5	5	2	0	0	*Time 1 Incident:* Episodes of perseveration. Coping strategy: Seeking Social Support	10	10	10	7	10
Time 2 Incidents: No additional incidents						*Time 2 Incidents:* Physical assault of carer		10	8	8	9
						Additional episodes of perseveration		10	6	10	4
						Pica		10	5	8	2
						Binge eating/choking		9	4	2	0
Time 3 Incidents: No additional incidents						*Time 3 Incidents:* Late return from day activities			7	6	8
						Argument with respite carer			8	9	10
Time 4 Incidents: Arranging for respite carer				10	0	*Time 4 Incidents:* No additional events					
Time 5 Incidents: No additional incidents						*Time 5 Incident:* Another set of perseverative behaviours					10

Table 4. Changes in care-giving demand and satisfaction measures across times 1-5

Carer	Measure and Score range	Time 1	Time 2	Time 3	Time 4	Time 5
Phillipa Robertson	CADI[a] (0-90)	40	26	15	21	28
	GHQ-28[b] (0-28)[c]	0	1	0	0	0
	CASI[d] (0-90)	59	67	75	71	70
	BAS[e] (0-10)	10	8	8	10	10
Pamela O'Rourke	CADI (0-90)	19	36	37	37	33
	GHQ-28 (0-28)	6	6	0	18	0
	CASI (0-90)	79	75	74	76	76
	BAS (0-10)	6	4	8	2	4
Camilla Williams	CADI (0-90)	29	31	32	27	44
	GHQ-28 (0-28)	11	8	4	18	12
	CASI (0-90)	64	70	71	67	67
	BAS (0-10)	10	8	8	6	6
Jackie Di Mattia	CADI (0-90)	66	63	58	60	69
	GHQ-28 (0-28)	13	11	6	8	16
	CASI (0-90)	52	35	33	36	29
	BAS (0-10)	6	8	2	6	8

[a] Carers' Assessment of Difficulties Index, [b] The General Health Questionnaire-28, [c] scores over 6 suggest levels of difficulty in the clinical range, [d] Carers' Assessment of Satisfactions Index, [e] Bradburn Affect Scale

Phillipa Robertson: A partnered carer dealing with high levels of challenging behavior

Stressful care-giving events. As discussed earlier, Bruce's respite workers not only provide him with positive care and attention across a range of activities he enjoys, but Phillipa remarked that the quality of care they provide reduces her stress level, as she does not have to worry about him when he is away from her. However, recent staffing changes led to changes in the respite care team and Phillipa nominated these changes at Time 1 as the care-giving incident that caused her the most stress within the seven days prior to her first interview. However, across subsequent months, the event ceased to be stressful to her (i.e., from a rating of 10 to four ratings of 0), as Bruce came to like the new team members and was comfortable staying over-night with them.

Across the four-month interview period, Phillipa dealt with eight additional stressful care-giving events, many of which were rated 10 at the time they occurred and at subsequent interviews. These incidents predominantly concerned Bruce's engagement in Pica and self-injurious behaviours. The high ratings Phillipa ascribed to these events may be attributable to a range of factors, including the persistent occurrence of these behaviours (e.g., after Phillipa had addressed one behaviour, it was replaced by another similar behaviour); the high risk to Bruce's personal safety associated with these events; and the possibility of the need to contact medical professionals to treat Bruce after the behaviour occurred.

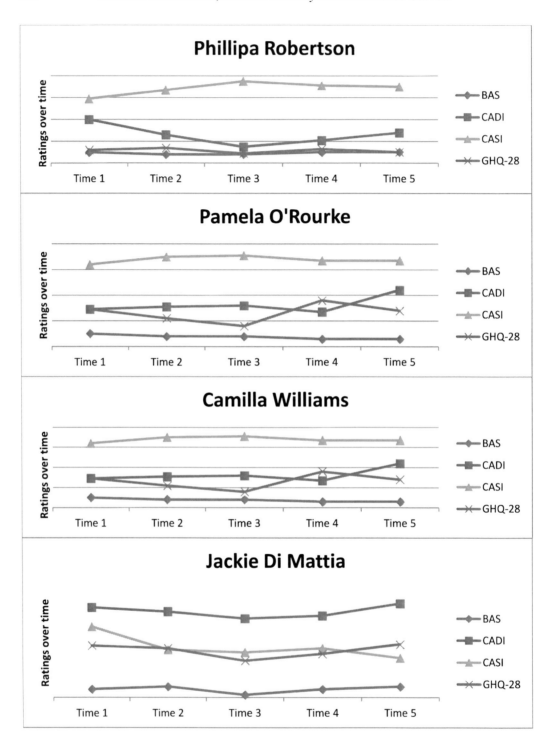

Figure 1. Changes across Times 1-5 in care-giving difficulties, satisfactions, psychological stress and positive affect.

One of the most difficult issues reported at each of her interviews concerned Bill's increased time away from the family. Phillipa acknowledged that, although she was grateful for Bill's continued employment and that he enjoyed his job, there were times when she felt quite lonely, especially on those occasions when Bruce was engaging in challenging behaviour. Phillipa reported on several FILEs that the strain of coping with Bruce's problems was another extremely difficult life event that she experienced. Despite the persistence of these behaviours, Phillipa's reports of care-giving difficulties (as measured by the CADI) remained fairly low, with her scores remaining below 30 for four of the five interviews. Given Phillipa's high ratings of stress associated with new instances of challenging/self-injurious behaviours, this suggests that Phillipa may have separated the ongoing duties associated with Bruce's care (e.g., personal care and housekeeping) from his episodes of challenging behaviour.

Psychological stress. Phillipa reported experiencing stress within the clinical range across the interviews (e.g., she reported at least five of the seven social dysfunction symptoms at each interview). However, Phillipa had no indicators within the severe depression clinical range across any of the interviews.

Care-giving satisfaction and positive affect. With respect to her levels of care-giving satisfaction, it is also interesting that Phillipa obtained immense gratification from caring for Bruce, even in the face of Bruce's high levels of challenging and self-injurious behaviours. Review of Figure 1 suggests a direct relationship between care-giving difficulties and satisfaction as care-giving difficulties decreased, Phillipa's care-giving satisfactions increased. Phillipa also reported high levels of positive affect at each interview.

Coping strategy usage. Phillipa's preferred set of coping strategies was Distancing, an emotion-focussed coping strategy, which she used only infrequently, as reflected in the ratings of 1 she assigned to usage of these particular strategies. Phillipa mentioned in her initial interview that she also found other forms of emotion-focussed coping useful, such as trying to remain calm when dealing with Bruce's behaviour, enabling her to focus on finding a solution to address the behaviour without making Bruce feel guilty or judged. Bill's emotional support was also instrumental in helping Phillipa to face these crises. One way he provided this support was in helping her to see the funny side of Bruce's behaviour, given that they both feel that there is little that they can do to stop him engaging in this behaviour. Phillipa also mentioned that she likes to garden, in order to relax.

Summary: Although Bruce's care involves a continued presentation of high-risk challenging behaviour that could involve permanent injury or death, his mother Phillipa still gains extremely high satisfaction from caring for him. Phillipa's capacity to cope may be due to the use of strategies that she finds effective in helping her manage her own emotional state while she assists Bruce, as well as to a relatively low level of ambient stressors and negative life events within her family. Phillipa reported high-level psychological stress associated with social dysfunction from meeting these demands. Phillipa acknowledged the continued love and support from Bill as being instrumental to her capacity to cope. Bruce's active lifestyle, which includes weekly social activities and respite care several times per year, also contributes to her sense of well-being.

Pamela O'Rourke: An unpartnered carer dealing with high levels of challenging behavior

Stressful care-giving events. Pamela nominated Clara's engagement in challenging behaviour as a stressful care-giving event at her first interview (e.g., wandering around the house in the early hours of the morning, opening cupboards and slamming doors shut). These behaviours interrupted Pamela's sleep, causing a range of secondary stressors (e.g., feelings of tiredness during the day and lowered energy levels, which affected Pamela's ability to undertake other duties, such as driving, shopping and attending appointments). Pamela also reported that constant interruptions to her sleep reduced her ability to cope, as she awoke most mornings feeling tired and with little energy. Pamela's ratings regarding this stressor declined from ratings of 10 at Times 1 and 2 to nil at Time 3, because Clara ceased engaging in the behaviour. The ratings slightly increased to ratings of 2 at Times 4 and 5. This is attributable to Clara's re-engagement with the behaviour, resulting in a re-emergence of some feelings of stress within Pamela.

Despite some fluctuation in her consecutive ratings of each of these additional events, Pamela reported the highest number of maximum stress ratings associated with these incidents (i.e., 20 of the 26 ratings she assigned to the subsequent stressful care-giving events she reported across the 5-month period were rated as 10, indicating maximum stress). This meant that Pamela was forced to cope with a continual high level of care-giving stress.

The stressfulness of these ongoing difficulties is also reflected in Pamela's CADI score, where she consistently rated at least one third of the items as being very stressful to extremely stressful for her. These items centred on issues concerning not receiving assistance from relatives, a deterioration in her standard of living and lack of emotional well-being, as well as a lack of understanding by professionals (e.g., Pamela commented during her interview that she had tried on several occasions to explain the dynamics of Clara's episodes of perseveration to her general practitioner (GP), but that he had simply commented that the behaviour would resolve itself.)

In addition to these stressful care-giving events, Pamela also reported several negative life events centred on issues to do with Clara's care and well-being (e.g., Clara's emotional issues, disagreements that they had had about Clara's friends, and her challenging behaviour which Pamela indicated on the FILE as an increased number of problems that don't get resolved). Pamela reported these same concerns in at least three of the five months. She also reported several stressful events that concerned her other children, such as break-ups in their relationships and coping with an unexpected pregnancy, as well as distress from the breakdown of one of her own personal friendships.

Psychological stress. As would be expected, Pamela's social dysfunction scores were within clinical range across Times 2-5. Her anxiety/insomnia scores all fell within clinical range at Times 2, 4 and 5. These ratings coincided with Clara's re-engagement in challenging behaviours (there were no additional episodes during the third month). This is also reflected in the re-emergence of feelings of stress associated with Clara's challenging behaviour. Pamela said that these behaviours "were the worst because you don't know what is going to happen next". Across the follow-up interviews, Pamela reported some difficulties on six of the seven social dysfunction items, indicating that this area of functioning presented continued difficulties to her. However, Pamela only indicated having two symptoms of severe depression across the entire five-month period.

Care-giving satisfaction and positive affect. In spite of all of these challenges, Pamela consistently rated her care-giving satisfaction as extremely high across all five months. Pamela said she derived great feelings of satisfaction when she overcame these challenges. Despite Pamela's high level of care-giving satisfaction, her positive affect scores were the lowest of all of the carers.

Coping strategy usage. Pamela's preferred strategy cluster was Confrontive, a set of problem-focussed strategies that involve identifying the problem but also taking immediate steps to address it, an approach that accords with the views expressed in her interview about meeting life's challenges. She used these strategies at quite a high level across four of the five months.

Summary: Pamela copes with a complex set of care-giving stressors, some of which result directly from Clara's challenging behaviour and some of which are factors extraneous to her care (e.g., issues relating to Clara's friendships and relationships with her carers). Although she has excellent support from a service provision agency that provides social and leisure activities for Clara, Pamela is facing concerns about what will happen to Clara if her own physical or psychological health deteriorates as a result of not being able to cope with these stressors. This is all the more difficult, given Pamela's pride in being able to face challenges, as is reflected in her preference for Confrontive coping strategies. Although Pamela reports gaining high levels of satisfaction from caring for Clara, her levels of positive affect were quite low.

Camilla Williams: A partnered carer dealing with multiple role demands

Stressful care-giving events. At the first interview, Camilla nominated arranging for Scott to be treated by a new doctor rather than his regular GP as the most stressful recent incident she had faced in the week of the first interview. Although coping with change is something that everyone faces, this issue was of concern as Scott's health issues have been fairly constant since childhood and will require treatment until the end of his life. Scott has become quite attached to certain specialists and has been known to refuse to see new staff. Despite this experience, Camilla's ratings reflected only a moderate level of concern.

Unlike the other carers in the study who encountered multiple stressors across the interview period, Camilla reported only one further incident at Time 4, concerning respite arrangements for Scott. Although she rated the incident at 10, out of concern that she would not be able to make suitable arrangements before the family left on holidays, this matter had been resolved by the following month.

The low occurrence of additional stressful care-giving incidents is also reflected in Camilla's CADI scores, which were generally just above 30, just within the Stressful range. This is also possibly attributable to Scott's adaptive behaviour: his ABS-RC:2 scores indicated that he relates well to others and has no challenging behaviour.

In comparison to the other families in the study, the major stressful events nominated by Camilla were not to do with Scott but instead centred on herself and other family members (e.g., the increased time she and her husband spent away from the home due to work commitments, increased conflict between herself and her husband, increased arguments between the children in the family and an increased number of chores that did not get done). These events were all reported on at least three of the five interviews.

Psychological stress. With respect to her psychological well-being, Camilla reported social dysfunction symptoms within the clinical range at each interview. Her anxiety/insomnia scores were within the clinical range at Times 4 and 5 and she reported somatic symptoms within the clinical range at Time 1. Camilla also indicated that she was experiencing several severe depression symptoms.

Care-giving satisfaction and positive affect. Camilla reported high levels of care-giving satisfaction and positive affect scores within average range. These scores reflect Camilla's observations of herself made during the interviews that she is an optimistic person who expects the best out of life.

Coping strategy usage. Camilla's preferred set of coping strategies was Problem Solving, which are problem-focussed strategies, although, she also used Self-Controlling, or emotion-focussed, strategies at a somewhat similar level. She used the Problem Solving strategies quite intensely, in response to the Time 1 care-giving event. This suggests that she found the strategies to be useful in reducing the stressfulness of the event, although it is interesting that Camilla maintained high strategy usage even after the event had ceased to be stressful to her. This may have represented a preventative focus (i.e., Camilla's continuing a course of action to prevent further incidents from occurring and/or to reduce their impact once they occurred).

Summary: Although Scott's care will involve continued support, particularly with respect to his health concerns, Camilla and her husband face a range of other life issues that cause them more stress. Despite the high level of stress she experienced, Camilla also reported high levels of positive affect and care-giving satisfaction. In the case of the Williams family, this stress not only comes from tensions amongst the adult siblings but also as a direct result of various partner, family and work role strains that they are facing as members of a couple with full-time work commitments.

Jackie Di Mattia: An unpartnered carer dealing with extreme challenging behaviour and multiple role demands

Stressful care-giving events. At the first interview, Jackie nominated Stella's episodes of perseveration as a stressful care-giving incident that had occurred within the last seven days. This event remained highly stressful for Jackie across the entire interview period. With the exception of the fourth month, further instances of challenging behaviour occurred, namely: Stella physically attacking Jackie; other episodes of perseveration; binge eating to the point of choking, lateness in leaving day activities which caused Jackie to be late back to her job; arguments with Stella's respite carer; and episodes of other perseverative behaviours. Jackie rated all of these behaviours, with the exception of the binge eating/choking incident which occurred only once and the lateness from day activities, as ranging from 8-10, representing episodes of severe stress for her.

Over the last 12 months, Jackie indicated on the FILE that she has also faced a number of stressful life events. Many of these concern Stella's care: reports of her emotional problems, Jackie's difficulty in coping with these problems, and increased medical expenses to manage these problems. Jackie also reported a range of secondary stressors arising from these care-giving difficulties: decreased work satisfaction, issues with her co-workers arising from the times she has unexpectedly had to leave work and take care of Stella; and an increased number of problems that do not get resolved and chores that do not get done. These difficulties imply stressors for Jackie across her care-giving, work and home duties roles.

With the exception of Month 3, Jackie's CADI scores indicated that she was experiencing significant care-giving difficulties. At all five interviews, Jackie provided responses to the CADI which were the highest across the four carers.

Psychological stress. Jackie experienced clinical levels of somatic, anxiety/insomnia and social dysfunction stress across each interview. Of particular concern was her report of experiencing clinical range severe depression at the first and second interviews. She continued to indicated that she was suffering symptoms of severe depression across the remaining interviews (i.e., that she felt life was hopeless, that life wasn't worth living and that she had thought about making away with herself).

Care-giving satisfaction and positive affect. Unlike the other carers, Jackie's CASI scores progressively declined over the interview period, from a score of 52 in the first month, indicating high satisfaction to a low of 29 in the last month, indicating low satisfaction. Jackie also reported the second lowest levels of positive affect.

Coping strategy usage. Jackie used all eight types of coping strategy over each of the five months. Seeking Social Support, which can be emotion- and/or problem-focussed, depending on the dynamics of the situation in which these strategies are used (Folkman & Moskowitz, 2004), was her preferred cluster of strategies; however, she reported infrequent use of these strategies.

Summary: Jackie is finding care-giving to be extremely stressful. This is not only apparent from her CADI ratings and continued high ratings of the stressful care-giving event that occurred at Time 1, her low CASI and positive affect scores but also from her clinical range GHQ-28 scores. Jackie continues to face a continuous stream of high-risk challenging behaviour from Stella, along with concerns that these episodes are becoming more frequent. Jackie mentioned in an interview that she was gravely concerned about whether she could continue to cope with these difficulties but that her investigation of alternate living arrangements for Stella with an organization for adults with disabilities had revealed the service to be unsatisfactory. This meant that not only was she faced with continuing challenges associated with her family and work roles but no current acceptable options for addressing them, resulting in a worsening of her psychological health.

DISCUSSION

The study provides support for both the adaptation and wear and tear hypotheses. Examination of Figure 1 shows direct relationships between care-giving difficulties and satisfactions across the 5-month period for Phillipa, Pamela and Camilla, according with the adaptation hypothesis (7). The reverse was true for Jackie, and when considered in conjunction with her reported clinical levels of psychological stress and low levels of positive affect, her experience is commensurate with the wear and tear hypothesis (6).

Examination of the carers' ratings of stressfulness of the Time 1 incident shows that some events continued to remain stressful for several months after their occurrence. This was true for Pamela and Jackie, who both nominated incidents involving challenging behaviour. In contrast, Phillipa and Camilla, who nominated incidents concerning medical and respite care arrangements, reported that these incidents ceased to be stressful because they were able to broker satisfactory arrangements for their adult child's care. However, Phillipa did mention during subsequent interviews that she had had to deal with several instances of challenging behaviour from Bruce across the interview period, and she rated each of these incidents as being extremely stressful for her.

Each carer attributed the stress associated with these incidents to a range of underlying causes: for Phillipa, it was the constancy of Bruce's challenging behaviour. In Pamela's case, Clara's episodes of difficult behaviour interfered with her sleep, which impacted upon her energy levels the following day. For Jackie, it concerned her attempts to balance work obligations and the demands associated with Stella's challenging/self-injurious behaviour. These findings support conclusions drawn by Pruchno and colleagues (14, 15) concerning the deleterious effects of challenging behaviour on carers of adults with intellectual disabilities.

In contrast, Camilla Williams was the only carer not to assign a high rating to her nominated Time 1 Incident. Across the interview period, she also experienced the lowest number of subsequent stressful care-giving incidents and, unlike the other carers, reported in her interviews that these incidents either caused her only moderate or no stress. However, she stated in several interviews and indicated on the FILE, that events concerning other members of the family, such as the pile-up of household chores and number of family problems that did not get resolved, caused her more stress than Scott's care. Camilla's experience accords with research by Baxter, Cummins and Yiolitis (24) who concluded that general life stressors or those associated with other family members may cause greater difficulties for parents than the care of a family member with disabilities. That is, that not all stress in these parents can be attributed to their role as parents of an individual with a disability.

The role of coping in stress management

In terms of the types of coping strategies used, Pamela and Camilla preferred Confrontive and Problem Solving, examples of problem-focussed coping (25) while Phillipa and Jackie preferred Distancing and Seeking Social Support respectively, which are examples of emotion-focussed coping (4). Phillipa also reported using other kinds of emotion-focussed coping to manage her stress levels, such as talking with her husband. As noted above, Camilla's self-reported stress ratings were the lowest of all the carers (see Table 3). Although the Time 1 incident remained moderately stressful for her during the second and third months, there were no further reports of stress during the final two months, indicating that the strategies were effective in reducing Camilla's stress. Pamela experienced high levels of stress again in the second month, no stress during the third month, followed by a slight recurrence during the last two months, suggesting that the problem-focussed Confrontive strategies reduced the negative impact of the incident on her well-being.

In comparison, while Phillipa reported no further reports of stress associated with the Time 1 Incident for the remainder of the study, Jackie continued to report high levels of stress each month. These results can be attributed to several factors: a complex behaviour problem that, unlike Phillipa's incident, was still unresolved by the conclusion of the study; low usage of coping strategies; and reliance on emotion-focussed strategies which have been shown to be less effective than problem-focussed strategies in reducing stress in carers of adults with intellectual disabilities (16,20). Furthermore, despite her reports of clinical levels of psychological stress and the continuance of Stella's challenging behaviour, Jackie did not express a preference for positive reappraisal, a meaning-based coping strategy. As subsequent research has identified additional forms of meaning-based coping (18), further investigation is required into their use by carers of adults with intellectual disabilities.

Carers at-risk: The relationship between psychological stress, care-giving satisfaction and positive affect

As mentioned above, each of these carers experienced psychological stress within the clinical range across the interview period. However, Phillipa, Pamela and Camilla all commented during their interviews that they still gained tremendous satisfaction from care-giving, this claim being supported by their reports of moderate to high levels of positive affect in each interview. In terms of the theories of care-giving stress, their accounts can be considered as examples of the adaptation hypothesis (7): despite coping with the care-giving and other role demands, they also reported ways in which they coped with these demands. For Phillipa and Pamela, this led to a sense of personal resilience that came from their extensive experience in coping with Bruce's and Clara's challenging behaviours. Pamela also remarked that she took pride in managing these demands on her own. Camilla derived satisfaction from meeting the demands of caring for all of her children and grandchildren, in addition to balancing work demands. These comments accord with the conclusions of Grant and colleagues (21, 22), and also other researchers (10) concerning the flow-on benefits of meeting the challenges associated with long-term care-giving.

In contrast, Jackie Di Mattia's account is consistent with the wear and tear hypothesis (6) and accounts of stress proliferation (11) and role burden (12, 13) in carers. Not only did she cope with Stella's regular episodes of challenging behaviour, she reported great difficulty balancing care-giving and work role demands. Jackie also reported the highest number of clinical range symptoms of psychological stress, including severe depression, as well the low levels of positive affect and lowest levels of care-giving satisfaction across the interview period. Jackie's account is also contradictory to that predicted by the dynamic model of affect (19), where carers who experience extremely high levels of stress would typically be expected experience high levels of positive affect in response to the psychological stress associated with the care-giving demands.

CONCLUSION

Although presenting the accounts of only several carers, the above study has shown that women carers of adults with intellectual disabilities have widely varying experiences, with respect to the number and type of demands and stressors they encounter. Support was found for both the wear and tear (6) and adaptation (7) hypotheses, indicating that care-givers vary not only in terms of their appraisals of care-giving demands and satisfactions over successive months but also in terms of coping strategy usage and personal resources, such as positive affect. Only problem-focussed coping was associated with a reduction in feelings of stress in carers of adults engaging in challenging behaviour.

Longitudinal analysis has also shown that carers' ratings of various stressors fluctuated over time, indicating that one-off measurement of stress levels, as undertaken in cross-sectional research, may not comprehensively capture the actual experiences of carers. Carers in this study reported somatic, anxiety/insomnia and social dysfunction symptoms within the clinical range on successive interviews. Current emphasis on reporting severe depression only as an index of psychological stress may therefore underestimate the impact of these other symptoms upon care-giver well-being. Concerns about the negative impact of long-term care-giving on carers like Jackie have already been identified (1, 2, 8); however, it remains to be determined what kinds of intervention can be offered to these carers. Consideration also needs to be given to a range of available options that take into account the wishes of these family carers, as well as the well-being of those for whom they care (22).

REFERENCES

[1]   Burton-Smith R, McVilly KR, Yazbeck M, Parmenter T, Tsutsui T. Quality of life of Australian family carers: implications for research, policy, and practice. J Policy Pract Intellect Disabil 2009;6(3): 189-98.

[2]   Hill C, Rose J. Parenting stress in mothers of adults with an intellectual disability: parental cognitions in relation to child characteristics and family support. J Intellect Disabil Res 2009; 53(12):969-80.

[3]   Bigby C. Beset by obstacles: A review of Australian policy development to support ageing in place for people with intellectual disability. J Intellect Dev Disabil 2008;33(1):76-86.

[4]   Folkman S, Moskowitz JT. Coping: pitfalls and promise. Ann Rev Psychol 2004;55:745-74.

[5]   Lazarus RS. Toward better research on stress and coping. Am Psychol 2000;55(6):665-73.

[6]   Johnson CL, Catalano DJ. A longitudinal study of family supports to impaired elderly. Gerontologist 1983;23(6):612-8.

[7]   Townsend A, Noelker L, Deimling G, Bass D. Longitudinal impact of interhouse caregiving on adult children's mental health. Psychol Aging 1989;4(3):393-401.

[8]   Edwards B, Higgins DJ, Gray M, Zmijewski N, Kingston M. The nature and impact of caring for a family member with a disability in Australia. Melbourne, Aust: Aust Inst Fam Stud, 2008.

[9]   Krauss MW, Seltzer MM. Coping strategies among older mothers of adults with retardation: a life-span developmental perspective. In: Turnbull AP, Patterson JM, Behr SK, Murphy DL, Marquis JG, Blue-Banning MJ, eds. Cognitive coping, families, and disability. Baltimore, MD: Brookes, 1993:193-82.

[10]   Smith LE, Seltzer MM, Tager-Flusberg H, Greenberg JS, Carter AS. A comparative analysis of well-being and coping among mothers of toddlers and mothers of adolescents with ASD. J Autism Dev Disord 2008;38:876-89.

[11]   Pearlin LI. The stress process revisited: Reflections on concepts and their interrelationships. In: Anesenshel CS, Phelan JC, eds. Handbook of the sociology of mental health. New York: Kluwer, 1999:395-416.

[12]   Essex EL, Hong J. Older caregiving parents: Division of labour, marital satisfaction, and caregiver burden. Fam Relat 2005;54: 448-60.

[13]   Gordon M, Rosenman L, Cuskelly MM. Constrained labour: maternal employment when children have disabilities. J Appl Res Intellect Disabil 2007;20(3):236-46.

[14]   Pruchno RA, Meeks S. Health-related stress, affect, and depressive symptoms experienced by caregiving mothers of adults with a developmental disability. Psychol Aging 2004;19(3):394-401.

[15]   Militiades HB, Pruchno, R. Mothers of adults with developmental disability: Change over time. Am J Ment Retard 2001;106(6): 548-61.

[16]   Kim HW, Greenberg JS, Seltzer MM, Krauss MW. The role of coping in maintaining the psychological well-being of mothers of adults with intellectual disability and mental illness. J Intellect Disabil Res 2003; 47(4-5):313-27.

[17]   Lazarus RS, Folkman S. Stress, appraisal, and coping. New York: Springer, 1984.

[18]   Folkman S. The case for positive emotions in the stress process. Anxiety Stress Coping 2008;21(1):3-14.

[19]   Zautra AJ, Smith B, Affleck G, Tennen H. Examinations of chronic pain and affect relationships: Applications of a dynamic model of affect. J Consult Clin Psychol 2001;69:786-95.

[20]   Essex EL, Seltzer MM, Krauss MW. Differences in coping effectiveness and well-being among aging mothers and fathers of adults with mental retardation. Am J Ment Retard 1999;104(6): 545-63.

[21]   Grant G. Invisible contributions in families with children and adults with intellectual disabilities. Can J Aging 2007;26(1):15-26.

[22]   Grant G, Ramcharan P, Flynn M. Resilience in families with children and adult members with intellectual disabilities: Tracing elements of a psychosocial model. J Appl Res Intellect Disabil 2007;20(6): 563-75.

SECTION TWO: CHRONIC DISEASE

In: Disability and Chronic Disease
Editors: J. Merrick, S. Aspler and M. Morad

ISBN: 978-1-62948-288-0
© 2014 Nova Science Publishers, Inc.

Chapter 11

MINDFULNESS TRAINING AND CHRONIC TENSION-TYPE HEADACHE

Stuart Cathcart, PhD[*1], *Vanessa Barone, MPsych*[1], *Maarten Immink, PhD*[2] *and Michael Proeve, PhD*[3]

[1]Centre for Applied Psychology, Faculty of Health, University of Canberra
[2]School of Health Sciences, University of South Australia
[3]School of Psychology, University of Adelaide, Australia

ABSTRACT

In this chapter we examine effects of mindfulness training on generalized hyperalgesia in chronic tension-type headache (CTH) sufferers. Method: Forty-three CTH sufferers participated in a randomized wait-list controlled trial of a mindfulness intervention for headache. Pressure and thermal (cold) pain detection thresholds, cold pain rating and tolerance, pericranial muscle tenderness, and conditioned pain modulation were assessed before and after intervention. Pain sensitivity was also measured in a sample of 56 healthy headache-free subjects and compared with the headache group. Results: Headache sufferers had increased pain sensitivity across multiple modalities and anatomical locations indicating generalized hyperalgesia. Repeated measures analysis of variance of the treatment vs wait-list data revealed no group or group x time effects for any pain sensitivity measure, although there were time effects indicating a reduction in muscle tenderness and cold pain sensitivity in treatment and wait-list control groups. Conclusions: Mindfulness training compared to a wait-list control condition does not reduce generalized hyperalgesia in CTH sufferers.

INTRODUCTION

Mindfulness training has been reported as beneficial for reducing symptoms in several chronic pain conditions (1-3) including headache (4). The mechanisms by which mindfulness

---

[*] Correspondence: Stuart Cathcart, PhD, Centre for Applied Psychology, University of Canberra, Bruce 2601, Australia. E-mail: stuart.cathcart@canberra.edu.au.

reduces chronic pain symptoms are unclear. One potential mechanism may be a reduction in pain sensitivity, which is increased across multiple stimulus modalities at symptomatic and non-symptomatic sites in many chronic pain conditions, including headache, reflecting generalized hyperalgesia (5-8). Mindfulness-based interventions have been shown to reduce pain sensitivity in healthy samples (9), however effects of mindfulness training on pain sensitivity in chronic pain sufferers have not been reported to date.

The present study sought to replicate previous findings of generalized hyperalgesia in chronic tension-type headache (CTH) (10, 11) and examine if this could be reduced by mindfulness intervention. We recently reported that the mindfulness intervention reported on here reduced headache activity in the present sample of CTH sufferers (12). Not reported was data on pain sensitivity in the CTH compared to a healthy control sample, nor effects of the mindfulness intervention on pain sensitivity in the CTH sample. The present study conducts such analyses. It was hypothesized that pain sensitivity would be increased in CTH sufferers compared with healthy control subjects, and that mindfulness training would reduce putatively increased pain sensitivity in CTH sufferers.

OUR STUDY

Participant information has been reported in detail elsewhere (12). Briefly, Fifty-eight volunteers satisfying diagnosis of CTH (13) were recruited from the general population and completed pre-treatment measures. Forty-three participants completed post-treatment measures (N=24 treatment, N=19 wait-list). Volunteers for the CTH sample were excluded if they reported any chronic pain (other than CTH), major medical, or psychiatric diagnoses concurrent or in the past 12 months. The healthy control group contained fifty-six volunteers who had no pain or psychiatric or major medical diagnoses currently or in the previous twelve months.

Measures

All pain assessments were conducted by one of the authors (SC), experienced in the techniques and blinded to group (healthy vs headache group) and condition (treatment vs wait-list control).

Muscle tenderness (MT)

Pericranial muscle tenderness was assessed by a standardised technique of manual palpation of 8 muscle and tendon insertions of the head, neck and shoulders, scored on a 0-3 point scale (14). The MT score is the sum of scores for all locations assessed.

Pressure pain detection threshold (PPT)

Pressure pain detection thresholds were assessed using a hand-held algometer (Wagner Instruments FBK-20) with a circular rubber tip measuring 0.79 cm^2. Thresholds were taken at the dorsal surface of the right-hand middle finger midway between the first and second distal joints (PPTF), and at the middle of the right side trapezius belly (PPTS). Pressure was increased at a rate of approximately 1 kg per second until subjects reported the onset of pain, with PPT recorded as the average of two measures taken 30 seconds apart.

Cold pressor test

Cold pressor responses were assessed by having subjects immerse their hand in a small 'water bath' containing circulating water at 2°C. Measures were; 1) pain detection threshold (CPTH); the duration (in seconds) of immersion at which subjects report pain onset, 2) pain intensity; the rating of pain at 10 (CP10) and 20 (CP20) seconds during immersion, 3) pain tolerance (CPTOL); the maximum amount of time subjects kept their hand immersed (up to 3 minutes).

Conditioned pain modulation (CPM)

Using a previously validated method for Conditioned Pain Modulation (15), an occlusion cuff was applied to the participant's left arm and inflated until subjects reported pain at an intensity of 3 out of 10 on a visual analogue scale. With the occlusion cuff inflated, PPT was taken at the finger contralateral to the occlusion cuff. CPM was calculated as the difference between PPTF before and PPTF during occlusion cuff stimulation.

Intervention

The intervention was based on Mindfulness-Based Stress Reduction (MBSR)(4) and Mindfulness Based Cognitive Therapy (MBCT)(16), and is detailed elsewhere (12). Delivered by one of the authors (MI), the intervention involved six 1-hour group classes held twice per week for three weeks, and 30mins daily home practice. The program was developed by some of the authors (SC, MP, MI) who are psychologists (SC, MP) with formal training and extensive teaching, practice, and research experience in mindfulness and/or meditation.

Three formal mindfulness meditation practices were taught: 1) body scan meditation, which involves focusing on each region of the body systemically from the foot to the head, and noticing the sensations that are present with openness and curiosity; 2) formal sitting meditation, focusing on mindfulness of breath and other experiences such as sounds and thoughts; 3) three-minute breathing space, which involves three sequential steps of a) focusing awareness of present internal experiences, b) focusing awareness on the breath, and c) expanding awareness to the body as a whole.

Home practice was supported by a written instruction manual and a compact disc containing audio-recorded instructions. The program also included other activities so that participants could practice applying concepts of mindfulness to activities of daily living, recognizing nourishing and draining activities, and documenting observations and reactions to pleasant and unpleasant events.

Procedures

The study was approved by the University of South Australia Human Research Ethics Committee. Following a screening interview and provision of written consent to participate, volunteers completed questionnaires and the pain assessment battery. Headache sufferers were then randomly assigned to either treatment or wait-list conditions. Post-treatment measures were recorded in all CTH participants in the week following completion of the intervention by the treatment group. The wait-list control group commenced mindfulness training the following week.

FINDINGS

The mean age of the total headache sample was 45.5 years (SD=13.8), 37% were male. The mean age of the healthy control group was 41.0 years (SD=10.5), 43% were male. Analysis of Variance and Chi Square test indicated no differences between groups (healthy controls, intervention, waitlist) on measures of age or gender respectively (all p>.05, two-tailed tests).

Descriptive data for pain sensitivity is presented in table 1. Independent groups t-tests revealed that CTH sufferers had increased pain sensitivity compared with healthy controls on measures of MT, PPTF, PPTS, CP10, CP20 and CPM (all p<.01). Differences between headache and control groups were not significant for CPTH or CPTOL (all p>.05).

Repeated measures analysis of variance examined effects of the intervention on pain sensitivity (table 2). Time effects were significant for MT ($F_{(1,41)} = 17.58$, $p < .01$, $\eta=.30$), CP20 ($F_{(1,41)} = 6.14$, $p = .02$, $\eta=.16$), and CPTOL ($F_{(1,41)} = 8.00$, $p < .01$, $\eta=.18$), indicating a reduction in MT, a reduction in cold pressor rating at 20 seconds, and an increase in cold pressor tolerance, in both the treatment and wait-list groups. Group, time, and group x time effects for treatment vs waitlist groups were not significant for all other variables (all p>.05).

DISCUSSION

Mindfulness training has previously been reported as effective in reducing chronic pain symptoms (1-4), however the mechanisms of this are unclear. Since chronic pain including CTH is often associated with increased pain sensitivity (5-8), and since mindfulness training has been shown to reduce pain sensitivity in healthy samples (9), we examined if mindfulness training could reduce increased pain sensitivity in CTH sufferers. Confirming previous work (10, 11), we found increased pain sensitivity across multiple stimulus modalities at symptomatic and non-symptomatic sites in CTH sufferers, indicating generalized hyperalgesia.

Table I. Pain sensitivity in healthy controls and headache sufferers before and after mindfulness or wait-list intervention

Measure	Mindfulness intervention headache group (N=24)		Wait-list headache group (N=19)		Healthy control group (N=56)	t-test value for healthy	p value for healthy
	Pre Mean (SD)	Post Mean (SD)	Pre Mean (SD)	Post Mean (SD)	Pre* Mean (SD)	control vs headache[#]	control vs headache
MT[1]	6.67 (5.4)	3.88 (4.3)	6.84 (4.9)	4.84 (3.0)	2.60 (2.5)	4.75	<.001
PPTF[2]	3.68 (0.9)	3.71 (1.0)	3.51 (0.9)	3.32 (0.9)	5.11 (1.2)	7.17	<.001
PPTS[3]	3.29 (1.3)	3.45 (1.2)	2.70 (1.0)	2.94 (0.9)	4.58 (1.2)	3.32	.001
CPTH[4]	8.38 (5.8)	7.46 (5.0)	10.05 (8.0)	8.53 (6.3)	12.79 (9.3)	1.61	.11
CP10[5]	5.36 (1.8)	5.50 (1.8)	5.58 (1.6)	4.95 (1.6)	4.34 (1.8)	3.29	.001
CP20[6]	7.05 (1.8)	6.58 (1.6)	6.93 (2.0)	6.53 (1.7)	5.72 (1.9)	3.31	.001
CPTOL[7]	92.38 (72.6)	109.67 (67.5)	77.47 (63.3)	93.26 (62.8)	99.88 (65.3)	1.40	.16
CPM[8]	0.09 (0.8)	0.06 (0.5)	0.06 (0.8)	0.03 (0.6)	.77 (0.9)	3.00	.003

* Pain sensitivity assessed only once in healthy control subjects as these subjects did not receive intervention.

\# Independent groups t-test comparing healthy controls vs headache subjects at pre-treatment (intervention and waitlist groups combined) df=97.

[1] Pericranial muscle tenderness (total of 8 locations bilaterally)

[2] Pressure pain detection threshold at the finger

[3] Pressure pain detection threshold at the shoulder

[4] Cold-pain detection threshold in seconds (cold pressor task at 2°C)

[5] Pain rating (0-10) at 10 seconds of cold pressor immersion

[6] Pain rating (0-10) at 20 seconds of cold pressor immersion

[7] Cold-pain tolerance in seconds (cold pressor task at 2°C)

[8] Conditioned Pain Modulation (PPTF during painful occlusion cuff - PPTF before occlusion cuff).

Table II. Repeated Measures Analysis of Variance for pain measures in mindfulness versus wait-list headache groups

	Group effects		Time effects		Group x Time effects	
Measure	F	p	F	p	F	p
MT[1]	.20	.65	17.58	<.01	3.32	.49
PPTF[2]	1.06	.31	.48	.49	.95	.34
PPTS[3]	3.12	.09	2.49	.12	.08	.79
CPTH[4]	.67	.42	1.70	.20	.11	.75
CP10[5]	.12	.73	1.12	.30	2.70	.11
CP20[6]	.10	.75	6.14	.02	.09	.78
CPTOL[7]	.63	.43	8.00	<.01	.02	.90
CPM[8]	2.67	.12	2.70	.11	.93	.34

[1] Pericranial muscle tenderness (total of 8 locations bilaterally).
[2] Pressure pain detection threshold at the finger.
[3] Pressure pain detection threshold at the shoulder.
[4] Cold-pain detection threshold in seconds (cold pressor task at $2°C$).
[5] Pain rating (0-10) at 10 seconds of cold pressor immersion.
[6] Pain rating (0-10) at 20 seconds of cold pressor immersion.
[7] Cold-pain tolerance in seconds (cold pressor task at $2°C$).
[8] Conditioned Pain Modulation (PPTF during painful occlusion cuff - PPTF before occlusion cuff).
All tests df=1,41.

However, pain sensitivity in CTH sufferers was not reduced following mindfulness training compared with a wait-list group. This was evident for every measure of pain sensitivity, strongly indicating that mindfulness training does not reduce generalized hyperalgesia in CTH sufferers.

Elsewhere we have reported that the present mindfulness training increased mindfulness and reduced headache activity in this sample of CTH sufferers (12). Although we did not examine relationships between headache activity and pain sensitivity, the present findings suggest that the therapeutic effect of the intervention previously observed in this sample was not due to a reduction in pain sensitivity in CTH sufferers.

Limitations to the present study include the use of subjective pain measures, the brief nature of our intervention, the relatively small sample size, the lack of an active control group, and the lack of longer-term follow-up. These issues withstanding, the present results indicate that mindfulness training, elsewhere shown to increase mindfulness and reduce headache activity, does not reduce generalized hyperalgesia in CTH sufferers. Replication and extension of the present results would further understanding of the importance of generalized hyperalgesia in, and the mechanisms of mindfulness intervention for, chronic pain.

ACKNOWLEDGMENTS

The authors are grateful to Nicola Galatis and Margaret Mitchell for assistance in data collection. This research was funded in part by a Medical Advances Without Animals Trust grant. This study is registered with the Australian and New Zealand Clinical Trials Registry, number ACTRN12610001039077.

REFERENCES

[1]   Sampalli T, Berlasso E, Fox R, Petter M. A controlled study of the effect of a mindfulness-based stress reduction technique in women with multiple chemical sensitivity, chronic fatigue syndrome and fibromyalgia. J Multidiscip Healthcare 2009;2:53-9.

[2]   Zautra A, Davis M, Reich J, Nicassio P, Tennen H, Finan P, et al. Comparison of Cognitive Behavioral and Mindfulness Meditation Interventions on Adaptation to Rheumatoid Arthritis for Patients With and Without History of Recurrent Depression. J Consult Clin Psychol 2008;76:408-21. doi:10.1037/0022-006X.76.3.408

[3]   Morone NE, Greco CM, Weiner DK. Mindfulness meditation for the treatment of chronic low back pain in older adults: a randomized controlled pilot study. Pain 2008;134:310-9.

[4]   Kabat-Zinn J, Lipworth L, Burney R. The clinical use of mindfulness meditation for the self-regulation of chronic pain. J Behav Med 1985;8:163-90.

[5]   Bendtsen L, Fernández-de-la-Peñas C. The role of muscles in tension-type headache. Curr Pain Headache Rep 2011;15:451-8. doi: 10.1007/s11916-011-0216-0.

[6]   Giesecke T, Gracely RH, Grant MA, Nachemson A, Petzke F, Williams DA, Clauw DJ. Evidence of augmented central pain processing in idiopathic chronic low back pain. Arthritis Rheum 2004;50:613–23.

[7]   Puta C, Schulz B, Schoeler S, Magerl W, Gabriel B, Gabriel HH, et al. Enhanced sensitivity to punctate painful stimuli in female patients with chronic low back pain. BMC Neurol 2012;12:98. doi: 10.1186/1471-2377-12-98.

[8]   Seifert F, Kiefer G, DeCol R, Schmelz M, Maihöfner C. Differential endogenous pain modulation in complex-regional pain syndrome. Brain 2009;132:788-800.

[9]   Zeidan F, Gordon N, Merchant J, Goolkasian P. The effects of brief mindfulness meditation training on experimentally induced pain. J Pain 2010;11:199-209. doi:10.1016/j.jpain.2009.07.015

[10]   Cathcart S, Petkov J, Winefield A, Lushington K, Rolan P. Central mechanisms of stress-induced headache. Cephalalgia 2010;30:285-95.

[11]   Ashina S, Bendtsen L, Ashina M, Magerl W, Jensen R. Generalized hyperalgesia in patients with chronic tension-type headache. Cephalalgia 2006;26:940-8.

[12]   Cathcart S, Galatis N, Immink M, Proeve M, Petkov J. Brief mindfulness-based meditation for chronic tension-type headache: A randomized controlled trial. Behav Cogn Psychother, in press.

[13]   International Headache Society. International Classification of Headache Disorders: 2nd Edition. Cephalalgia 2004;24(suppl 1):9-160.

[14]   Langemark M, Olesen J. Pericranial tenderness in tension headache. Cephalalgia 1987;7:249-55.

[15]   Cathcart S, Winefield A, Rolan P, Lushington K. Reliability of temporal summation and diffuse noxious inhibitory controls. Pain Res Manage 2009;14:433-8.

[16]   Segal Z, Williams J, Teasdale J. Mindfulness-based cognitive therapy for depression: A new approach to preventing relapse. New York: Guilford, 2002.

In: Disability and Chronic Disease
Editors: J. Merrick, S. Aspler and M. Morad

ISBN: 978-1-62948-288-0
© 2014 Nova Science Publishers, Inc.

Chapter 12

MINDFULNESS TRAINING AND INFLAMMATORY CYTOKINE LEVELS IN CHRONIC TENSION-TYPE HEADACHE

Stuart Cathcart, PhD[*,1], *Chris Della Vedova, PhD*[2], *Maarten Immink, PhD*[3], *Michael Proeve, PhD*[4] *and John Hayball, PhD*[2]

[1]Centre for Applied Psychology, Faculty of Health, University of Canberra
[2]School of Pharmacy and Medical Sciences, University of South Australia
[3]School of Health Sciences, University of South Australia
[4]School of Psychology, University of Adelaide, Australia

ABSTRACT

In this chapter we examine the effects of mindfulness training on serum pro-inflammatory cytokine levels in chronic tension-type headache (CTH) sufferers. Method: Forty-three CTH sufferers participated in a randomized wait-list controlled trial of a mindfulness intervention for headache. Serum concentrations of cytokines IL1-β, IL-2, IL-6, IL-8, IL-12, IL-18, IFN-γ, MCP-1 and TNF-α were measured before and after treatment/wait-list control conditions. Results: Repeated Measures Analysis of Variance revealed that IL1-β, IL-6, IL-8, MCP-1 and TNF-α decreased from pre to post assessments in the treatment and wait-list groups, with no group or group x time effects. Conclusions: Mindfulness training compared to a wait-list control condition does not reduce serum cytokine levels in CTH sufferers.

---

[*] Correspondence: Stuart Cathcart, PhD, Centre for Applied Psychology, University of Canberra, Bruce 2601, Australia. E-mail: stuart.cathcart@canberra.edu.au.

INTRODUCTION

Mindfulness training has been reported as beneficial for reducing symptoms in several chronic pain conditions, including headache (1, 2). One potential mechanism for the therapeutic effects of mindfulness may be a reduction in pro-inflammatory cytokine (PIC) levels. Cytokines are regulatory proteins secreted by numerous cells including immune cells in the periphery and microglia in the Central Nervous System (CNS). Pro-inflammatory cytokines are involved in both stress and pain processing (3, 4), and are increased in several chronic pain conditions, including headache (5, 6). Mindfulness-based interventions have been shown to reduce PIC levels in healthy and clinical samples (7, 8), however this has not been examined in CTH sufferers to date.

Elsewhere we reported elevated PIC levels in the present sample of CTH sufferers (9), and a reduction in headache activity following mindfulness intervention (10). The present study examines if the mindfulness intervention reduced PIC levels in that sample of CTH sufferers.

OUR STUDY

Participant information has been reported in detail elsewhere (9, 10). Briefly, Fifty-eight volunteers satisfying diagnosis of CTH were recruited from the general population and completed pre-treatment measures. Forty-three participants completed post-treatment measures (N=24 treatment, N=19 wait-list). Volunteers were excluded if they reported any chronic pain other than CTH, satisfied other headache diagnoses including migraine or suspected Medication Overuse Headache, or had major medical or psychiatric diagnoses concurrent or in the past 12 months. The mean age of the total sample was 45.5 years (SD=13.8), 37% were male.

Measures

Blood samples (9mL) were collected via venepuncture by a phlebotomist nurse at the School of Psychology, University of South Australia. All participants had their blood taken between 9am and 11am, to control for circadian variation in cytokine levels. Samples were collected in ethylenediaminetetracetic acid (EDTA) and serum clotting tubes, and transported in biohazard containers to the Experimental Therapeutics Laboratory, Hanson Institute. The tubes were centrifuged at 2,500 x g for 10 minutes at room temperature, and the blood components (serum, plasma, buffy coat cells) were aliquoted separately (500µL) into labelled 1.8mL cryovials (Nunc, Roskilde, Denmark). The cryovials were placed into liquid nitrogen to snap freeze, and stored at -70oC before analysis.

Determination of cytokine levels

Cytokine levels in serum samples were analyzed using an established cytometric bead array kit (FlowCytomix; Bender MedSystems, Vienna, Austria) according to the manufacturers' instructions. The kit reagents were diluted 1:2 for each run, and all samples were run in duplicate. Standard curves for each cytokine were included in each run, and sample concentrations were calculated using FlowCytomix Pro software.

Intervention

The intervention was based on Mindfulness-Based Stress Reduction (MBSR) and Mindfulness Based Cognitive Therapy (MBCT), and is detailed elsewhere (10). Delivered by one of the authors (MI), the intervention involved six 1-hour group classes held twice per week for three weeks, and 30mins daily home practice. The program was developed by some of the authors (SC, MP, MI) who are psychologists (SC, MP) with formal training and teaching, practice, and research experience in mindfulness and/or meditation.

Three formal mindfulness meditation practices were taught: 1) body scan meditation, which involves focusing on each region of the body systemically from the foot to the head, and noticing the sensations that are present with openness and curiosity; 2) formal sitting meditation, focusing on mindfulness of breath and other experiences such as sounds and thoughts; 3) three-minute breathing space, which involves three sequential steps of a) focusing awareness of present internal experiences, b) focusing awareness on the breath, and c) expanding awareness to the body as a whole.

Home practice was supported by a written instruction manual and a compact disc containing audio-recorded instructions. The program also included other activities so that participants could practice applying concepts of mindfulness to activities of daily living, recognizing nourishing and draining activities, and documenting observations and reactions to pleasant and unpleasant events.

Procedures

The study was approved by the University of South Australia Human Research Ethics Committee. Following a screening interview and provision of written consent to participate, volunteers completed questionnaires and had blood drawn for cytokine analysis. Headache sufferers were then randomly assigned to either treatment or wait-list conditions. Post-treatment measures were recorded in all CTH participants in the week following completion of the intervention by the treatment group. The wait-list control group commenced mindfulness training the following week.

FINDINGS

Repeated Measures Analysis of Variance results (table 1) yielded significant Time effects indicating a decrease from pre to post assessments for IL1-β (F $(1,41) = 9.65$, p $< .01$, $\eta=.15$), IL-6 (F $(1,41) = 15.56$, p $< .01$, $\eta=.22$), IL-8 (F $(1,41) = 5.13$, p $< .04$, $\eta=.10$), MCP-1 (F $(1,41) = 10.66$, p $< .01$, $\eta=.17$) and TNF-α (F $(1,41) = 11.54$, p $< .01$, $\eta=.18$). Group and Group x Time effects were not significant for any measure (all p>.05).

Table 1. Cytokine levels before and after mindfulness intervention and wait-list control conditions in chronic tension-type headache sufferers

Measure[1]	Mindfulness group N=24				Wait-list group N=19				Test value[2]		
	Pre		Post		Pre		Post		Group effect	Time effect	G x T effect
	Mean	SD	Mean	SD	Mean	SD	Mean	SD			
IL-1β	3.59	.53	2.57	1.95	3.56	.62	3.03	1.48	.42	9.65**	.98
IL-2	2.53	1.19	1.81	1.89	2.26	.50	2.17	1.10	.05	3.11	1.93
IL-6	15.22	1.95	10.09	7.59	14.77	1.97	12.12	5.66	.65	15.56**	1.57
IL-8	35.08	110.9	24.32	85.17	14.46	9.59	11.85	9.11	.62	5.13*	1.91
IL-12	1.74	.46	1.27	.98	1.70	.46	1.65	.88	1.27	3.63	2.28
IL-18	1.05	.93	.85	.95	.92	1.01	.70	.92	.48	1.43	.01
IFN-γ	1.66	.38	1.31	1.03	1.62	.48	1.63	.88	.91	1.44	1.57
MCP-1	223.76	99.68	159.38	151.11	278.10	153.70	230.79	203.74	2.81	10.66**	.25
TNF-α	6.40	.81	4.41	3.30	6.21	.83	5.31	2.56	.66	11.54**	1.67

1. Serum cytokine levels (mean fluorescent intensity) IL-1β; Interleukin 1-beta, IL-2; interleukin-2, IL-6; interleukin-6, IL-8; interleukin-8, IL-12; interleukin-12p70, IL-18; interleukin-18, IFN-γ; interferon-γ, MCP-1; Monocyte Chemoattractant Protein-1, TNF-α; Tumour Necrosis Factor-alpha.

2. Repeated measures analysis of variance F value, all df=1,41.

*p<.05, **p<.01.

DISCUSSION

To our knowledge, this is the first study to examine effects of mindfulness training on pro-inflammatory cytokines in CTH sufferers. The results indicate a pre to post treatment reduction in several of the PIC's examined, in both the treatment and wait-list groups, with no difference between groups. This indicates that mindfulness training compared to a wait-list control group does not reduce PIC levels in CTH sufferers. Elsewhere we have reported that the mindfulness training reduced headache activity in this sample of CTH sufferers (10). Although we did not presently examine relationships between headache activity and PIC's, the findings suggest the therapeutic effect of the intervention previously observed was not due to a reduction in PIC levels. The results also call in to question previous uncontrolled findings of effects of mindfulness training on cytokines (e.g., 8). The cause of the decrease in PICs in the treatment and wait-list groups is unclear. One possibility is non-specific effects common to both treatment and wait-list conditions (e.g., expectancy). Alternatively, the reduction in PIC levels may be coincidental.

Limitations to the present study include the brief nature of our intervention, the lack of an active control group, and the lack of longer-term follow-up. The lack of significant findings is unlikely due to low power associated with the small sample size, since time effects were observed and there were no trends indicating a group x time effect. The above limitations withstanding, the present results indicate that mindfulness training, elsewhere shown to reduce headache activity in this sample of CTH sufferers, does not reduce PIC levels in the same sample. Replication and extension of the present results would further understanding of the importance of PICs in, and the mechanisms of mindfulness intervention for, CTH.

ACKNOWLEDGMENTS

The authors are grateful to Nicola Galatis and Margaret Mitchell for assistance in data collection. This research was funded in part by a Medical Advances Without Animals Trust grant. This study is registered with the Australian and New Zealand Clinical Trials Registry, number ACTRN12610001039077

REFERENCES

[1]   Morone NE, Greco CM, Weiner DK. Mindfulness meditation for the treatment of chronic low back pain in older adults: a randomized controlled pilot study. Pain 2008;134:310-9.

[2]   Kabat-Zinn J, Lipworth L, Burney R. The clinical use of mindfulness meditation for the self-regulation of chronic pain. J Behav Med 1985;8:163-90.

[3]   Chapman C, Tuckett R, Song C. Pain and stress in a systems perspective: Reciprocal neural, endocrine, and immune interactions. J Pain 2008;9(2):122-45.

[4]   Marchand F, Perretti M and McMahon SB. Role of the immune system in chronic pain. Nat Rev Neurosci 2005;6:521-32.

[5]   Bazzichi L, Rossi A, Massimetti G, Giannaccini G, Giuliano T, De Feo F, Ciapparelli A, Dell'Osso L, Bombardieri S. Cytokine patterns in fibromyalgia and their correlation with clinical manifestations. Clin Exp Rheumatol 2007;25:225–30.

[6]   Koçer A, Koçer E, Memişoğullari R, Domaç FM, Yüksel H. Interleukin-6 levels in tension headache patients. Clin J Pain 2010;26(8):690-3.

[7]   Koh KB, Lee Y, Beyn KM, Chu SH, Kim DM. Counter-stress effects of relaxation on proinflammatory and anti-inflammatory cytokines. Brain Behav Immun 2008;22(8):1130-7.

[8]   Carlson LE, Speca M, Faris P et al. One year pre-post intervention follow-up of psychological, immune, endocrine and blood pressure outcomes of mindfulness-based stress reduction (MBSR) in breast and prostate cancer outpatients. Brain Behav Immun 2007 21(8):1038-49.

[9]   Della-Vedova, C. Cathcart, S. Dohnalek, A., Immink, M. & Hayball, J. Peripheral interleukin-1 Beta and Interleukin-18 levels are elevated in Chronic Tension-Type Headache. Pain Res Manage, in press.

[10]   Cathcart S, Galatis N, Immink M, Proeve M, Petkov J. Brief mindfulness-based meditation for chronic tension-type headache: A randomized controlled trial. Behav Cog Psychother, in press.

In: Disability and Chronic Disease
Editors: J. Merrick, S. Aspler and M. Morad

ISBN: 978-1-62948-288-0
© 2014 Nova Science Publishers, Inc.

Chapter 13

PHYSICAL THERAPY MANAGEMENT OF OLDER ADULTS WITH CHRONIC LOW BACK PAIN

Katja Ehrenbrusthoff, MSc[1,2], Cormac G Ryan, PhD[*1], Patricia A Schofield, RGN, PhD, PGDipEd, DipN[3] and Denis J Martin, PhD[1]*

[1]Health and Social Care Institute, Teesside University, Middlesbrough, UK
[2]Hochschule fur Gesundheit, University of Applied Sciences, Bochum, Germany and [3]School of Health and Social Care, Avery Hill Campus, Grey Building, Eltham, Greenwich University, UK

ABSTRACT

Chronic low back pain (CLBP) is common in older adults. Findings from younger patients may not be generalizable to older adults with this condition. Objective: To investigate the evidence from RCTs for the effectiveness of physiotherapeutic interventions on pain and function in older adults with non-specific CLBP. Study group: Studies including older adults (≥65years) with non-specific CLBP of ≥3 month's duration were included. Methods: The Cochrane Back Research Groups' guidelines were used as a methodological template for this systematic review. A literature search of EMBASE, CENTRAL, Medline, AMED, CINAHL and PEDro was performed up to November 2010. Two reviewers assessed the quality of included articles and the evidence for interventions was qualified using the GRADE system. Results: Three moderate quality RCTs were included. They investigated the following: mindfulness meditation, Percutaneous Electrical Nerve Stimulation [PENS], Exercise, and PENS and Exercise combined. Outcome measures for pain and function were reported for the short and medium-term only. There was limited evidence that compared to control/placebo interventions mindfulness meditation, exercise, and PENS combined with exercise have no effect on pain or function in older adults with non-specific CLBP. There was conflicting evidence that PENS compared to placebo is effective for pain and function. Conclusions: This systematic review identified only three studies that have investigated

---

[*] Correspondence: Cormac Ryan, PhD, School of Health and Social Care, Teesside University, Middlesbrough, TS1 3BAUnited Kingdom. E-mail: c.ryan@tees.ac.uk.

the effect of physiotherapeutic interventions on older adults with CLBP. There was insufficient research upon which to make firm clinical recommendations. Further research is needed on this severely under investigated and growing clinical population, to guide clinical practice.

INTRODUCTION

Chronic low back pain (CLBP) affects 30-40% of UK older adults and the prevalence of severe CLBP increases with age (1-3). Currently 17% of the UK population are over 65years of age, and this is predicted to increase to 23% by 2035 as the population continues to age. Thus, the number of adults with CLBP is likely to steadily increase over the coming years (4). CLBP can be disabling, reducing independence and quality of life for older people (5). Biological, psychological and social factors associated with aging influence how older people are affected by chronic pain (6-8). For example, changes in the structure and function of peripheral and central nociceptive pathways may place the older adult at greater risk for the development of chronic pain and render them especially vulnerable to associated negative effects (8). As such, older adults should be given particular consideration (9) while recognising that chronological age is a crude categorisation. Findings from studies which have looked at younger adults may not be generalisable to older adults. Physical therapy is strongly indicated for CLBP yet guidelines are based upon data from younger adults [18-65years] (10). This may partly explain why physical therapy is less likely to be prescribed for older adults with CLBP compared to their younger counterparts (3). There is a need to review the evidence for physical therapy treatments for CLBP in this growing clinical population in order to guide clinical practice.

The aim of this systematic review, therefore, was to examine the evidence from RCTs for the effectiveness of physical therapy interventions in comparison to control/placebo interventions on pain and function in older adults with non-specific CLBP.

OUR STUDY

The Cochrane Back Review Group's [CBRG] guidelines (11, 12) were used as a methodological template for this review. A literature search of EMBASE, CENTRAL, Medline, AMED (Allied and Complementary Medicine), CINAHL (Cumulative Index to Nursing and Allied Health Literature) and PEDro (Physiotherapy Evidence Database) was conducted up to November 2010. The reference lists of key trials were hand searched for additional studies. Keywords used were low back pain, sciatica, older adults, elderly, seniors, complementary therapies, acupuncture therapy, mind-body therapies, musculoskeletal manipulations, electric stimulation therapy, physical therapy and rehabilitation. Keywords and search strings were combined using Boolean operators. A detailed description of the search strategy used for Medline, CINAHL and AMED is shown in table 1. A detailed description of the search strategies used for EMBASE, CENTRAL and PEDro are shown in Appendix 1 and 2 which are available online.

Only RCTs involving participants aged ≥65years, consistent with the WHO's definition of an older adult, were included (13). Participants had to be diagnosed with non-specific

CLBP of ≥3 months duration. The interventions had to be deliverable by physiotherapists. Studies were included if they measured pain and/or function (14). The timing of outcome measurement follow-up was categorised as 'short-term' (~4weeks), 'intermediate' (~6months) and 'long-term' (~1year) (11).

Table 1. Search Strategy for MEDLINE, CINAHL, AMED (via EBSCO)

Last run: November 21st 2010

1.	randomized controlled trial
2.	controlled clinical trial
3.	TI randomized or AB randomized
4.	TI randomly or AB randomly
5.	TI trial or AB trial
6.	TI groups
7.	1 or 2 or 3 or 4 or 5 or 6
8.	animals NOT humans
9.	7 NOT 8
10.	(MM"Low Back Pain/TH")
11.	(MM"Sciatica/TH")
12.	10 OR 11
13.	older N2 adult*
14.	elderly N3 patient*
15.	13 OR 14
16.	12 AND 15
17.	9 AND 16
18.	(MH"Physical Therapy Modalities+")
19.	(MM" Complementary Therapies+")
20.	18 OR 19
21.	15 AND 20
22.	12 AND 20
23.	12 AND 21
24.	Limiters: Publication Type: Randomized Controlled Trial; Clinical Trial
	Narrowed by Subject Age: 65+ years

Legend:
TI   =   denotes a word in the title.
AB =   denotes a word in the abstract.
MM=   denotes Major Concept.
/TH =   denotes subheading 'Therapy'.
* = denotes truncation.
+= denotes headings are exploded to retrieve all references indexed to the   search term.
N2 =denotes Near operator: word within 2/3 words of one another.
MH = denotes major heading.

The study selection process comprised of two stages. In the first stage titles and abstracts of the search results were examined and obviously irrelevant or duplicate trials were removed. The full text of potentially relevant trials were accessed and screened for compliance with the eligibility criteria, leading to removal or full inclusion in the review. Data was then extracted by KE from the included trials using the CBRG validated extraction forms. The extraction forms sought to obtain the following information; Study title, author affiliation, verification of study eligibility (correct population, intervention, outcome, and study design), study design, unit of allocation, method of randomisation, allocation concealment, blindedness, recruitment of patients, place, enrollment dates, inclusion criteria, exclusion criteria, age, sex, ethnicity, work status, diagnosis of low back pain, duration of pain, previous treatments, cause of pain, total number of patients recruited, number of patients who met inclusion criteria, total number of patients randomised, total number of patients followed, Interventions, who carried out measurements, what was measured at baseline, how was it measured is the tool validated, what was measured immediately after the intervention, when were the follow-up measurements taken, statistical techniques used, intention to treat analysis, does technique adjust for confounding, number followed-up from each group, quantitative results, adverse effects or complications. The CBRG criteria for assessing the risk of bias were used to assess the methodological quality of individual trials (11). Studies were rated as high, moderate or low quality [table 2]. (15) Each selected article was independently assessed for quality by two of the authors C.R. and K.E. The initial agreement between both reviewers was good (κ = 0.69, p<0.01) and a third reviewer was not needed. Risk of bias across studies such as publication bias or selective outcome reporting was assessed qualitatively.

Table 2. The quality of evidence grading system

Quality of Individual trials

Quality of RCT	*Rating Criteria*
High	>75% of the criteria have been met [> 9/12]. Where they have not been met the conclusions of the study or review are thought very unlikely to alter.
Moderate	50-75% of the criteria have been met [6 – 9/ 12]. Those criteria that have not been met or not adequately described are thought unlikely to alter the conclusions.
Low	Less than 50% of the checklist criteria were fulfilled [< 6/12]. The conclusions of the study are thought likely or very likely to alter.

Synthesis: Grading the Quality of Evidence [GRADE]

Grading Level	*Rating Criteria*
Strong	Consistent findings from multiple high quality RCTs.
Moderate	Consistent findings among multiple moderate quality RCTs and/or one high quality RCT.
Limited	One Moderate quality RCT
Conflicting	Inconsistent findings among multiple RCTs
No evidence	No RCTs were identified

Legend: This table was adapted from Van Tulder et al. 2003[11] and Clarke et al. 2011[14].

Data synthesis and analysis

The principal summary method for individual studies was difference in means. Pooling of results for quantitative analysis was not possible, as the studies lacked homogeneity, thus results were compared descriptively using best evidence synthesis. A modified version of the

CBRG's GRADE system was used to rate the quality of evidence for each intervention across all studies [table 2] (12).

FINDINGS

The electronic search identified 495 potentially relevant papers. Following a screening process (detailed in Figure 1) the full text of 17 papers were examined. Of these, nine were excluded because they did not meet the definition of non-specific CLBP (16-24). One study was excluded as it was not a physical therapy intervention (25) another because it included participants with knee pain and the relevant data for people with back pain only could not be extracted (26). Three studies, one of which was published in two parts, did not meet the age criteria of ≥65years (27-30). In total, three studies (31-33) were included in the final review (table 3). The quality assessment of each of these studies is shown in table 4. The only evidence of risk of bias identified across studies was that all three papers included in the final review were published by the same research group/institute.

Methodological quality summary

The three trials included in the review were of moderate methodological quality with scores ranging from 6/12 to 9/12. The three studies investigated different types of physical therapy interventions and have been categorized as: 1) Mindfulness meditation 2) PENS 3) Exercise 4) PENS & Exercise combined.

Mindfulness meditation

One moderate quality study (31) (n=37) compared the effects of an 8-week mindfulness-based meditation program to a waiting-list control.

Pain

Pain intensity was measured using the McGill Pain Questionnaire short-form [MPQ-SF] and the SF-36 Pain Scale (less pain indicated by higher scores). Only short-term measures were obtained. A decrease in pain of >5 points on the MPQ-SF (35) and ≥30 points on the SF-36 Pain Scale (36) was considered clinically relevant.

Mean (SD) MPQ-SF scores changed from 15.5 (10.0) at baseline to 13.7 (7.9) post intervention; and control group scores changed from 15.2 (7.0) to 15.7 (9.1). In the same period SF-36 pain scores changed from 35.5 (6.0) at baseline to 39.9 (7.7) in the meditation group; and from 35.7 (7.2) to 38.8 (8.3) in the control group. The differences between groups were neither statistically nor clinically significant.

Table 3. Characteristics of included studies

Author	Population	n	Intervention	Comparison	Assessment Timing	Outcome Measures
Morone et al., 2008[29]	Characteristics: older adults with CLBP, moderate intensity occurring daily or almost every day, aged 65 years or older. Mean age: 74.9 years Setting: community-dwelling (USA) Recruitment: telephone	37 ♀= 16 ♂= 21	8-week mindfulness-based meditation programme, once a week for 90 minutes (Three techniques were used 1) bodily scan – In a lying position the individual places their attention, non-judgementally, to each body area beginning at the toes and ending at the head 2) sitting practice – the individual focuses on their breathing while sitting on a chair or the floor 3) walking meditation – mindful slow walking where the individual focuses their attention on bodily sensations and/or breathing (n=19)	wait list control group (n=18)	Pre treatment Short-term follow-up: immediately post intervention (8 weeks)	*Pain* 1.MPQ-SF *Function* 1.SF-36 2.RMDQ
Weiner et al., 2003[30]	Characteristics: adults aged 65 and older with CLBP of at least moderate intensity almost every day Mean age: 73.8 years Setting: community-dwelling (USA) Recruitment: newspaper advert	34 ♀= 16 ♂= 18	Twice weekly PENS for 6 weeks, PENS sessions lasted 30 minutes and stimulation frequency ranged from 2-200Hz. The electrical stimulation was maintained below the pain threshold. Participants also received physical therapy including; exercise programmes, pain management techniques and manual therapy modalities (n=17)	Twice weekly sham PENS for six weeks. Participants also received physical therapy including; exercise programmes, pain management techniques and manual therapy modalities(n=17)	Pre treatment Short-term follow-up: immediately post intervention (6 weeks), and at 3 months post intervention	*Pain* 1.MPQ-SF 2.MPI *Function* 1.RMDQ 2.Physical performance battery (balance, gait speed, chair rise time)
Weiner et al., 2008[31]	Characteristics: adults aged 65 and older with CLBP mean age: 73.9 years Setting: outpatient(USA) Recruitment: telephone-screening	200 ♀= 114 ♂= 86	PENS twice weekly for 6 weeks, electrical stimulation provided for 30 minutes (n=50)	1. Sham PENS (n=50) 2. PENS + Exercise (n=50) 3.Sham PENS + Exercise (n=50)	Pre treatment Short-term follow-up: immediately post intervention (6 weeks) Intermediate follow-up: 6 months post intervention	*Pain* 1.MPQ-SF 2.Pain thermometer *Function* 1.RMDQ 2.Physical performance battery (gait speed, chair rise time, stair climb time)

Legend: CLBP = Chronic low back pain , RCT = randomized controlled trial; n = number of participants; ♀= Females; ♂=Males; PENS = Percutaneous Electrical Nerve Stimulation; RMDQ= Roland Morris Disability Questionnaire; MPI=Multidimensional Pain Inventory; MPQ-SF = McGill Pain Questionnaire Short-Form.

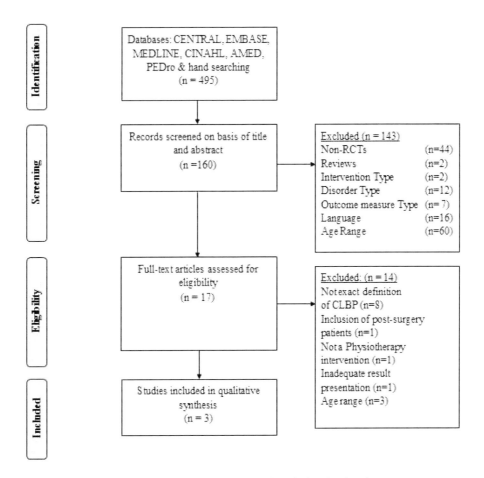

Figure 1. RCTs = randomised controlled trials; CLBP = chronic low back pain.
(Adapted from Moher et al. 2009 (34).

Function

Function was measured using the SF-36 Physical Function scale, the Roland Morris Disability Questionnaire (RMDQ) and a short physical performance battery (balance, gait speed and ability to rise from a chair). A difference of ≥2 points on the RMDQ (11) and ≥15 points on the SF-36 Physical Function scale (36) was considered clinically relevant.

Mean (SD) RMDQ scores improved in the meditation group from 11.5 (3.7) at baseline to 9.4 (5.1); and from 11.8 (4.6) to 10.6 (5.3) in the waiting-list control group. The difference between groups was neither statistically nor clinically significant. SF-36 physical function score improved in the meditation group from 42.0 (10.9) to 45.7 (9.2), while the score deteriorated in the control group from 45.1 (9.5) to 44.5 (10.1). The difference between groups was statistically significant (p = 0.03) but not clinically significant.

The authors stated that there was no statistically significant difference between the two groups on the physical performance battery measure but provided no raw data.

Quality of evidence statement

There was limited evidence that mindfulness-based meditation has no immediate effect on pain or function in older adults with CLBP compared to a waiting list control.

Percutaneous Electrical Nerve Stimulation (PENS)

Two moderate quality RCTs, undertaken by the same research group, investigated the effect of PENS compared to a placebo PENS intervention (32, 33). In the first study (n=34) (32) participants were seen twice weekly for six weeks. In the control group the acupuncture needles were applied as in the intervention but without electrical current. Both groups also received advice, education and exercise.

In the second study (n = 100) (33) participants were seen twice weekly for six weeks. The control group received minimal electrical stimulation (applied at T-12 dermatome for 5 minutes) compared to the intervention. There were two other groups within this study which combined exercise with PENS and control PENS. These two groups will be discussed in the sections on exercise.

Pain

In the earlier study (32) pain intensity was measured by the MPQ-SF and the Pain Severity Scale of the Multidimensional Pain Inventory (MPI-PS) collected immediately post treatment (short-term) and 3 months after its completion (medium-term). An effect size (ES) of 0.42 on the MPI was considered clinically relevant (37).

Mean (SD) MPQ-SF scores decreased in the PENS group from 13.06 (1.31) to 6.66 (0.87) immediately post intervention and increased from 12.24 (1.69) to 12.47 (2.04) in the control group. After three months, scores decreased in the intervention group to 6.19 (0.88) and to 11.82 (1.90) in the control group. The difference between groups was statistically and clinically significant in both the short and medium term.

Mean (SD) MPI-PS scores decreased in both the PENS group from 3.21 (0.25) to 2.00 (0.20) [ES = 4.84] and the control group from 3.28 (0.28) to 3.22 (0.23) [ES = 0.21] immediately after the intervention period. At three months, the intervention group score was 2.16 (0.30) [ES = 4.20] compared to 3.10 (0.16) [ES = 0.39] in the control group. The difference between groups was statistically and clinically significant in both the short and medium term.

In the more recent study (33), pain intensity was measured by the MPQ-SF and a pain thermometer measuring average and strongest pain in the past week, collected post treatment (short-term) and 6 months after completion of treatment (medium-term). Difference data rather than pre and post data were presented in the paper. The difference in pain, as measured by the MPQ-SF between groups was 0.5 (1.4) and 1.0 (1.5) at short and medium term follow up respectively. The difference between groups was neither statistically or clinically significant. Pain thermometer scores showed similar results.

Function

In the 2003 study (32) function was measured using the RMDQ, the MPI pain interference scale and a series of physical performance tests including timed chair rise, lower extremity strength, postural control and standing balance.

In the intervention group mean (SD) RMDQ scores decreased from baseline to post-treatment and short-term follow-up from 12.63 (1.13) to 7.81 (1.02) to 9.25 (1.08) compared to 11.24 (1.47) to 11.06 (1.17) to 12.18 (1.21) in the control group. The difference between groups was statistically and clinically significant.

Similarly, mean (SD) MPI function decreased in the intervention group from 3.52 (0.37) at baseline to 2.44 (0.33) post-treatment and 2.61 (0.26) at short-term compared to 3.30 (0.37) to 3.10 (0.40) to 2.97 (0.37) in the control group. The difference between groups was statistically and clinically significant. Of the physical performance tests, the chair rise test and the lifting endurance test showed statistically significant improvements in favour of the intervention group.

In the 2008 (33) study function was measured using the RMDQ and three physical performance tests; usual pace gait speed, chair rise time and stair climb time.

The difference in function, as measured by the RMDQ between groups was 0.1 (0.9) and 1.1 (0.9) at short and medium-term follow-up respectively. The difference between groups was neither statistically or clinically significant. Physical performance test scores showed similar results.

Quality of evidence statement

There is conflicting evidence that PENS is effective for pain and function in older adults with CLBP, compared to placebo PENS.

Exercise

The nature of the subgroups in the design of the moderate quality RCT by Weiner et al., (33) provided an analysis of the effects of exercise on pain and function in older adults with persistent CLBP, by way of comparison of placebo PENS to placebo PENS combined with exercise (n = 100). The exercise was described as weekly supervised aerobic exercise combined with a home program of daily stretching and walking.

Pain

The difference in pain, as measured by the MPQ between groups was -0.3 (1.4) and -0.6 (1.5) at short and medium-term follow-up, respectively. The difference between groups was neither statistically or clinically significant. Pain thermometer scores showed similar results.

Function

The difference in function, as measured by the RMDQ between groups was -0.2 (0.9) and 0.3 (0.9) at short and medium-term follow-up respectively. The difference between groups was neither statistically or clinically significant. Physical performance test scores showed similar results.

Quality of evidence statement

Thus, there is limited evidence that exercise combined with placebo PENS has no effect on pain or function in older adults with CLBP compared to placebo PENS only.

Exercise and PENS Combined

Weiner et al. (33) also investigated the effects of exercise and PENS combined (n = 50) against the other three subgroups of placebo PENS, active PENS, and placebo PENS and Exercise. There were no statistically or clinically significant effects of the combined treatment when compared to any of the other groups for pain or function at either the post treatment or 6-month follow-up point.

Quality of evidence statement

There was limited evidence that exercise combined with PENS has no effect on pain or function in older adults with CLBP.

Adverse effects

One study (33) which looked at the effects of PENS and exercise combined reported no significant intervention-associated adverse effects, though it was stated that one participant dropped out due to increased pain. The comparison between PENS and exercise (32) did not report whether or not adverse events occurred. The study on mindfulness meditation stated that no serious side effects were reported (31).

DISCUSSION

The aim of this systematic review was to examine the effectiveness of physiotherapeutic interventions on pain and function in older adults (≥65years) with non-specific CLBP. There was limited evidence that mindfulness meditation, exercise, and PENS combined with Exercise have no effect on pain or function in older adults with non-specific PLBP CLBP compared to a control/placebo. There was conflicting evidence that PENS is effective for pain and function, compared to placebo PENS.

Perhaps the most striking finding of the study was that only three RCTs met the inclusion criteria. Not only that but two were by the same research team and the other from a team in the same institute. The interventions in those studies are limited compared to the range of interventions that fall within the scope of physical therapy. This shortage of direct research explains why guidelines for chronic pain management for older adults have had to make inferences from studies on younger adults or samples that partially comprised ≥65's (38). That carries some validity but does not extrapolate directly to the ≥65 population. Aging can affect how pain affects an individual and those effects are more likely to be seen in people of advanced years (It is worth repeating that chronological age can be a crude indicator of biological age).

The findings about exercise are somewhat conflicting with the literature for younger adults with back pain. There is strong evidence that exercise therapy is beneficial for back pain (39) and as such it is a cornerstone of physiotherapeutic management. The lack of effect of the exercise intervention on pain should not have been wholly unexpected as that outcome is less of a primary target of exercise than function. An effect on function would have been more expected. The lack of effect of the specific exercise programme on function, as measured by the RMDQ, could indicate that older adults with CLBP are less susceptible to the benefits of exercise than younger adults. However, without a wider body of evidence with which comparison can be made this is very speculative and other studies have shown a positive effect of exercise in older adults with persistent pain not specific to the back (40). It may just as well be that the specific exercise regime was insufficient for this particular group. It is known that there are particular internal and external barriers to exercising for older people, and as recommended in the British Geriatric Society guidelines on chronic pain management for older people, these should be considered in implementing any programme (41) It may be that the exercise programme delivered was less than optimal in some dimensions for this sample of older adults with CLBP. It should also be noted that the exercise did show an effect on secondary psychological outcome measures, which are important and, in themselves, provide support for exercise interventions to be used with this patient group.

There was conflicting evidence for the benefit of PENS from two studies produced by the same research group (32, 33). Studies were deemed of insufficient homogeneity for a meta-analysis. Although both studies were rated as moderate quality the study showing no effect was arguably more robust as it had a more credible placebo intervention and a larger sample size (n=37 vs.100).

Strengths and limitations

The main limitation of this review was the lack of literature with only three studies, all of moderate quality, included in the final review, all of which were produced from the same research institute in Pennsylvania, USA. The scope for extrapolation out with the population directly described by the samples is limited. Importantly, within that context, all three studies excluded individuals with comorbidities even though comorbidity is common in older adults. This questions, to some extent, the external validity of the findings to the full population of older adults with CLBP. The primary strengths of this systematic review is that it follows the methods recommended by the Cochrane Back Review Group. The search was extensive including the key search engines recommended by the Cochrane group along with hand searching and all included studies were reviewed by two reviewers to minimise reviewer bias.

Table 4. The Methodological Quality Assessment of individual trials (n=3) included in this review

	A	B	C			D		E	F				Scoring	Methodological Quality
	1	2	3	4	5	6	7	8	9	10	11	12		
Morone et al., 2008	+	+	-	-	+*	+	+	+*	+	-	+	+	9/12	moderate
Weiner et al., 2003	+	-	-	-	+	+	+	+	+	+	-	+	8/12	moderate
Weiner et al., 2008	+	-*	-*	-	+	+	?	+	+	-*	-	+	6/12	moderate

Legend:

A 1   Was the method of randomization adequate?   + criterion achieved
B 2   Was the treatment allocation concealed? - criterion not achieved
C   Was the knowledge of allocated interventions adequately prevented during the study? *Assessors initially disagreed
   3   Was the patient blinded to intervention?
   4   Was the care provider blinded to intervention?
   5   Was the outcome assessor blinded to the intervention?
D   Were incomplete data adequately addressed?
   6   Was the drop-out rate described and acceptable?
   7   Were all randomized participants analysed in the group to which they were allocated?
E 8   Are reports of the study free of suggestion of selective outcome reporting?
F   Other sources of potential bias
   9   Were the groups similar at baseline regarding the most important prognostic factors?
   10 Were co-interventions avoided or similar?
   11 Was the compliance acceptable in all groups?
   12 Was the timing of outcome assessment similar in all groups?

Implications for policy/practice

Considering the restricted literature base that this review draws upon no firm clinical recommendations can be made. The lack of positive findings for an effect of exercise on pain or function are far from sufficient to question current physiotherapeutic guidelines that strongly endorse exercise for people with CLBP (10) and exercise should still play an important role in the management of older adults with non-specific CLBP. The paucity of literature investigating the use of exercise in older adults has implications for policy and practice and may partly explain why older adults with CLBP are more likely to just be prescribed medication and less likely to be prescribed physical therapy or exercise than younger adults (3). The lack of adverse events identified support the safety of these physiotherapeutic interventions and highlights their potential advantages over pharmacological interventions in older adults often associated with adverse effects (42, 43).

Unanswered questions and future research

There is an urgent need for firm physiotherapeutic guidelines for older adults with CLBP. This review, in highlighting the lack of research in this patient sub-group shows the need for robust RCTs to investigate the effects of various different interventions specifically for older adults with non-specific CLBP. This includes standard therapies which have been researched relatively thoroughly in younger adults e.g., advice, education and exercise. This research should be undertaken by different research groups in different countries, cultures and health care settings.

CONCLUSION

Despite a high prevalence of non-specific CLBP in older adults this systematic review identified only three studies that have investigated the effect of physiotherapeutic interventions on this patient group. There was limited evidence that mindfulness meditation, exercise, and PENS combined with Exercise, have no effect on pain or function in older adults with non-specific CLBP compared to control/placebo. There was conflicting evidence that PENS is effective for pain and function in this patient group compared to placebo. Due to the paucity of evidence there is insufficient information upon which to make firm clinical recommendations. Further research is needed on this severely under investigated and growing clinical population.

APPENDIX 1: SEARCH STRATEGY FOR EMBASE AND CENTRAL (VIA OVID)

Last run: November 21st, 2010

1.	randomized controlled trial.pt.
2.	controlled clinical trial.pt.
3.	randomized.ab.
4.	placebo.ab.
5.	clinical trials as topic.sh.
6.	randomly.ab.
7.	trial.ti.
8.	1 or 2 or 3 or 4 or 5 or 6 or 7
9.	exp animals/ not humans.sh.
10.	8 not 9
11.	exp Low Back Pain/px, rh, th [Psychology, Rehabilitation, Therapy]
12.	exp Sciatica/px, rh, th [Psychology, Rehabilitation, Therapy]
13.	11 or 12
14.	(older adj3 adult*).mp. [mp=ti, ot, ab, tx, ct, sh, kw, de, hw, tn, dm, mf]
15.	(elderly adj3 patient*).mp. [mp=ti, ot, ab, tx, ct, sh, kw, de, hw, tn, dm, mf]

Appendix 1. (Continued)

16.	14 or 15
17.	13 and 16
18.	exp complementary therapies/ or acupuncture therapy/ or auriculotherapy/ or mind-body therapies/ or musculoskeletal manipulations/ or reflexotherapy/ or spiritual therapies/ or electric stimulation therapy/ or physical therapy modalities/ or exp rehabilitation/
19.	10 and 13 and 18
20.	16 and 19

Legend:

pt   =   denotes the publication type term

ab   =   denotes a word in the abstract

fs.   =   denotes a floating subheading

sh.   =   denotes a Medical Subject Heading (MeSH) term

ti.   =   denotes a word in the title

adj3 =   operator indicates within three words

*.   =   indicates truncation

.mp. =   indicates a search of title, original title, abstract, name of substance word and subject heading word

exp. =   expands the search results of terms entered and include more specific related topics.

APPENDIX 2: SEARCH STRATEGY FOR PEDRO

Last run: November 1st 2010

(via: http://search.pedro.org.au/pedro/findrecords.php?-type=new_search)

1. Search Option	Advanced Search
2. Abstract & Title	Back pain (Chronic low back pain) Non-pharmacological AND treatment Non-pharmacological AND intervention (Older adults) Elderly Elderly patients
3. Therapy	No selection
4. Body Part	Lumbar spine, sacro iliac joint or pelvis
5. Sub discipline	Gerontology Musculoskeletal
6. Method	Clinical trial Systematic Review
7.When Searching	Match all search terms (AND)

REFERENCES

[1]   Papageorgiou AC, Croft PR, Ferry S, Jayson MI, Silman AJ. Estimating the prevalence of low back pain in the general population. Evidence from the South Manchester back pain survey. Spine 1995;20:1889-94.

[2]   Rusteon T, Wahl AK, Hanestad BR, Lerdal A, Paul S, Miaskowski C. Age and the experience of chronic pain. Clin J Pain 2005;21:513-23.

[3]   Macfarlane GJ, Beasley M, Jones EA, Prescott GJ, Docking R, Keeley P, McBeth J, Jones GT. The Prevalence and management of low back pain across adulthood: results from a population-based cross sectional study (the MUSICIAN study). Pain 2012;153:27-32.

[4]   UK National statistics. Topic guide to older people. Accessed 2013 Febr 15. URL: www. Statistics.gov.uk/hub/population/ageing/older-people

[5]   Smith BH, Elliot AM, Chambers WA, Smith WC, Hannford PC, Penny K. The impact of chronic pain in the community. Fam Pract 2001;18:292-99.

[6]   Gibson SJ. IASP global year against pain in older persons: highlighting the current status and future perspectives in geriatric pain. Expert Rev Neuro ther 2007;7:627-35.

[7]   Gibson SJ, Helme RD. Age-related differences in pain perception and report. Clin Geriatr Med 2001;17:433-56.

[8]   Gibson SJ, Farrell M. A Review of age differences in the neurophysiology of nociception and the perceptual experience of pain. Clin J Pain 2004;20:227-39.

[9]   Ryan CG, Ryan HE. Persistent pain in older adults: A brief overview. J Physiother Pain Assoc 2011;31:10-5.

[10]   Chartered Society of Physiotherapy. Clinical guidelines for the physiotherapy management of persistent low back pain (LBP). London: Chartered Society Physiotherapy, 2009.

[11]   Furlan AD, Pennick V, Bombardier C, van Tulder MW. 2009 Updated method guidelines for systematic reviews in the cochrane back review group. Spine 2009;34:1929-41.

[12]   Van Tulder M, Furlan A, Bombardier C, Bouter L. Updated method guidelines for systematic reviews in the cochrane collaboration back review Group. Spine 2003;28:1290-9.

[13]   Kowal P, Peachey K. Information needs for research, policy and action on Ageing and Older Adults. Indicators for the Minimum Data Set Project on Ageing: A critical review in sub-Saharan Africa. Bethesda, MD: National Institute Aging, 2001.

[14]   Deyo RA, Battie M, Beurskens AJHM. et al. Outcome measures for low back pain research: a proposal for standardized use. Spine 1998;23:2003-13.

[15]   Clarke CL, Ryan CG, Martin D. Pain neurophysiology education for the management of individuals with chronic low back pain: a systematic review and meta-analysis. Man Ther 2011;16:544-9.

[16]   Basler H, Bertalanffy H, Quint S, Wilke A, Wolf U. TTM-based counselling in physiotherapy does not contribute to an increase of adherence to activity recommendations in older adults with chronic low back pain-a randomised controlled trial. Eur J Pain 2007;11:31-7.

[17]   Hondras MA, Long CR, Cao Y, Rowell RM, Meeker WC. A randomized controlled trial comparing 2 types of spinal manipulation and minimal conservative medical care for adults 55 years and older with subacute or chronic low back pain. J Manipulat Physiol Ther 2009;32:330-43.

[18]   Itoh K, Katsumi Y, Kitakoji H. Trigger point acupuncture treatment of chronic low back pain in elderly patients -a blinded RCT. Acupunct Med 2004;22:170-7.

[19]   Itoh K, Katsumi Y, Hirota S, Kitakoji H. Effects of trigger point acupuncture on chronic low back pain in elderly patients-a sham-controlled randomised trial. Acupunct Med 2006;24:5-12.

[20]   Itoh K, Itoh S, Katsumi Y, Kitakoji H. A pilot study on using acupuncture and transcutaneous electrical nerve stimulation to treat chronic non-specific low back pain. Complement Ther Clin Pract 2009;15:22-5.

[21]   Koc Z, Ozcakir S, Sivrioglu K, Gurbet A, Kucukoglu S. Effectiveness of physical therapy and epidural steroid injections in lumbar spinal stenosis. spine 2009;34:985-9.

[22]   Liu-Ambrose TY, Khan KM, Eng JJ, Lord SR, Lentle B, McKay H. Both resistance and agility training reduce back pain and improve health-related quality of life in older women with low bone mass. Osteoporos Int 2005;16:1321-9.

[23]   Zambito A, Bianchini D, Gatti D, Rossini M, Adami S, Viapiana O. Interferential and horizontal therapies in chronic low back pain due to multiple vertebral fractures: a randomized, double blind, clinical study. Osteoporos Int 2007;18:1541-5.

[24]   Zucco F, Orlandi B. Very low frequency and low intensity magnetic fields in a different treatment of disease: chronic low back pain in senile degenerative arthritis. Bioelectrochem Bioenerg 1985;14:187-95.

[25]   Brockow T, Dillner A, Franke A, Resch KL. Analgesic effectiveness of subcutaneous carbon-dioxide insufflations as an adjunct treatment in patients with non-specific neck or low back pain. Complement Ther Med 2001;9:68-76.

[26]   Nguyen M, Revel M, Dougados M. Prolonged effects of 2-week therapy in a spa resort on lumbar spine/knee and hip osteoarthritis: follow-up after 5 months: a randomised controlled trial. Br J Rheumatol 1997;36:77-81.

[27]   Grant DJ, Bishop-Miller J, Winchester DM, Anderson M, Faulkner S. A randomized comparative trial of acupuncture versus transcutaneous electrical nerve stimulation for chronic back pain in the elderly. Pain 1999;82:9-13.

[28]   Meng CF, Wang D, Ngeow J, Lao L, Peterson M, Paget S. Acupuncture for chronic low back pain in older patients: a randomized, controlled trial. Rheumatology (Oxford) 2003;42:1508-17.

[29]   Suen LKP, Wong, EMC. Longitudinal changes in the disability level of the elders with low back pain after auriculotherapy. Complement Ther Med 2008;16:28-35.

[30]   Suen LKP, Wong TKS, Chung JWY, Yip VYB. Auriculotherapy on low back pain in the elderly. Complement Ther Clin Pract 2007;13:63-9.

[31]   Morone NE, Greco CM, Weiner D. Mindfulness meditation for the treatment of chronic low back pain in older adults: a randomized controlled pilot study. Pain 2008;134:310-9.

[32]   Weiner DK, Rudy TE, Glick RM, Boston JR, Lieber SJ, Morrow LA, et al. Efficacy of percutaneous electrical nerve stimulation for the treatment of chronic low back pain in older adults. J Am Geriatr Soc 2003;51:599-608.

[33]   Weiner DK, Perera S, Rudy TE, Glick RM, Shenoy S, Delitto A. Efficacy of percutaneous electrical nerve stimulation and therapeutic exercise for older adults with chronic low back pain: a randomized controlled trial. Pain 2008;140:344-57.

[34]   Moher D, Liberati A, Tetzlaff J, Altman DG, The PRISMA Group. Preferred reportingitems for systematic reviews and meta-analyses: The PRISMA statment. Plos Medicine 2009;6(7):e1000097. doi:10.1371/journal.pmed.1000097.

[35]   Inger Strand L, Ljunggren AE, Bogen B, Ask T, Johnsen TB. The short-form mcgill pain questionnaire as an outcome measure: test-retest reliability and responsiveness to change. Eur J Pain 2008;12:917-25.

[36]   Lauridsen HH, Hartvigsen J, Manniche C, Korsholm L, Grunnet-Nilsson N. Responsiveness and minimally clinically important difference for pain and disability instruments in low back pain patients. BMC Musculoskeletal Disord 2006;7:82.

[37]   Angst F, Verra ML, Lehmann S, Aeschlimann A. Responsiveness of five condition-specific and generic outcome assessment instruments for chronic pain. BMC Med Res Methodol 2008;8:26.

[38]   Ferrell B, Casarett D, Epplin J, Fine P, Gloth FM, Herr K, Katz P, Keefe F, Koo PJS, O'Grady M, Szwabo P, Vallerand AH, Weiner D. The management of persistent pain in older persons: AGS panel on persistent pain in older persons. J Am Geriatr Soc 2002;50:S205-24.

[39]   Hayden J, van Tulder MW, Malmivaara A, Koes BW. Exercise therapyfor treatment of non-specific low back pain. CochraneDatabase Syst Rev 2005;3:CD000335.

[40]   Ferrell BA, Josephson KR, Pollan AM, Loy S, Ferrell BR. A randomised trial of walking versus physical methods for chronic pain management. Aging Clin Exp Res 1997;9:99-105.

[41]   Schofield PA, Abdulla A, Adams N, Bone M, Elliott AM, Gaffin J, JonesD, Knaggs R, Martin D, Sampson L. Guidelines for the management of pain in older adults. London: British Pain Society, British Geriatric Society, 2012.

[42]   Griffin MR, Yared A, Ray WA. Nonsteroidal anti-inflammatory drugs and acute renal failure in elderly persons. Am J Epidemiol 2000;151:488-96.

[43]   Smalley WE, Ray WA, Daugherty JR, Griffin MR. Nonsteroidal anti-inflammatory drugs and the incidence of hospitalizations for peptic ulcer disease in elderly persons. Am J Epidemiol 1995;141:539-45.

In: Disability and Chronic Disease
Editors: J. Merrick, S. Aspler and M. Morad

ISBN: 978-1-62948-288-0
© 2014 Nova Science Publishers, Inc.

Chapter 14

THE LONG-TERM EFFECTIVENESS OF PAIN MANAGEMENT PROGRAMS

Laura Chipchase, DHealthPsy[*]*, David Sheffield, PhD and Patrick Hill, DClinPsy*

Multidisciplinary Pain Service, Birmingham Community Healthcare NHS Trust and
Centre for Psychological Research, University of Derby, Birmingham, UK

The short-term efficacy of pain management programmes (PMPs) is well established. However, their ability to demonstrate long-term benefits for people with chronic pain remains a key question for both the application and evolution of PMPs. Objective: To evaluate the long-term treatment gains of pain management programme (PMP) interventions on self efficacy, catastrophic thinking, and pain perceptions in patients with chronic pain. Methods: Electronic databases, key journals and reference lists of included studies were scrutinized for inclusion. The search process revealed a total of eleven studies for inclusion. Assessment of study quality was made based on length of follow-up period, the validity of measures used and information regarding the intervention. Results: Six studies included a 12 month follow-up, four studies included a 6 month follow-up, and a single study included a 9 month follow-up. Meta-analyses revealed treatment gains across pain perceptions are maintained at 12 months post-treatment. However, gains in self-efficacy significantly decreased at 12 months follow-up. There were significant improvements in pain-perception, self efficacy and pain perceptions at 6 month follow-up compared to baseline. Conclusion: The review provides some support for the long-term efficacy of PMP interventions. There is a need for pragmatically designed follow-up studies to measure the long-term efficacy of PMPs on psychological variables, especially self-efficacy. Further research is warranted into the observed loss in treatment gains in self-efficacy over time; booster sessions delivered at 6 months post-treatment aimed at enhancing self efficacy may help aid self-management of chronic pain.

---

[*] Correspondence: Laura Chipchase, DHealthPsy, Birmingham Community Healthcare NHS Trust, Multidisciplinary Pain Service, The Dove Primary Care Centre, Dovedale Road, Birmingham, B23 5BG United Kingdom. E-mail: laurachipchase@nhs.net.

INTRODUCTION

In the United Kingdom, the number of multidisciplinary Pain Management Programmes (PMPs) has sharply increased in the last few decades (1). Whilst the short-term efficacy of PMPs has been established through systematic review and meta-analytic studies (2, 3), the ability to demonstrate long-term benefits in patients with chronic pain remains a key factor in evaluating the effectiveness of these interventions (4). Establishing whether PMPs are effective in the long-term relies on verifying whether clinically meaningful gains are maintained over time, and not diminished or lost after treatment. This is a critical question for both the application and evolution of PMPs.

Ideally, a body of evidence using high quality randomized control trials incorporating long-term follow-ups, and comparisons with both wait list and control treatments would provide evidence for the long-term efficacy of PMPs.

However, undertaking such studies in practice is problematic. For example, since consecutive samples of pain patients are studied and long-term follow-ups included, no untreated or control treatment group data is accessible. Thus, high quality controlled studies evaluating the long-term efficacy of pain management interventions are rare as this methodology is not useful for evaluation of treatment where there is no control group, as typical in clinical practice. Despite these barriers in establishing the long-term efficacy of PMPs, efforts should be made to provide evidence of their long-term effectiveness; whether the benefits PMPs are maintained over time. What is needed is evidence from clinical practice i.e., practice-based evidence (5) such as long-term follow-up data, to demonstrate whether patients report clinically significant changes over time (6).

There are several follow-up studies of PMPs that appear to show that initial treatment gains are largely maintained at one-year follow-up (7,8). However, the majority of these follow-up studies have focused on patients' functional ability and have reported treatment gains in terms of pain intensity, physical functioning, return to work and hospital visits, with little attention paid to psychological outcomes. The lack of follow-up research focusing on the psychological benefits of PMPs is surprising given that the BPS (1) guidelines highlight that a core aim of the intervention is the normalising of psychological processes. PMPs target unhelpful pain perceptions, which are the internal representations patients develop about their pain (9) for example; the perception that pain is necessarily indicative of tissue damage; catastrophic thought processes, defined as an exaggerated negative orientation toward the threat of actual or anticipated pain (10); and self efficacy, which describes confidence in ability to manage pain (11). As PMP treatment programmes aim to address all such aspects of the pain experience, effective evaluation strategies should also endeavour to evaluate all aspects of the programme, including treatment gains in terms of self-efficacy, pain perceptions and catastrophic thinking in addition to improvements on physical functioning measures.

The importance of psychological traits in the maintenance of effective pain management have been documented (12). In particular, there is growing evidence that improvements in self-efficacy are related to positive long-term outcomes of pain coping skills training and educational self-help interventions (13, 14). Some authors have suggested self-efficacy is a mechanism of behavioural change able to predict and enhance long-term effects of rehabilitation (15). Pain catastrophizing has emerged as a powerful predictor of pain-related outcomes, with evidence indicating that catastrophizing can be changed over the course of psychosocial interventions, and that these changes are related to long-term improvements in pain, psychological functioning, and physical disability (13). Pain perceptions are also important determinants of long-term coping and self management behaviour; for example, there is an association between unhelpful pain perceptions (such as extended timelines, severity and a large number of symptoms associated with the condition) and poorer clinical outcome six months after consultation (16). Findings point to the importance and clinical relevance of achieving long-term changes in these psychological variables, and suggest that this may maintain effective self-management over time.

A number of studies (6, 8, 17) have demonstrated the short-term efficacy of PMPs on self efficacy, catastrophic thinking and pain perceptions, and have reported that gains are maintained up to one month post treatment. However, despite research documenting short-term benefits, studies assessing the long-term treatment gains of PMP interventions with regard to these psychological variables have not been reviewed. Given that there is increasing advocacy for their role in the maintenance of effective pain management, it is important that these psychological variables are reviewed as primary outcome measures, to establish whether there are long-term changes in these measures following PMP intervention. This review aims to systematically assess the long-term effect of PMPs on self-efficacy, catastrophizing and pain perceptions in patients with chronic pain.

OUR STUDY

The updated guidelines for systematic reviews of the Centre for Reviews and Dissemination Group (CRD) (19) were consulted to determine the quality criteria used in this systematic review; some aspects (i.e., intervention content) were tailored according to the recent literature such as the PMP Guidelines for Adults (1).

Searching

Relevant publications were identified from a comprehensive search strategy of electronic bibliographic databases [Medline (PubMed), PsyArticles, PsycINFO, CINHAL & SportsDiscus, and Web of Knowledge], hand searches of subject relevant journals [PAIN, European Journal of Pain, Journal of Pain, The Clinical Journal of Pain, Journal of Pain Research, Journal of Pain and Symptom Management], and references lists. In addition, key authors were contacted to obtain details of relevant unpublished studies in an attempt to address publication bias. All the databases were searched for relevant publications since the development of the British Pain Society (BPS) guidelines in 1999.

Selection

The inclusion criteria were kept fairly broad in order to capture all relevant articles. Initially, titles and abstracts were included and full manuscripts were retrieved for future inspection if the study was an intervention that focused on the long-term follow-up of Pain Management Programmes and appeared to measure at least one of the primary outcomes. If these initial inclusion requirements were unable to be extracted from the titles and abstract, the full manuscript was retrieved to enable a judgement about inclusion. The inclusion and exclusion criteria were defined in terms of the intervention, outcome measure, and study design (19). The full manuscripts were then scrutinized and included in the systematic review if the following criteria were met:

1. Participants were adult patients (>18-yrs old) with chronic (non cancer) non-specific musculoskeletal pain (e.g., chronic low back or back pain, FM) who had completed a PMP
2. The sample of chronic pain patients did not report any other ongoing health problems (e.g., cancer).
3. The intervention was a PMP, based on BPS guidelines, and included multidisciplinary treatment with at least physiotherapy and patient education as part of the programme. Interventions described as pain education programmes were excluded, unless they were part of a programme that fulfilled BPS criteria for PMP intervention (1).
4. The study reported PMP treatment outcomes in at least one of these psychological variables; self-efficacy, catastrophic thinking or pain perceptions, and include pre-intervention (baseline) data to enable comparisons.
5. Finally a follow-up of at least 6 months was reported

Data extraction

Extracted data included year, participant information (age range, pain nature and duration), type and length of Pain Management Programme and treatment components (e.g., inpatient or outpatient, weeks/hours, facilitators, location), results (outcome measures, effect size, significance) and duration of follow-up. All papers were independently reviewed by a co-author (DS) to ensure accuracy and reliability. Reviewers met to confirm agreement of extraction and reliability was established.

Quality assessment

All included studies were subjected to a quality assessment to limit potential bias, to allow for potential comparisons between individual studies to be made, and to allow for meaningful conclusions to be drawn (20). Quality criteria were developed, based on recommendations elsewhere (1). Each study was assessed according to clear aims, study design, sample size, description of intervention provided to allow repetition, attrition, effect size, details of long-term follow-up and sustained change, measured with reliable measurement tools and results provided for each, and appropriate statistical analysis. A score of 0-3 was awarded for each item (0= no detail, 1 = poorly described, 2 = partially described, 3 = fully and adequately described): these scores were summated to create a score between 0 and 48. Studies were considered well-conducted and reported if they scored 32 +, average between 16 and 31, and poor if they scored less than 15. The ranges were adapted from recommendations of quality criteria (21). Studies did not have to be RCTs or include comparator (control) groups, but this would have been reflected in the quality assessments.

Data analysis

The included studies reported similar research aims, but utilised a variety of outcome measures and research design. Six studies reported treatment outcomes in terms of self efficacy (6, 22-26), three in terms of catastrophic thinking (6, 27, 28) and two reported pain perceptions (29,30). The six studies that measured self efficacy utilised validated measurement tools; two studies used the Pain Self- Efficacy Questionnaire (PSEQ) (6, 22), other studies utilised the Self-Efficacy Measure (SEM) (26), Pain Cognitions List (PCL) [30], Chronic Pain Self Efficacy Scale (CPSES) (24), and a single study used a measure of posture-related and pain-related self efficacy which had been developed and validated by the authors (25). All three studies measuring catastrophic thinking utilised the catastrophizing subscale of the Coping Strategies Questionnaire (CSQ) (6, 27, 31). Measures used in the three studies reporting pain perception data included Pain Cognition List (PCL) (30), the Illness Perception Questionnaire – Revised (IPQ-R) (28), and the Pain Interference subscale of the Multidimensional Pain Inventory (MPI) (29).

FINDINGS

The search strategy retrieved 868 articles overall. Thereafter, 139 abstracts were selected on the basis of the title, abstract and keywords. Of those 139 abstracts, 21 articles were obtained in full-text version. Searching the reference list of included papers helped identify five further citations of which two were abstracts (32, 33). Authors of those abstracts were contacted but no study details were obtained. Fifteen studies were excluded because; they had no PMP intervention (n=2); had no follow-up (n= 3); did not report outcome data that it was possible to extract (n=2); did not report baseline data (n=1); did not measure any of the primary outcomes (n=4); or were not available in English full-text version (n=3). As a result a total of 11 studies (see table 1) were included in this review. Figure 1 summarises study selection.

Study design

All included studies were longitudinal. Six studies included a 12 month follow-up (22-24, 29-31), four studies included a 6 month follow-up (25-28), and a single study included a 9 month follow-up (6).

Table 1. Characteristics of Included Studies (n = 11)

Author, Country Year of Publication	Total (N)	Sample Characteristics	Pain Nature	Nature of Intervention	Outcome(s) Measured	Measurement Tools	Follow up Period(s)
Altmaier et al. (1993), USA	45	A sample of low back pain patients. No further specific demographic details reported.	Low Back Pain	3 week pain management programme delivered in secondary care	Self Efficacy	Self Efficacy Measure	6 months
van Wilgen et al. (2009), Netherlands	32	All patients referred by GP. 27% were male, and 73% were female. The mean age was 42 yrs (SD 11.0). The sample had a pain duration of 8 years (SD 7.0).	Chronic pain or sever disuse syndrome	Inpatient pain management programme delivered at a pain management treatment centre	Pain Perceptions	Pain Cognitions Checklist (PCL)	6 & 12 months
Angst et al., (2009), Netherlands	164	Patients referred by GPs, rheumatologists, psychiatrists and hospitals. 21 % of patients were male, and 79% were female. Mean age was 45 years, (SD 10.6). with a range of 19.7 – 72.7 years. Mean duration of pain was 72.0 months (SD 42.1).	Chronic non-specific low back pain or fibromyalgia or wide spread pain	Inpatient pain management programme at a Rehabilitation clinic with over a 100 hours input.	Catastrophic thinking	The Coping Strategies Questionnaire (CSQ)	6 months
Wells-Federman et al., (2003), USA	110	The sample consisted of 53 patients with fibromyalgia syndrome and 57 patients with chronic low back pain. Of the patients with fibromyalgia, 4% were male, and 96% female. 57 % of the chronic low back pain patients were female, and 43 % were male. The mean age of the fibromyalgia patients was 45 years, and 42 years for the chronic low back pain patients. The mean pain duration for fibromyalgia was 82 months (SD = 60), and 66 months (SD = 42) for chronic low back pain.	Chronic Low Back Pain or Fibromyalgia	10 week outpatient pain management programme	Self Efficacy	The Chronic Pain Self-Efficacy Scale	12 months
Henriksson et al, (2004), Sweden	191	The 4 programmes included 57, 53, 40 and 41 participants respectively. 64% of the participants were referred from primary care, 21% from occupational health or specialist at secondary care level, and 15% by private doctors, insurance agencies, or had applied directly to pain of rheumataology units. The overall mean age was 42.7 years (SD =10.0), with an age range of 22 - 74.	Fibromyalgia	The pain management programmes were delivered at specialist rheumatology or pain rehabilitation units at 3 hospitals across Sweden. All programmes were outpatient programmes and ranged in duration from 6 months, 3 months, 10 weeks, and 6 weeks respectively. The scheduled staff/participants hours ranged from about 18-70 hours. The resources in number of professional hours varied considerably.	Catastrophic Thinking Self Efficacy	The Coping Strategies Questionnaire (CSQ) (Swedish Version) The Arthritis Self Efficacy Scale (ASES) (Swedish Version)	12 months

Author, Country Year of Publication	Total (N)	Sample Characteristics	Pain Nature	Nature of Intervention	Outcome(s) Measured	Measurement Tools	Follow up Period(s)
Moss-Morris et al., (2007), New Zealand	76	Participants were recruited from the Auckland Regional Pain Service pain management programme. Patients had been referred onto the programme from hospital services, general practices, and insurance and compensation agencies across a wide geographical area. 65% of participants were female, and 35 % were male. The mean age of the sample was 42.4 years (SD = 9.49). Participants had experienced their pain problem for a mean length of 7.05 years (SD = 6.88) and 57% were unemployed because of their pain.	Chronic Pain Problem	4 week outpatient pain management programme which patients attended 5 days a week from 8.15am to 3.00pm.	Catastrophic Thinking Pain Perceptions	Pain Catastrophizing Scale (PCS) Illness Perception Questionnaire Revised (IPQ-R)	6 months
Johansson et al., (1998), Sweden	85	Patients were mainly referred to the Department of Rehabilitation Medicine at Sandviken Hospital from the surrounding areas by their general practitioners or medical specialists at other hospitals. At their initial visit the patients underwent a screening procedure to see if they met the criteria of participation. 32 % of the participants were male, and 68 % were female. The average time since pain onset was 11 years (SD = 9.0) and 49% of people had multiple pain sites. The mean age of the sample was 42 years (SD = 8.6).	Chronic musculoskeletal pain	4 week outpatient pain management programme conducted in a hospital setting, compromising 5 full days. About half the patients lived at the hospital during the week due to the long distances home. The rest of the patients were only in the department during the daytime.	Catastrophic Thinking	The Coping Strategies Questionnaire (CSQ)	12 months
Morley et al., (2008), UK	1013	The sample consisted of patients who had attended an NHS pain management service between 1989 and 1998. Primary assessment for participation on the pain management programme was made by anaesthetists and clinical psychologists. 38 % of the participants were male, and the remaining 62% were female. The primary sites of pain amongst the sample were low back, shoulder and upper limb, lower limb, and neck. The mean time since onset was 113 months (SD = 108.3 months; range = 3 – 677, median = 74 months).	Chronic Pain	4 week inpatient pain management programme	Self Efficacy Catastrophic Thinking	Pain Self Efficacy Questionnaire (PSEQ) The Coping skills Questionnaire (Catastrophizing Subscale) (CSQ-cat).	9 months

Table 1. (Continued)

Author, Country Year of Publication	Total (N)	Sample Characteristics	Pain Nature	Nature of Intervention	Outcome(s) Measured	Measurement Tools	Follow up Period(s)
Keller et al., (1997), Germany	35	The sample consisted of patients who were referred by physicians and other patients who were self-selected for programme participation. 74 % of the sample were female and 25% were male. The average pain duration was 9.6 years (SD = 7.1).	Chronic Low Back Pain	Outpatient pain management programme conducted at PROMOTIO Health Centre in Gottingen, Germany. The programme consisted of 18 2 hour group meetings (three per week) in addition to 18 individualized training sessions	Self Efficacy	Pain-related Self efficacy Posture-related Self efficacy	6 months
Man et al., (2007), Hong Kong	45	The sample was compromised of patients had been referred to the pain management centre between 2002 and 2005. All patients were assessed by a pain medicine specialist and a clinical psychologist, and suitable patients were referred onto the pain management programme.33% of the sample were male, and the remaining 67% were female. The median pain duration was 46 months (range = 12 to 333). The commonest pain Location was the back followed by the upper limbs. The mean age of the sample was 42 years with an age range of 23 -75years (Median = 42).	Chronic Pain	6 week outpatient pain management programme	Self Efficacy Catastrophic Thinking	Pain Self Efficacy Scale (PSEQ) (Chinese Version) Pain Catastrophizing Scale (PCS) (Chinese Version)	6 &12 months
Oslund (2009), Texas	108	The sample consisted of a 108 Patients who had attended a comprehensive pain program at Baylor University Medical Centre. 70 % of the sample were female, and the remaining 30 % were male. The mean duration of pain was 110months (SD = 136.73) Commonest pain location was lower back.	Chronic Pain	4 week outpatient pain management programme conducted at Baylor University Medical centre. The programme compromised 6 hours per day for 5 days per week.	Pain Perceptions	Multidimensional Pain inventory (perceived control of pain subscale) (MPI)	6 & 12 months

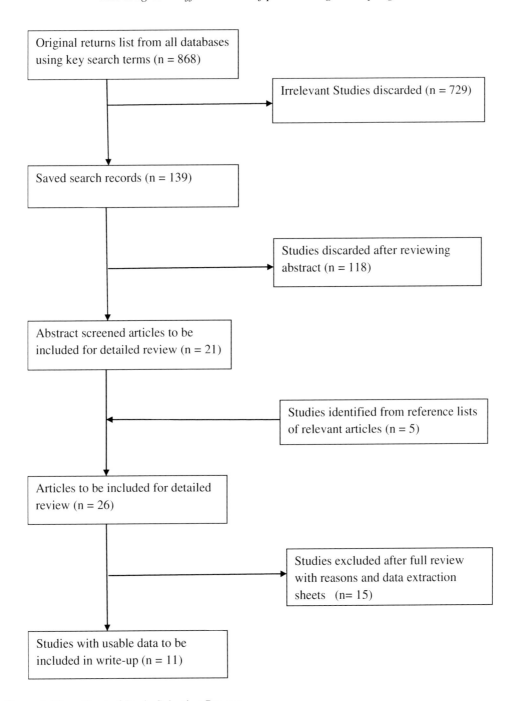

Figure 1. Flow Chart of Study Selection Process.

Participants

All studies utilised a clinical population of patients with chronic pain. Seven studies included patients with chronic musculoskeletal pain (6, 22, 25, 26, 28, 29, 31), three studies included mixed chronic pain patients and patients with severe disuse syndrome (27, 30, 33), and one study (23) included patients with Fibromyalgia, diagnosed according to the criteria proposed by the American College of Rheumatology (ACR; 22).

The number of patients in each study varied between 32 and 1013 (median = 81), totalling 1,860 patients. Of these, a total of 1,118 were female and 611 were male. The female: male ratio was not reported in one study (23). The percentage of female participants ranged from 47% to 96%. The size of the individual treatment groups varied between 3 and 10 patients, but was mostly between 5 and 7. The mean age of all participants was 43 years ranged from 22 to 75. Based on the available data, the mean pain duration was 7.6 years, and the commonest pain location was the back. Participants were commonly referred for the PMP by their GPs. Three studies (6, 22, 30) reported that patients had been assessed by a multi-disciplinary team, one study (23) stated that patients had self-referred, and in a single study patients had been randomly allocated to PMP intervention or waiting list (25).

Three studies were based in the USA (24, 26, 29), two were conducted in the Netherlands (27, 30), two were undertaken in Sweden (23,31), and the remaining four studies were conducted in the United Kingdom (6), New Zealand (28), Germany (25) and Hong Kong (22).

Interventions

Seven of eleven programmes were performed in an outpatient setting (22-25, 28, 29, 31), and three of eleven took place in an inpatient setting (6, 27, 30). The nature of one of the programmes was not reported (26). The content of the PMP interventions commonly included education, pacing, relaxation, and goal setting (1). However, the time and input devoted to each principle varied markedly amongst the programmes. The duration of the programmes varied between 4 and 15 weeks for outpatient programmes and between 3 and 8 weeks for inpatient programmes. Based on the available data reported in the studies, the median duration of all treatments was 35 hours.

Quality assessment of included studies

A number of methodological factors were assessed for quality. Due to the nature of the studies, randomisation procedures were not used, as all studies used samples of LBP patients going through the treatment process; in some cases waiting list controls were used. Similarly, interventionist and patients could not be blinded to treatment allocation; thus no studies reported on treatment allocation concealment (34). Quality scores for study design depended on: whether clinically relevant outcomes were measured, the comparability of the sample to typical pain patients, the length of follow-up, and how clear these procedures were reported. Attrition rates were not reported in two of the included studies (22, 30). From the data that was extracted, 427 participants were lost from 1,860 assigned participants due to not wanting to participate, medical reasons, non-attendance, and unable/inability to complete.

The quality of the interventions was good, with few points lost on assessment. Details of what the interventions were, how they were delivered, and their duration were clearly reported for each study. In line with the BPS PMP guidelines, all studies involved multidisciplinary teams but these varied: four studies involved psychologists in the delivery of the intervention (6, 22, 30, 31); three of the interventions were delivered by a combination of physiotherapists, nurses, physicians and occupational therapists (23-25) and the remaining four studies described the facilitators as 'interdisciplinary' (26-29). Not all studies reported where the intervention had taken place although the majority were based in primary care pain clinics or secondary care hospital settings. All of the interventions were reported in sufficient detail to enable replication. Three studies were considered well-conducted (scoring 32+); the remaining eight were considered of average quality. Those of higher quality had clearer aims and objectives and better defined inclusion criteria.

Quantitative analysis

The studies used similar statistical methods to assess the research questions, specifically ANOVA, ANCOVA, and t-tests, which were judged to be appropriate for the study designs utilised. One study used Wilcoxon's test for Bivariate comparisons of effect analysis (27).

Self efficacy measures were reported in six studies (6, 22-26). Two of three studies that measured self efficacy at 6 month follow up reported that significant treatment gains had been maintained at 6 months post-treatment (6, 26). One study (25) reported mixed results at follow up; significant post-treatment gains for posture related self-efficacy were reported at 6 month follow up, but not for pain efficacy. Of the six studies that measured self efficacy at 12 months post-programme, three studies reported significant long-term treatment gains (24, 30, 31), but this was not confirmed in two studies (22, 23).

Three studies reported catastrophic thinking data (6, 27, 28). One study measured catastrophic thinking at 6 months post-treatment (27), a further study reported 12 month follow-up date (28) and a single study measured catastrophic thinking at nine months post programme (6). Findings from these three studies reported that significant treatment gains in catastrophic thinking had been maintained at 6 and 9 months post-treatment.

Significant long-term treatment gains were reported in both studies which measured pain perceptions at 12 months post treatment (29, 30). However, one study (29) reported that although gains had been maintained at follow-up, they had begun to decrease in the longer term.

Meta analysis

Eleven meta-analyses were conducted for each of the primary outcome at 6 and 12 month follow-up where data was available. Between subjects data were calculated for self efficacy, catastrophic thinking and pain perception outcomes at 6 and 12 month follow-up points.

Two studies (22, 28) were initially excluded from all analysis; Man et al. (22) did not report standard deviation for group means, and as such no measures of variance were available to calculate the appropriate statistics for meta-analysis; Moss-Morris et al. (28) did not descriptively summarise reported statistics and therefore data comparisons at different follow-up points could not be meaningfully interpreted. The authors of both studies were contacted; additional descriptive statistical data provided by Moss-Morris enabled the study to be included in the analysis, but no further data was obtained from Man and colleagues.

Initial analysis included data from all appropriate studies. Within group analysis was performed on the scores for each outcome. Due to the nature of the research question control group data was not included in the analysis. The included studies did not report all statistical data. All studies except one (29) reported pre-post and follow-up mean scores and standard deviations could be calculated. Data calculated for each individual study comprised: Estimate of t (within subjects), z score (measure of probability), r (measure of effect size), and r' (Fisher's transformation of r). Combined effect size was calculated from r' (weighted by sample size), which was transformed to a combined r score to give an overall measure of effect size. Combined probability was calculated from z scores for each study.

Sensitivity analysis was carried out to identify contributors to heterogeneity. In such cases, data was recalculated on the basis of a random effects model. Random effects data is also reported for homogeneous set of studies to enable comparison of effect size. Findings are synthesised in both a statistical and descriptive form.

Self efficacy

i Pre intervention – 12 months follow-up

Analysis of the 6 studies using self report measures of self efficacy at baseline and 12 months post PMP produced a combined effect size (r) of 0.025 (CI: 0.019 to 0.324, p <.05). Tests for heterogeneity of effect size indicated significant differences amongst these studies (p < .001). Re-calculation of the data using a random effects model reported a combined effect size (r) of 0.131 (CI: -0.230 to 0.518, p >.05), suggesting that there is no significant difference in self-efficacy at 12 months post-programme compared to baseline.

ii Post – 12 months

The four studies reporting data for self efficacy at post-intervention and at 12 months follow-up were analyzed, and a combined r effect size of 0.103 (CI: -0.075 to 0.281, p>.05) reported. For comparison, data was re-calculated using a random effects model which reported a combined effect size (r) of 0.103 (CI: -0.081 to 0.280, p>.05). Interpretation of these statistics show a non-significant small effect, suggesting that any treatment gains in self efficacy observed immediately after completing PMP remain unchanged at 12 month follow-up.

iii Pre intervention – 6 months follow-up

Analysis of the 3 studies reporting self-efficacy data at baseline and 6 months post-treatment produced a combined r effect size of 0.264 (CI: 0.200 to 0.296, p<.05). However, heterogeneity of this effect size was found (p < .001). Data were recalculated using a random effects model, which revealed a combined effect size (r) of 0.549 (CI: 0.467 to 0.940, p<.05), and so it can be concluded that a positive medium effect of PMPs on self efficacy is maintained up to 6 months after completing the programme.

iv Post intervention – 6 months follow-up

The three studies reporting data for self efficacy at post-intervention and at 6 months follow-up were analyzed, and a combined r effect size of -0.709 (CI: -0.736 to -0.668, p<.05) reported. Calculations for heterogeneity revealed significant differences amongst the studies (p<.001). Re-calculation of the data using a random effects model produced a combined effect size (r) of -0.927 (CI: -0.977 to -0.775, p<.05), suggesting that there is a significant reduction in treatments gains in self-efficacy between post intervention and 6 month follow-up.

Catastrophic thinking

i   Pre intervention – 6 months follow-up
Two studies reported data for catastrophic thinking at baseline and at 6 month follow-up, and a further study reported data at 9 month follow-up. For the purpose of this meta-analysis these studies were combined as 6 month follow-ups are often overdue in practice. This was confirmed by Morley et al.'s initial meta-analysis which reported that the mean time of initial follow-up time of United Kingdom PMPs was 9 months. Analysis of these studies produced a combined effect size (r) of 0.282 (CI: 0.223 to 0.338, p<.05), although tests for heterogeneity indicated that the two studies were significantly different (p< .001). Re-calculation of the data using a random effects model revealed a combined effect (r) of 0.486 (CI: 0.217 to 0.721, p<.05), and so it can be concluded that at least a positive medium effect of treatment gains in catastrophic thinking is maintained 6 months after completing PMP.

ii   Post intervention – 6 months follow-up
Two studies reported data for catastrophic thinking at post treatment and 6 months, and a single study reported 9 months post-treatment data. Analysis of these studies produced a combined effect size (r) of -0.687 (CI: -0.919 to -0.653, p<.05), although tests for heterogeneity indicated that the studies were significantly different (p<.001). Data was re-calculated using a random effects model which revealed a combined effect (r) of -0.792 (CI: -0.999 to -0.628, p<.05), and so it can be concluded that there is a significant large reduction in treatments gains self efficacy between post intervention and 6 month follow-up.

Pain perceptions

i   Pre intervention – 12 months follow-up
The two studies reporting data for pain perceptions at baseline and at 12 months follow-up were analyzed, and reported a combined r effect size of 0.550 (CI: 0.369 to 0.691, p<.05). Calculations for heterogeneity revealed significant differences between the two studies (p < .001). For comparison, data was re-calculated using a random effects model which revealed a combined effect size of 0.611 (CI: 0.513 to 0.655, p<.05), and so it can be concluded that there is a medium effect of PMPs on improvements in pain perceptions for up to 12 months after completing the programme.

ii   Post intervention – 12 months follow-up
The two studies which reported data for pain perceptions at post treatment and 12 month follow-up, were analysed and produced a combined r of 0.087 (CI: -0.143 to 0.308, p>.05). Test for heterogeneity revealed that studies were not significantly heterogeneous (p lies between .70 and .50), and therefore conclusions can be made.

For comparison, data was re-calculated using a random effects model, which reported a combined effect size (r) of 0.136 (CI: -0.068 to 0.203, p>.05). Interpretation of these statistics demonstrates a non-significant small effect, indicating that pain perceptions at post-treatment remain unchanged at 12 months post-programme.

iii   6 months follow-up – 12 months follow-up

The two studies reporting both 6 and 12 monthly follow-up data for pain perceptions were analysed and produced a combined effect size of 0.257 (CI: 0.055 to 0.439, p<.05). Tests for heterogeneity of this effect indicated that studies were homogenous (p lies between .50 and .30). For comparison, data was re-calculated using a random effects model which reported a combined effect size (r) of 0.259 (CI: 0.062 to 0.437, p<.05), suggesting that the reported statistics are reliable and that there is a medium effect of PMPs on improvements in pain perceptions for 6 to 12 months after completing the programme.

iv   Pre intervention – 6 months follow-up

Analysis of the data from the three studies reporting pain perception scores at baseline and 6 months post-treatment produced a combined r effect size of 0.336 (CI: 0.156 to 0.495, p<.05). Tests for heterogeneity of this effect indicated that studies were homogenous (p>.99) suggesting the reported statistics are reliable and conclusion can be drawn. Data was re-calculated using a random effects model for comparison which revealed an effect size of 0.334 (CI: 0.188 to 0.465, p<.05). Reported statistics indicate a positive medium effect of PMPs on pain perceptions, and these treatment gains are maintained at 6 months post programme.

v   Post intervention – 6 months follow-up

The three studies which reported pain perceptions scores at post treatment and 6 month follow-up, were analysed and produced a combined r of 0.069 (CI: -0.033 to 0.155, p>.05). Calculations for heterogeneity revealed significant differences amongst the studies (p< .001), and so data was re-calculated using a random effects model, which revealed an effect size of 0.291 (CI: -0.840 to 0.553, p>.05). Interpretation of these statistics demonstrates a non-significant small effect, indicating that pain perceptions at post-treatment remain unchanged at 6 months post-programme.

DISCUSSION

The literature evaluating the long-term efficacy of pain management programme interventions on psychological variables is relatively sparse, with this systematic review identifying only eleven studies for inclusion; however one of these did not provide sufficient detail to be included in meta-analyses.

Favourable results were observed for the longer-term (12 month follow-up) efficacy of PMP interventions in only one of the outcome measures: pain perceptions. Observed treatment gains in pain perceptions remained stable from post-intervention to 6-month follow-up, and through to 12-month follow-up. Interestingly, pain perceptions were more favourable at 12-month compared to 6-month follow-up suggesting that they continue to evolve over time. In contrast, treatment gains in self efficacy decreased over time. Pre-treatment to 12-month post-treatment data showed that self-efficacy had returned to baseline levels at longer-term follow-up. However, post to 12 month follow-up data indicated that treatment gains in self-efficacy remained unchanged from post-intervention to 12-month follow-up; making the patterning of these self-efficacy findings difficult to interpret. This is likely to have been due to the varying number of studies reporting self-efficacy data at each follow-up point. Future studies reporting measures at multiple follow-ups would allow for easier comparison. Data was favourable for short-term follow-up for self-efficacy; there was significant improvement in self-efficacy at 6 months follow-up, compared to pre-treatment. However, these treatment gains had begun to decrease since post-treatment. Long-term follow up data (12 month follow-up) were not available for catastrophic thinking. Overall, these findings suggest that initial treatment gains are weaker but present at 6-month follow-up, and return to baseline for self-efficacy but are still improving for pain perception at 12 month follow-up.

A number of controlled trials and RCTs (6, 17, 18) have demonstrated the short-term efficacy of PMPs on self efficacy, catastrophic thinking and pain perceptions up to three months post treatment. The findings from this review build on existing research, and demonstrate that treatment gains in pain perceptions are maintained up to 12 months after completing PMP, and gains in catastrophic thinking and self-efficacy are maintained up to 6 months post-treatment. Interestingly, treatment gains in self efficacy appeared to significantly decrease over the 12 month follow-up period and returned to baseline levels. The loss of treatment gains in self-efficacy over time is an area that warrants further investigation as this may have implications for effective self-management of chronic pain over time. Previous studies have suggested that self-efficacy is a mechanism of behavioural change, which is able to predict changes in pain, distress, and beliefs about pain, independent of changes in medical regimens or adherence to specific behaviours in patients with chronic pain (5). As gains in efficacy were favourable up to 6 months post-intervention, undertaking booster sessions at 6 month follow-up which are specifically targeted at patients' own beliefs in their ability to perform specific self-management behaviours or change specific thinking patterns may be effective way of sustaining effective self-management of chronic pain.

The quality assessments revealed that the majority of studies included in this review were of moderate quality. A comparison of the outcomes of studies deemed to be of good quality (score of greater than or equal to 32) with those of moderate quality (score of 16-31) indicated small differences. Those studies with an average quality score had a shorter term follow-up period than those with a good quality score. The variation in quality score can be attributed to a number of factors including differences in length of follow-up, sampling method and variation in measures. Not all of the included studies included long-term follow-up: only six studies included a long-term follow up of 12 months post-treatment, and four studies included a shorter-term follow-up at 6 months post-treatment. There were differences in methodology and sampling methods amongst the studies included in the analysis, and in some, these differences were more profound. The study by Henriksson et al. (23) was the only study in which patients self-referred onto the PMP. Furthermore, the tools used to measure self-efficacy, catastrophic thinking, and pain perceptions were diverse, particularly in regards to self-efficacy as in one study measures were split into further measures of posture-related and pain-related self efficacy.

If the effectiveness of PMP interventions is going to be evaluated adequately, long-term follow-up needs to be included in all interventions in addition to pre-and post intervention scores. Research recommendations made in a previous review encourage evaluative follow-up studies, which include standardised follow-up periods and use standardised measures to build up a body of literature so that the long-term outcomes of PMP could be accurately evaluated (35). Assessment of the included studies showed that more recent studies had longer follow-up periods, making them of a higher standard. However, although validated, a variety of measures were used making it difficult to combine the results of the studies. Further, different studies were included in each of the meta-analyses due to the relatively small number of studies that were available; this made the patterning of the self-efficacy findings hard to interpret. Including measures at multiple follow-ups would allow for easier comparison. Therefore, the current review reiterates the recommendations that long-term follow-ups must be systematically evaluated through studies including standardised follow-up and standardised measures in order to establish the clinical effectiveness of PMP interventions over time.

In conclusion, findings provide some support for the long-term effectiveness of PMP interventions in the self-management of chronic pain. Treatment gains in pain perceptions were maintained up to 12 months post treatment. However, gains in self-efficacy appeared to significantly decrease back to baseline at long-term follow-up. Treatment gains were favourable across all variables at 6 months post-programme. More follow-up research is needed in this area to establish the long-term clinical effectiveness of multidisciplinary pain treatment programmes, especially with regard to self-efficacy, in supporting patients to manage chronic pain. Incorporating longer term follow-ups (e.g., 2 years+) into existing desirable criteria and agreeing on core outcome measures are two options available to service providers. In addition, booster sessions delivered at 6 months post-treatment aimed at maintaining gains in patients' self-efficacy may be an effective way of sustaining effective self–management of chronic pain.

REFERENCES

[1]   British Pain Society (BPS). Recommended guidelines for pain management programmes for adults. London: British Pain Society, 2007.

[2]   Morley S, Eccleston C, Williams A. Systematic review and meta-analysis of randomized controlled trials of cognitive behaviour therapy for chronic pain adults, excluding headache. Pain 1999;80:1-13.

[3]   Flor H, Fydrich T, Turk DC. Efficacy of multidisciplinary pain treatment centers: a meta-analytic review. Pain 1992;49:221-30.

[4]   Melzack RA, Wall, PD. The challenge of pain. London: Penguin, 1996.

[5]   Barkham M. Mellor-Clark J. Bridging evidence-based practice and practice-based evidence: developing a rigorous and relevant knowledge for the psychological therapies. Clin Psychol Psychother 2003;10:319-27.

[6]   Morley S, Williams A, Hussain S. Estimating the clinical effectiveness of cognitive behavioural therapy in the clinic: Evaluation of a CBT informed pain management programme. Pain 2008;137:670-80.

[7]   Robbins H, Gatchel RJ, Noe C. A prospective one-year outcome study of interdisciplinary chronic pain management: Compromising its efficacy by managed care policies. Anesth Analg 2003;97:156-62.

[8]   Becker N, Sjogren P, Bech P, Olsen AK, Jorgen E. Treatment outcome of chronic non-malignant pain patients managed in a Danish multidisciplinary pain center compared to general practice: a randomized controlled trial. Pain 2000;84:203-11.

[9]   Leventhal H, Nerenz DR, Steele DJ. Illness representations and coping with health threats. In: Baum A, Taylor SE, Singer JE, eds. Handbook of psychology and health: Social psychological aspects of health, Vol 4. Hillsdale, NJ: Earlbaum, 1984:219-52.

[10]   Sullivan MJL, Thorn B, Haythornthwaite JA, Keefe FJ, Martin M, Bradley LA. et al. Theoretical perspectives on the relation between catastrophizing and pain. Clin J Pain 2001;17:52–64.

[11]   Nicholas MK. The pain self-efficacy questionnaire: Taking pain into account. Eur J Pain 2007;11(2):153-63

[12]   Eccleston C. Role of psychology in pain management. Br J Anaesth 2001;87:144-52.

[13]   Keefe FJ, Rumble ME, Scipio CD, Louis AG, Perri LCM. Psychological Aspects of Persistent Pain: Current State of the Science. J Pain 2004;5(4):195-211.

[14]   Lorig K, Mazonson P, Holman H. Evidence suggesting that health education for self-management in patients with chronic arthritis has sustained health benefits while reducing health care costs. Arthritis Rheum 1993;36:439-46.

[15]   Burckhardt CS. Educating patients: Self-Management approaches. Disabil Rehabil 2005;27:703-9.

[16]   Foster NE, Bishop A, Thomas E, Main C, Horne R, Weinman J, Hay E. Illness perceptions of low back pain in primary care: What are they, do they change and are they associated with outcome? Pain 2008;136:177-87.

[17]   Gatchel RJ, Okifuji A. Evidence-based scientific data documenting the treatment and cost-effectiveness of comprehensive pain programs for chronic non-malignant pain. J Pain 2006;7:779-93

[18]   Williams AC de C, Richardson PH, Nicholas MK. Inpatient vs. Outpatient pain management: results of a randomised controlled trial. Pain 1996;66:13-22.

[19]   Centre for Reviews and Dissemination (CRD) Group. Systematic reviews: CRD's guidance for undertaking reviews in healthcare. York: University York, 2009.

[20]   Higgins JPT, Green S (editors). Cochrane Handbook for Systematic Reviews of Interventions Version 5.0.2. The Cochrane Collaboration, 2009. Accessed 2013 Aug 01. URL: www.cochrane-handbook.org.

[21]   Khan KS, ter Riet G, Popay J, Nixon J, J K, editors: Undertaking systematic reviews of research on effectiveness (CRD Report No 4). York: University York, 2001.

[22]   Man AKY, Chu MC, Chen P, Ma M, Gin T. Clinical experience with a chronic pain management programme in Hong Kong Chinese patients. Hong Kong Med J 2007;13:372-8.

[23]   Henriksson C, Carlberg U, Kjallman M, Lundberg G, Henriksson KG. Evaluation of four outpatient educational programmes for patients with longstanding Fibromyalgia. J Rehabil Med 2004;36:211-9.

[24]   Wells-Federman C, Arnstein P, Caudill-Slosberg M. Comparing patients with fibromyalgia and chronic low back pain participating in an outpatient cognitive-behavioural treatment program. J Musculoskelet Pain 2003;11:5-12.

[25]   Keller S, Ehrhardt-Schmelzer S, Herda C, Schmid S, Basler H-D. Multidisciplinary rehabilitation for chronic back pain in an outpatient setting: A controlled randomized trial. Eur J Pain 1997;1:279-92.

[26]   Altmaier EM, Russell, DW, Kao CF, Lehmann TR, Weinstein JN. Role of self-efficacy in rehabilitation outcome among chronic low back pain patients. J Couns Psychol 1993;40:335-9.

[27]   Angst F, Verra ML, Lehmann S, Brioschi R, Aeschlimann A. Clinical effectiveness of an interdisciplinary pain management programme compared with standard inpatient rehabilitation in chronic pain: a naturalistic, prospective controlled cohort study. J Rehabil Med 2009;41:569-75.

[28]   Moss-Morris R, Humphrey K, Johnson MH, Petrie KJ. Patients' perceptions of their pain condition across a multidisciplinary pain management program: do they change and if so does it matter? Clin J Pain 2007;23:558-64.

[29]   Oslund S. Long-term effectiveness of a comprehensive pain management program: strengthening the case for interdisciplinary care. Baylor University Medical Center Proceedings 2009;22:211-4.

[30]   van Wilgen CP, Dijkstra PU, Versteegen GJ, Fleuren MJT, Stewart R, van Wijhe M. Chronic pain and severe disuse syndrome: long-term outcome of an inpatient multidisciplinary cognitive behavioural programme. J Rehabil Med 2009;41:122-8.

[31]   Johansson C, Dahl J, Jannert M, Melin L, Andersson G. Effects of a cognitive-behavioural pain-management program. Behav Res Ther 1998;36:915-30.

[32] Benrud-Larson L, Bruce BK, Sletten, CD, Hodgson JE, Rome JD. Predictors of 6-month post treatment changes in pain, depression and activity level following a multidisciplinary pain treatment program. Pain Med 2002;3:184-5.

[33] Wells-Federman C, Arnstein P, Caudill-Slosberg M. Comparing patients with fibromyalgia and chronic low back pain participating in an outpatient cognitive-behavioural treatment program. J Musculoskelet Pain 2003;11:5-12.

[34] Altman DG. Concealing treatment allocation in randomised trials. BMJ 2001;323:446-7.

[35] Peat GM. Pain management program follow-ups. A national survey of current practice in the united kingdom. J Pain Symptom Manag. 2001;21:218-26.

In: Disability and Chronic Disease
Editors: J. Merrick, S. Aspler and M. Morad

ISBN: 978-1-62948-288-0
© 2014 Nova Science Publishers, Inc.

Chapter 15

IMPACT OF OXYGEN THERAPY IN PATIENTS WITH ADVANCED LUNG DISEASE

Kaitlin Koo, BSc, Justin Kwong, BSc, MD,
Janet Nguyen, BSc, MD, Florencia Jon, MRT(T), Liang Zeng, MD,
Kristopher Dennis, MD, Lori Holden, MRT(T),
Shaelyn Culleton, BSc, MD, Luluel Khan, MD,
Amanda Caissie, MD, PhD and Edward Chow, MBBS*

Rapid Response Radiotherapy Program, Department of Radiation Oncology, Odette
Cancer Centre, Sunnybrook Health Sciences Centre, University of Toronto, Toronto,
Ontario, Canada

ABSTRACT

Due to the poor prognosis associated with cancerous and non-cancerous advanced lung disease, the main intention of treatment is to improve the patient's quality of life (QOL). A treatment option that may achieve this goal is oxygen therapy. Currently, there is little literature analyzing the QOL of patients with advanced lung cancer receiving oxygen therapy for dyspnea. However, research has been conducted on patients with chronic obstructive pulmonary disease (COPD) suffering from dyspnea. The similarities of symptoms and underlying pulmonary function between patients with advanced lung cancer and COPD suggest that these populations could be similarly impacted by oxygen therapy. A systematic, computerized literature search was performed using the Ovid search engine for the following databases: MEDLINE® (1950 to September Week 1, 2010), EMBASE (1980 to 2010 Week 37) and PsychINFO (1967 to September Week 2, 2010). Search strands were designed to retrieve articles on patients with advanced lung cancer or COPD, oxygen therapy, QOL and survival. Based on the 12 articles reviewed, studies have contrasting conclusions with regards to the patients' QOL when using

* Correspondence: Professor Edward Chow MBBS, MSc, PhD, FRCPC, Department of Radiation Oncology, Odette Cancer Centre, Sunnybrook Health Sciences Centre, 2075 Bayview Avenue, Toronto, ON M4N 3M5, Canada. E-mail: Edward.Chow@sunnybrook.ca.

oxygen therapy. Further research is suggested to explore the impact of oxygen therapy on patients with advanced lung disease.

INTRODUCTION

As defined by the American Thoracic Society, dyspnea is the subjective experience of breathing discomfort that consists of qualitatively distinct sensations that vary in intensity (1). The prevalence of severe dyspnea has been reported in palliative patients with heart failure (65%), lung cancer (70%) and chronic obstructive pulmonary disorder (90%) (2). Some of the etiologies of dyspnea include: muscle weakness, anemia, restrictive and obstructive lung changes, brochospasm, anxiety and hypoxia (3). Dyspnea often intensifies during the dying process thereby eroding one's quality of life, psychological well-being and social functioning (4).

Dyspnea is a common symptom that accompanies a diagnosis of chronic obstructive pulmonary disorder (COPD) and often interferes with the patient's health-related quality of life (QOL) (4). More specifically, COPD is a devastating respiratory disease common amongst the elderly that causes significant morbidity and mortality (5). It is the fourth leading cause of death worldwide and is predicted to be the third leading cause of death worldwide by 2020 (6). Patients with COPD also commonly suffer from co-morbid conditions that produce a variety of symptoms. Therefore, the symptoms of COPD can vary greatly between patients; however, some of the common symptoms of COPD include cough, dyspnea and sputum production (7). Similarly, patients with advanced malignant lung disease (patients with primary lung cancer or metastatic lung cancer) often exhibit dyspnea, which can reduce their QOL (8).

Due to the poor prognosis associated with advanced lung disease, the main intention of treatment is to improve the patient's QOL. Improving dyspnea may be a means to achieve this goal. A treatment option that may reduce dyspnea would be the use of oxygen therapy. The proposed benefit of oxygen therapy is the provision of supplementary oxygen to the patient as room air consists of about 21% oxygen (9). Oxygen is transported into our tissues via binding to hemoglobin (97%) and dissolving in plasma (3%) (9). Oxygen therapy may relieve dyspnea by depressing the hypoxic drive mediated by peripheral chemoreceptor, improving respiratory musculature function, altering the level of awareness of oxygen uptake or by stimulating non-specific nasal receptors (10).

Currently, there is little literature analyzing the QOL of patients with advanced lung cancer receiving oxygen therapy for dyspnea. However, research has been conducted on patients with COPD suffering from dyspnea. The similarities of symptoms and underlying pulmonary function between patients with advanced lung cancer and patients with COPD suggest that these populations could be similarly impacted by oxygen therapy, and that the influence of therapy on the QOL of one group may be of reference to the other.

OUR STUDY

A systematic, computerized literature search was performed using the Ovid search engine for the following databases: MEDLINE® (1950 to September Week 1, 2010), EMBASE (1980 to 2010 Week 37) and PsychINFO (1967 to September Week 2, 2010).Search strands were designed to retrieve articles on patients with advanced lung cancer or COPD, oxygen therapy, quality of life and survival. To search for article abstracts pertaining to the quality of life in patients with advanced lung cancer using oxygen therapy, the following strand of subject headings was used: ("lung neoplasms" OR "advanced lung cancer" OR "lung metastases") AND ("oxygen inhalation therapy" OR "oxygen therapy") AND ("quality of life" or "survival"). To search for articles assessing quality of life in COPD patients receiving oxygen therapy, the following search strand was used: ("chronic obstructive pulmonary disease" OR "chronic obstructive lung disease" OR "chronic obstructive airway disease" OR "chronic airflow limitation" OR "chronic obstructive respiratory disease" or "COPD") AND ("oxygen inhalation therapy" OR "oxygen therapy") AND ("quality of life" OR "survival").

The abstracts from the references produced by these literature searches were read by two independent authors (KK and JK), to select full articles for subsequent review according to the predetermined criteria that the abstract must contain detailed assessments of quality of life in patients with COPD or advanced lung cancer receiving oxygen therapy.

Inclusion criteria included published journal articles and review articles. Abstracts from articles within the reference lists of articles meeting the inclusion criteria were searched according to the same criteria. Exclusion criteria included duplicate articles, articles not written in English and articles without published abstracts.

OUR FINDINGS

A total of 925 article references were identified by the literature searches. Three hundred and fifteen citations were reviewed in detail to determine which articles were related to the question of interest. Editorials and articles unrelated to quality of life in COPD patients receiving oxygen therapy, based on their respective abstracts, were excluded. Upon further investigation, these articles were assessed and further exclusions were made based on the relevance of the article to the systematic review. At the end, 10 of the most relevant articles were included in the review.

When the literature search was conducted regarding: patients with advanced lung cancer, oxygen therapy and quality of life, 15 papers were identified and 13 articles were excluded as they were unrelated to oxygen therapy in patients with advanced lung cancer. Overall, two papers were retrieved and analyzed. All of the studies reviewed are listed in table 1.

Amongst the 12 articles reviewed, some of the assessment tools used to assess the patient's quality of life included: the St. George's Respiratory Questionnaire (SGRQ), the Sickness Impact Profile (SIP), Hospital Anxiety and Depression Scale (HADS), EORTC QLQ-C30, Chronic Respiratory Questionnaire (CRQ) and the Medical Outcomes Study 36-item Short-Form Health Survey (SF-36).

Table 1. Outlining all of the studies reviewed in this paper. The authors, year, country, title, number in the sample, age, sex, design interventions and findings are presented in this table

Author, Year, Country, Title	Number in Sample, Age, Sex	Design Interventions	Findings: Positive Improvements	No Improvements/ Worse Outcome
Crockett et al., 2001 Australia Survival on long-term oxygen therapy in chronic airflow limitation: from evidence to outcomes in the routine clinical setting	N=505 Age mean: Male-69.9± 9.1 years Female-71.0± 9.4 years 249 males and 256 females	A list of patients prescribed domiciliary oxygen therapy for Chronic Airway Limitation was generated from Respiratory Unit records and hospital financial records for the supply of this therapy. Survival was compared with that reported for the original randomized control trials, and for Swedish and Belgian COPD patients. Factors influencing survival were studied.	Improvements in QOL and survival greater in female patients with hypoxia and oxygen therapy compared to males.	
Lai et al., 2007 Hong Kong China Perceptions of dyspnea and helpful interventions during the advanced stages of lung cancer: Chinese patients' perspective	N=11 51-80 years 3 women and 8 men	Semi-structured and open-ended interactive interviews (20-35 minutes) conducted in Cantonese. Interviews were: 1. Transcribed verbatim 2. Transcripts were read again to acquire overall feeling of what participants were recounting 3. Significant phrases and sentences were extracted 4. Coding was assigned and grouped	All 11 participants were on oxygen therapy. Most participants verbalized that oxygen therapy was essential for them.	5 participants expressed that oxygen therapy was a burden and caused inconveniences as they could not move freely without oxygen therapy

Author, Year, Country, Title	Number in Sample, Age, Sex	Design Interventions	Findings	
			Positive Improvements	No Improvements/ Worse Outcome
Jaturapatporn et al., 2010 Canada Patients' experience of oxygen therapy and dyspnea: a qualitative study in home palliative care.	N=8	8 patients from a specialty home Palliative program were approached. A qualitative in-depth interview, using an interview guide, was conducted with each participant in their respective homes in Toronto, Canada from January to June 2008. A framework approach was used for qualitative data analysis as follows: 1. Familiarization 2. Identifying a thematic framework 3. Indexing and charting 4. Mapping and interpretation	In 4 out of 8 patients, shortness of breath persisted but was improved on oxygen. The other four patients reported that using oxygen therapy completely reversed their shortness of breath.	
Bruera et al., 1992 Canada Symptomatic benefit of supplemental oxygen in hypoxemic patients with terminal cancer: the use N of 1randomized controlled trial.	N=1 Age=53 years Female	A before and after study was conducted on an advanced ovarian cancer patient. Double blind crossover, six randomized trials of 6-minute trials of oxygen or air by mask. Measurements were taken at rest and then after the intervention. Patient rated dyspnea by Dyspnea VAS (0-100). The difference between interventions was also rated on a scale of: 1 (not important) to 6 (great importance).	VAS: Baseline versus Air $p<0.01$ VAS: Baseline versus oxygen $p<0.01$ VAS: Air versus oxygen $p<0.01$ Patient chose oxygen over air $p=0.09$ Patient rating effect of 4.8/6	Baseline versus air was not statistically significant.

Table 1. (Continued)

Author, Year, Country, Title	Number in Sample, Age, Sex	Design Interventions	Findings — Positive Improvements	No Improvements/ Worse Outcome
Swinburn et al., 1993 United Kingdom Symptomatic benefit of supplemental oxygen in hypoxemic patients with chronic lung disease.	N=22 Age Mean=58 years 13 Males & 9 Females	A before and after, prospective, two double blind random trial period of oxygen and air involving 10 interstitial lung disease and 12 patients with COPD. Measurements were taken at rest and post- intervention. Patient rated dyspnea using VAS (0-100).	Based on the VAS, oxygen was better than air for ILD, COPD p<0.05 Both air and oxygen were reported as helpful but oxygen was more consistent and frequent than air p<0.01	Not all significant differences for patients with ILD and COPD were observed.
Bruera et al., 1993 Canada Effects of oxygen on dyspnea in hypoxic terminal cancer patients.	N=14 Age mean=64 years 8 Males & 6 Females	Before and after, crossover trial, prospective, double blind of patients with advanced cancer-lung primary and metastatic, no COPD. 2 trials each of oxygen or air by mask. Then cross over to the other intervention. 2 blinded trials of more effective treatment	Baseline to oxygen, and air to oxygen, statistical significance for all measures. Patient chose oxygen as most effective gas twice in 12 cases. The investigator chose oxygen as most effective gas twice for same 12 patients.	Baseline to air-no statistical significance in any measures.

Author, Year, Country, Title	Number in Sample, Age, Sex	Design Interventions	Findings	
			Positive Improvements	No Improvements/ Worse Outcome
Currows and Agar, 2009 Australia Does palliative home oxygen improve dyspnoea?	N=413	A 4-year consecutive cohort from a regional community palliative care service was used to compare baseline breathlessness before oxygen therapy with dyspnea sub-scales on the symptom assessment scores (SAS; 0-10) 1 week and 2 weeks after the introduction of oxygen.	150 out of 413 people had more than a 20% improvement in mean dyspnea scores.	There were no significant differences overall 1 or 2 weeks (p=0.28) nor for any sub-groups.
Okubadejo et al., 1996 UK Does long-term oxygen therapy affect quality of life in patients with chronic obstructive pulmonary disease and sever hypoxaemia?	N=23 47-82 years 15 females and 8 males	Patients were selected from out-patient chest clinics. Used the SGRQ, the SIP and the Hospital Anxiety and Depression Scale (HADS) to evaluate QOL. Patients were prescribed oxygen concentrators and assessed at baseline. Patients were reassessed after 2 weeks, 3 and 6 months.	After six months of treatment, the study group had small improvements that were not significant. (p=0.69)	Start of the study, the study group with more severe hypoxaemia had a significantly worse quality of life (SGRQ and SIP). Two weeks, the study group had a mean improvement in SGRQ Total score of 6.8 compared to an improvement of 4.0 in the control group. The improvement was not significant (p=0.48). Therefore, significant correlations between changes in oxygen use and quality of life scores were not observed.

Table 1. (Continued)

Author, Year, Country, Title	Number in Sample, Age, Sex	Design Interventions	Findings	
			Positive Improvements	No Improvements/ Worse Outcome
Abernethy et al., 2010 Australia, USA and UK Effect of palliative oxygen versus room air in relief of breathlessness in patients with refractory dyspnoea: a double-blind, randomized controlled trial	N=239	Double-blind randomized control. Patients with life-limiting illness, refractory dyspnoea, and partial pressure of oxygen in arterial blood. Patients were randomly assigned to receive oxygen or room air and were instructed to use for 15h/day. Breathlessness was measured twice a day (morning and evening) on a numerical rating scale of 0-10.		Breathlessness did not differ between groups at any time during the study period. 58 (52%) of 112 patients assigned to oxygen and 40 (40%) of 101 patients assigned to room air responded to interventions. QOL did not differ between groups. 43(18%) of participants did not want to receive oxygen after the study. 63 (26%) said that they derived no benefit from the intervention. 41 (17%) requested and received unblended oxygen after the study. 74 (31%) requested oxygen but did not receive it.

Author, Year, Country, Title	Number in Sample, Age, Sex	Design Interventions	Findings	
			Positive Improvements	No Improvements/ Worse Outcome
Eaton et al., 2006 New Zealand Short-burst oxygen therapy for COPD patients: a 6-month randomised, controlled study	N=78 subject available for rando-mization 36 males and 42 females	A 6-month randomised, double-blind, placebo-controlled, parallel study group of cylinder oxygen versus cylinder air versus usual care was performed. Health-related questionnaires use for this study include: Chronic respiratory questionnaire (CRQ), Medical Outcomes Study 36-item Short-Form Health Survey (SF-36) and the Hospital Anxiety and Depression (HAD) scale		There were no significant differences between patients groups in any of the HRQOL measures (CRQ, SF-36, HAD) over the 6-month period.
Booth et al., 1996 United Kingdom Does oxygen help dyspnea in patients with cancer?	N=38 Age mean=71 years 16 Males & 22 Females	Study was conducted on patients with advanced cancer (20-lung, 2-mesothelioma, 16-lung metastases, 13-COPD and 4-CHF). Before and after, single blind random trial, one trial of each oxygen and airflow. Measures were taken at rest and post intervention using VAS (0-100), Modified Borg Scale and Arterial O_2 saturation & pulse oximetry.		VAS & Borg revealed no significant difference between oxygen and air effect. No difference in sequencing of intervention. No correlation between baseline saturation and change in VAS after O_2. No difference in benefits between cancer and cardiopulmonary disease. No significant difference in initial levels of dyspnea between any subgroups.

Table 1. (Continued)

Author, Year, Country, Title	Number in Sample, Age, Sex	Design Interventions	Findings	
			Positive Improvements	No Improvements/ Worse Outcome
Tsara et al., 2008 Greece Quality of life and social-economic characteristics of Greek male patients on long-term oxygen therapy	N=85 Age means: LTOT Group- 70.7± 8.4 years Control Group- 63.5± 10.6 years All male subjects, no female subjects	Quality of life was evaluated with the 36-question Medical Outcomes Study Short Form (SF-36). The SF-36 HRQOL data from the study subjects was compared to published SF-36 assessments of normal Greek persons.		The HRQOL measurements were low in most SF-36 domains compared to the normal Greek subjects. Patients with COPD using LTOT experience marked impairments of HRQOL and psychological status. Suggest that patients with COPD perceive dyspnea as the leading symptom of the disease that affects their QOL.

Articles showing benefit with the use of oxygen therapy

The aim of the Crockett et al. study was to determine whether the survival of chronic airflow limitation (CAL) patients prescribed long-term oxygen therapy (LTOT) at Flinders Medical Centre (FMC) was gender-and-age related, and equivalent to that reported in randomized trials. A total of 505 participants (249 males and 256 females) were prescribed LTOT for CAL in this study. Concentrator oxygen information was obtained from the 3 to 6 monthly service reports to estimate compliance with the therapy. The amount of continuous oxygen therapy received was compared to the patients' survival rates. The authors concluded that improvements in survival were greater in female patients with hypoxia and oxygen therapy compared to males (11).

A qualitative descriptive design was used in Lai et al.'s study to explore, describe, interpret and understand the perceptions of dyspnea in patients with advanced lung cancer. Eleven patients (eight men and three women) with a medical diagnosis of terminal lung cancer were studied. The participants were interviewed in Cantonese using semi-structured and open-ended interactive interviews that were 20-35 minutes in duration. The interviews were all tape-recorded, transcribed verbatim, reviewed for overall feeling of the patients' accounts, significant phrases and sentences were extracted from the transcripts and then coded into categories. Based on the results, most of the participants verbalized that oxygen therapy was essential for their management of dyspnea. However, five out of the eleven participants expressed that oxygen therapy was a burden to them and caused inconveniences (12).

A recent study by Jaturapatporn et al. (13) reported the prevalence and described the experiences of dyspnea, pattern of oxygen use and burdens of oxygen therapy in home palliative care patients receiving oxygen. Qualitative in-depth interviews were conducted using an interview guide on eight participants from a specialty home palliative program. Qualitative data analysis included: familiarization, identifying a thematic framework, indexing and charting, and mapping and interpretation. Conclusions from this study indicated that five out of eight participants perceived oxygen therapy was a tool that increased their functional capacity and was a life-saving intervention. Some of the disadvantages mentioned in this study included: decreased mobility, discomfort in the nasal and ear cavity due to the nasal prongs and the noise related to the equipment. The authors concluded that the participants identified more advantages than disadvantages of oxygen therapy use (13).

Moreover, Bruera et al. (14) conducted a before and after, double blind crossover clinical trial to determine the symptomatic effects of supplementary oxygen by mask in one hypoxic, dyspneic patient with cancer. The clinical trial compared two interventions by administering the two conditions (airflow and oxygen use) in a random order. The subjects' rating of dyspnea by Visual Analogue Scale (VAS) using a scale of 0-100mm, after six randomized trials of oxygen versus airflow, showed a significant difference. This paper concluded that the benefits demonstrated by oxygen use were significantly better than air flow in this patient (14).

Swinburn et al. (15) investigated 22 hypoxic patients with chronic obstructive and interstitial lung disease with dyspnea at rest. A before and after, prospective, double blind random trial of oxygen and air was measured at rest and post intervention. Patients rated their dyspnea using the VAS (0-100mm). After two trial of both airflow and oxygen by mask, patients revealed that oxygen relieved their dyspnea to a greater degree and more consistently than air (15).

Finally, in 1993, a study by Bruera et al. (16) was conducted with a sample of 14 hypoxic patients with advanced cancer involving the lung with dyspnea at rest. A before and after, double blind, crossover prospective trial concluded that there was no significant improvement in dyspnea from baseline to intervention with airflow. However, significant improvements were demonstrated in relief with oxygen by mask (16).

Studies that revealed no effect on QOL when using oxygen therapy

Currowand Agar (17) conducted a four-year consecutive cohort study from a regional community palliative care service in Western Australia. They defined any symptomatic benefit of the provision of home oxygen by recording baseline breathlessness before oxygen therapy; dyspnea sub-scales in the symptom assessment scores1 and 2 weeks after the introduction of oxygen were also analyzed. Currow and Agar concluded that oxygen prescribed, on the basis of breathlessness alone, across a population predominantly with cancer does not improve breathlessness for the majority of people (17).

Okubadejo et al. (18) studied a group of 23 patients (15 males and 8 females) with a diagnosis of COPD from an out-patient chest clinic in the East London area. The SGRQ, SIP, and the Hospital Anxiety and Depression Scale (HADS) were used to evaluate patient QOL. The patients were assessed at baseline and were then prescribed oxygen concentrators for the provision of LTOT for at least 15 hours per day. At the start of the study, the study group with more severe hypoxemia had a significantly worse quality of life (SGRQ and SIP). At the two week data collection, the study group had a mean improvement in SGRQ total score of 6.8 compared to an improvement of 4.0 in the control group. The improvement was not significant (p=0.48). After six months of treatment, the study group had small improvements that were not significant (p=0.69). This study suggests that LTOT provided by an oxygen concentrator does not adversely affect quality of life, but provides little benefit (18).

In the Abernethy et al. study (19), 239 participants were randomly assigned by a central computer-generated system to receive oxygen or room air via a concentrator (oxygen, n=120; room, n=119) as well as complete seven dates of assessment. "Breathlessness right now" was recorded by the patient twice a day (morning and evening) in a diary with a scale of 0 (not breathless at all) to 10 (breathlessness as bad as you can imagine). The patients' QOL was assessed everyday using the McGill quality of life questionnaire. Their findings suggested that breathlessness did not differ between groups at any time (morning or evening) during the study period. In addition, the change in quality of life did not differ between the control and study group. The distribution of preferences was similar between the two groups since: 43(18%) of participants did not want to receive oxygen after the study, 63 (26%) stated that they derived no benefit from the intervention, 41 (17%) requested and received unblended oxygen after the study, 74 (31%) requested oxygen but did not receive it. Therefore, oxygen did not provide any additional symptomatic benefit for relief of refractory breathlessness as both groups (oxygen and room air) did not demonstrate any significant changes in breathlessness or QOL (19).

One of the objectives of Eaton et al. (20) study was to determine whether short-burst oxygen therapy improved health-related quality of life. They conducted a 6-month randomized, double-blind, placebo-controlled parallel study group of cylinder oxygen versus cylinder air versus usual care with a sample size of 78 patients. Health-related quality of life questionnaires used included: the Chronic Respiratory Questionnaire (CRQ), Medical Outcome Study 36-item Short-Form Health Survey and the Hospital Anxiety and Depression Scale. There were no significant differences between patient groups in any of the HRQOL measures over the 6-month period except for the CRQ emotion domain occurring in the usual care group. The availability of short-burst oxygen did not improve health-related QOL nor did it reduce acute healthcare utilization (20).

Booth et al. (21) conducted a before and after, single-blind random trial with 38 dyspneic subjects with advanced cancer. Measurements of patients' dyspnea were taken at rest and post intervention using the VAS (0-100). This study concluded that there was no correlation between baseline oxygen saturation and change in dyspnea score by VAS after administration of oxygen (21).

Negative effect on QOL when using oxygen therapy as a treatment for COPD

Tsara et al. investigated health-related QOL in Greek male patients with COPD using LTOT. A group of 85 patients with COPD and hypoxemia on LTOT, and a control group of 48 patients with stable COPD but without hypoxemia were analyzed. The quality of life was evaluated using the 36-question Medical Outcomes Study Short Form (SF-36) and psychological status was evaluated using the Greek version of the 30-question General Health Questionnaire for mental status. Eighty percent of the LTOT group had severe COPD, and 20% had moderate COPD. In the control group, 30% had severe COPD, 36% had moderate COPD and 34% had mild COPD. Results from the SF-36 indicated that patients with COPD using LTOT experienced noticeable impairment of HRQOL and psychological status(22).

DISCUSSION

Based on the articles reviewed, studies have demonstrated a range of varying effects in the patients' QOL when using oxygen therapy. Crockett et al., Jaturapatpron et al., Bruera et al., Swinbrun et al. and Lai et al. studies (11-16) demonstrated an increase in quality of life when oxygen therapy was used. Patients involved with these studies included: CAL patients, palliative care patients, dyspneic patient with cancer, patients with chronic obstructive and interstitial lung disease and patients with advanced stage lung cancer. Several studies by Currow and Agar, Okubadejo et al., Eaton et al., Abernethy et al. and Boothet al. (17-21) concluded that oxygen did not affect the patients' QOL nor did it cause any adverse effects. One study conducted in Greece by Tsara et al. (22) concluded that oxygen therapy had a negative impact on the patients' QOL.

Based on the articles reviewed, patients' quality of life in several of the studies demonstrated an increase in overall quality of life. In the study by Okubadejo et al. significant correlations between changes in oxygen use and quality of life scores were not observed (18). However, patients receiving LTOT had a slightly greater improvement in their quality of life compared to the control group; this was not statistically significant during the study period. It was suggested that the questionnaires used were not appropriate for the population of interest. Therefore, selection of an appropriate QOL questionnaire is crucial to the success of any successive study analyzing the effects of oxygen therapy in patients.

Patients receiving oxygen therapy often have chronic obstructive pulmonary disease, hypoxemia, advanced lung cancer or a condition that limits the uptake of oxygen. Greater than 80% of patients with lung cancer die within a year and fewer than 15% achieve long-term survival (8). Therefore due to the poor prognosis associated with these patients, potential benefits in treatment are often short-lived and only aid in ensuring that the patient is comfortable during the terminal stages of their disease.

Oxygen therapy is a central component of the routine treatment of COPD patients with chronic severe hypoxemia (18, 19). Many of the symptoms experienced by COPD patients such as cough, dyspnea and sputum production (7) are also experienced by patients with advanced lung cancer. Therefore, the possible impact associated with the use of oxygen therapy in COPD patients could be applied to patients with advanced lung disease due to the similar characteristics of both conditions.

As suggested, the use of oxygen therapy in patients with advanced lung cancer should be further investigated to determine the potential effects of patients' QOL. Lai et al.'s study regarding advanced lung patients receiving home oxygen therapy is limited due to the small sample size and lack of standardized assessment tools to evaluate quality of life. It was the first study to investigate the benefit of oxygen in patients with cancer; therefore there is lack of information regarding these patients and further investigation is required specific to this patient population

Although there is some evidence that supports the benefits of using oxygen therapy, it becomes difficult to distinguish the sources of improvement. Abernethy et al. randomly assigned patients to receive room air or oxygen by concentrator and nasal cannula. Their results demonstrated that there was no change in quality of life between the two groups. Therefore, benefits may be observed due to: the movement of gas across the nasal passage which affects the sensation of dyspnea, the mere presence of intervention which may alleviate the patient's anxiety, the concentrator as a placebo thereby inducing the expectation of some benefit, and finally the additional attention may improve psychological status thereby reducing breathlessness (19). Hence, these factors should be considered when analyzing the benefits and effects that oxygen therapy has on QOL in patients with advanced lung disease.

One of the problems with comparing quality of life for patients with advanced lung cancer was the numerous variations of QOL questionnaires used; this created inconsistent methods of comparing patients' quality of life. Patients requiring oxygen therapy may be on other medications which can affect the outcomes of oxygen therapy as well as the patient's QOL. Some patients may be sedated failing to potentially benefit from this treatment. The only study by Lai et al. which analyzed patients with cancer had a sample size of 11 participants. This study may be biased due to the limited number of participants and collection of data from one care unit in Hong Kong (12).

It is suggested that the use of an appropriate assessment tool to analyze the population of interest and obtain a comprehensive idea of the patients' QOL is required to properly analyze the benefits associated with oxygen therapy. To accurately measure the benefit associated with the use of oxygen therapy in patients with advanced lung cancer, follow-ups should be conducted soon after the initial administration of oxygen therapy. Based on the current literature for patients with COPD and the wide-ranging effects of using oxygen therapy, further research is suggested regarding the possible benefits of oxygen therapy use in patients with advanced lung cancer.

The benefits of oxygen therapy are unknown and could possibly decrease patients' quality of life due to the additional limitations of being confined to a portable oxygen machine. This may present additional problems as the patients may be limited in activities they would normally carry out on a day-to-day basis. Moreover, the additional oxygen could possibly increase tumor growth as more oxygen is being provided in the blood allowing for an increase in uptake of oxygen in the tissues. Therefore, further research is suggested to explore if oxygen therapy may help in providing the patient with more comfort and an increased quality of life when living with advanced lung cancer. Their QOL should also be evaluated since these patients often have a poor prognosis. The main objective of treatment at this stage of their disease is to improve their quality of life. Therefore, further investigation into the effects of oxygen therapy in patients with advanced lung cancer on quality of life would be urgently needed.

ACKNOWLEDGEMENT

This study was supported by the Michael and Karyn Goldstein Cancer Research Fund and we thank Mrs. Stacy Yuen for her administrative assistance.

REFERENCES

[1]   American Thoracic Society Board of Directors. Dyspnea. Mechanisms, assessment, and management: A consensus statement. American thoracic society. Am J Respir Crit Care Med 1999;159(1):321-40.

[2]   Lynn J, Teno JM, Phillips RS et al. Perceptions by family members of the dying experience of older and seriously ill patients. SUPPORT investigators. Study to understand prognoses and preferences for outcomes and risks of treatments. Ann Intern Med 1997;126(2):97-106.

[3]   Gallagher R, Roberts D. A systematic review of oxygen and airflow effect on relief of dyspnea at rest in patients with advanced disease of any cause. J Pain Palliat Care Pharmacother 2004;18(4):3-15.

[4]   Tanaka K, Akechi T, Okuyama T, et al. Prevalence and screening of dyspnea interfering with daily life activities in ambulatory patients with advanced lung cancer. J Pain Symptom Manage 2002;23(6):484-9.

[5]   Nazir SA, Redland ML. Chronic obstructive pulmonary disease: An update on diagnosis and management issues in older adults. Drugs Aging 2009;26(10):813-31.

[6]   Rocker G, Horton R, Currow D, et al. Palliation of dyspnoea in advanced COPD: Revisiting a role for opioids. Thorax 2009;64(10):910-5.

[7]   Jablonski A, Gift A, Cook K. Symptom assessment of patients with chronic obstructive pulmonary disease. West J Nurs Res 2007;29(7):845-63.

[8]   8. Ozturk A, Sarihan S, Ercan I, et al. Evaluating quality of life and pulmonary function of long-term survivors of non-small cell lung cancer treated with radical or postoperative radiotherapy. J Clin Oncol 2009;32(1):65-72.

[9]   Pruitt WC, Jacobs M. Breathing lessons: Basics of oxygen therapy. Nursing 2003; 33(10):43-5.

[10]   Spector N, Connolly MA, Carlson KK. Dyspnea: Applying research to bedside practice. AACN Adc Crit Care 2007;18(1):45-58.

[11]   Crockett AJ, Cranston JM, Moss JR, et al. Survival on long-term oxygen therapy in chronic airflow limitation: From evidence to outcomes in the routine clinical setting. Intern Med J 2001;31(8):448-54.

[12]   Lai YL, Chan CW, Lopez V. Perceptions of dyspnea and helpful interventions during the advanced stage of lung cancer: Chinese patients' perspectives. Cancer Nurs 2007;30(2):E1-8.

[13]   Jaturapatporn D, Moran E, Obwanga C, et al. Patients' experience of oxygen therapy and dyspnea: a qualitative study in home palliative care. Support Care Cancer 2010;18:765-70.

[14]   Bruera E, Schoeller T, MacEachern T. Symptomatic benefit of supplemental oxygen in hypoxemic patients with terminal cancer: The use of N of 1 randomized controlled trial. J Pain Symptom Manage 1992;7(6):365-8.

[15]   Swinburn C, Mould H, Stone T, et al. Symptomatic benefit of supplemental oxygen in hypoxemic patients with chronic lung disease. Am Rev Respir Dis 1991;143:913-5.

[16]   Bruera E, de Stoutz N, Velasco-Leiva A, et al. Effects of oxygen on dyspnea in hypoxaemic terminal-cancer patients. Lancet 1993;342:13-4.

[17]   Currow DC, Agar M, Smith J, et al. Does palliative home oxygen improve dyspnoea? A consecutive cohort study. Palliat Med 2009;23(4):309-16.

[18]   Okubadejo AA, Paul EA, Jones PW, et al. D and severe hypoxaemia? Eur Respir J 1996; 9(11):2335-9.

[19]   Abernethy AP, McDonald CF, Frith PA et al. Effect of palliative oxygen versus room air in relief of breathlessness in patients with refractory dyspnea: a double-blind randomized controlled trial. Lancet 2010:376:784-93.

[20]   Eaton T, Fergusson W, Kolbe J, et al. Short-burst oxygen therapy for COPD patients: A 6-month randomised, controlled study. Eur Respir J 2006;27(4):697-704.

[21]   Booth S, Kelly M, Cox N, et al. Does oxygen help dyspnea in patients with cancer? Am J Respir Crit Care Med 1996;153:1515-8.

[22]   Tsara V, Serasli E, Katsarou Z, et al. Quality of life and social-economic characteristics of greek male patients on long-term oxygen therapy. Respir Care 2008;53(8):1048-53.

[23]   Plywaczewski R, Sliwinski P, Nowinski A, et al. Incidence of nocturnal desaturation while breathing oxygen in COPD patients undergoing long-term oxygen therapy. Chest 2000; 117(3):679-83.

[24]   Stoller JK, Panos RJ, Krachman S, et al. Long-term Oxygen Treatment Trial Research, Group. Oxygen therapy for patients with COPD: Current evidence and the long-term oxygen treatment trial. Chest 2010;138(1):179-87.

In: Disability and Chronic Disease   ISBN: 978-1-62948-288-0
Editors: J. Merrick, S. Aspler and M. Morad   © 2014 Nova Science Publishers, Inc.

Chapter 16

AUTOGENIC TRAINING IN PATIENTS TREATED FOR CHRONIC HEADACHE

Gisèle Pickering[*], MD, PhD, DPharm[1,2,3], Christel Creac'h, MD[4],
Françoise Radat, MD[5], Jean-Michel Cardot, DPharm[1],
Jean-Pierre Alibeu, MD[6], Gilbert André, MD[7], Sylvie Chaib, MPsy[8],
Ludovic Douay, MD[9], Françoise Hirsch, MPsy[10],
Véronique Malochet, MD[7], Malou Navez, MD[4],
Pascale Picard, MD[8], Eric Serra, MD[9], Marc Sorel, MD[11],
Estelle Simen, Msc[1], Anne-C Sergent, MD [10],
Claude Dubray, MD[1,2,3] and Bernard Laurent, MD[4]

[1]CHU Clermont-Ferrand, Centre de Pharmacologie Clinique, Clermont-Ferrand, [2]Inserm, CIC 501, UMR 766, Clermont-Ferrand, [3]Clermont Université, Laboratoire de Pharmacologie, Faculté de Médecine, Clermont-Ferrand, [4]Centre d'Evaluation et traitement de la Douleur, CHU Saint-Etienne, [5]Centre d'Evaluation et traitement de la Douleur, CHU Bordeaux, [6]Centre d'Evaluation et traitement de la Douleur, CHU Grenoble, [7]Unité d'Evaluation et traitement de la Douleur, CH Puy-en-Velay, [8]Centre d'Evaluation et traitement de la Douleur, CHU Clermont-Ferrand, [9]Centre d'Evaluation et traitement de la Douleur, CHU Amiens, [10]Centre d'Evaluation et traitement de la Douleur, CHU Toulouse, [11]Unité d'Evaluation et traitement de la Douleur, CH Nemours and [12]Unité d'Evaluation et traitement de la Douleur, CHU Brest, France

ABSTRACT

Randomised clinical trials on autogenic training (AT) in headaches are scarce. This multi-centre, randomised, controlled study in two parallel groups studies the impact of AT in headaches. Method: 60 patients, 30 with treatment (ST), 30 having also AT (8

[*] Correspondence: Gisèle Pickering, MD, PhD, DPharm, Clinical Pharmacology Centre, Bâtiment 3C, CHU, Hopital G Montpied, 63001 Clermont-Ferrand cedex, France. E-mail: gisele.pickering@u-clermont1.fr.

sessions for 2 months) were compared at inclusion, 2 and 4 months for : response rate to treatment, headache score(HS), Number of headaches(NH), analgesics consumption (AC) and health-related outcomes, using ANOVA and t-test (significance <0.05). Results: 36 patients were analysed: the number of patients with a reduction of > 33% of HS is significantly larger at V3 (p=0.050) and V4 (0.039) in AT than in ST group. In both groups, NH, HS and analgesics consumption tend to diminish with an improved quality of life, and coping with pain. Conclusion: Although not all significant, the results are pertinent, as the addition of AT to ST tends to improve HS, AC and coping strategies.

INTRODUCTION

The concept of the headache as a psychophysiological disorder has led to the development of treatments acting on behaviour, like cognitive-behavioral therapy, or on physiological responses like relaxation training. Relaxation methods such as autogenic training (AT), progressive muscle relaxation, relaxation–biofeedback, and relaxation–hypnosis are frequently used in many psychological treatment approaches. Meta-analytic reviews have indicated that relaxation training (all techniques combined) was more effective in headache than waitlist control, reaching 35% improvement versus 5% in the waitlist controls (1). AT is a self-help relaxation technique invented by a German psychiatrist, Johannes Schultz (2), and is the relaxation method most frequently used in German-speaking countries and in Europe. The AT technique consists of exercises and is usually learned in groups over a period of 6-8 weeks with home practice. An analysis of the interest of AT in clinical outcome studies has shown positive effects of AT and of AT versus control in several studies on headache in adults (3). Most of the included studies however, using AT for headache, had a few methodological caveats, among which a small number of patients, no randomisation, patients with various types of headaches, tension-headache (TH) or migraine(M), and mixed TH/M, patients receiving a mixed therapy, and in the largest study (4) the so-called "autogenic training" group combined different components.

A more recent non-randomised study (5) included 25 patients (11 with mixed headache, 8 with migraine, and 6 with tension-type headache) and showed that AT may lead to a reduction in both headache frequency and in the use of headache medication. There is today a growing awareness of the importance of methodological issues in clinical trials on pharmacological and non-pharmacological treatments of migraine in order to provide quality information to clinicians. Guidelines on clinical trials in chronic migraine have been published and are intended to assist in the design of well-controlled clinical trials of chronic migraine in adults (6).

The International Association for the Study of pain recently published a pain clinical update (7) on the methodological issues in non pharmacological trials for chronic pain. Non pharmacological studies may be difficult to design, as regards the choice of the "control" arm or the impossibility of "blinding" the intervention. Placebo responses in clinical trials for pain may be very high and for example studies on acupuncture for chronic low back pain have showed that patient expectations of a positive result are related to the outcome (8). The placebo response can be higher in non pharmacological trials than in pharmacological trials, all the more than trials on pain rely most of the time on a subjective assessment of pain intensity or pain relief.

Considering on the one hand the fact that AT is frequently offered to patients with migraine (9,10) and on the other hand the paucity of clinical trials with AT in migraine and their heterogeneous methodological quality, a randomised controlled study of AT in migraine patients could bring valuable information. Therefore, this 4-month study aims at studying 1-the impact of AT on pain in a homogeneous group of well defined migraine patients and to compare it to waitlist patients, 2-Health-related outcomes and quality of life.

OUR STUDY

This is a prospective, randomised, multicenter, controlled study with two parallel groups of patients suffering from headache. Both groups have the same prophylactic treatment, one group combining this treatment with relaxation training. The study follows standardized ethical and safety guidelines. It has been approved by the French Ethics Committee and is in accordance with Good Clinical Practice Guidelines; subjects have provided informed consent. It was declared on clinicaltrials.gov (NCT00904527)

Inclusion and exclusion criteria

Male or female patients, 18 to 60 years old should comply with diagnostic criteria established by the International Headache Society (IHS) in the 2002 International Classification of Headache Disorders (ICHD-I), including paragraphs 1.1 to 1.7 of the IHS classification (ICHD) (11). Patients must have experienced headaches for at least three months occurring 5 to 14 days per month before the first visit. At the second visit they will be prescribed the background treatment recommended in France, a beta-blocker or oxytoron, if they have no contraindication.

Exclusion criteria were patients with probable or confirmed medication-overuse headache (codes IHS 8.2.6 and IHS 8.2.7), who cannot distinguish migraines from tension headaches, with face vascular algia, or other types of headaches (codes HIS 3, 4 and 5) or with tension headache (code IHS 2.3.1 et 2.3.2) or a combination of tension headache (2.2) and migraines (1.1 ou 1.2) reaching a cumulated number of days of less than 5 or at least 15 days per month. Will also be excluded patients who cannot communicate, who have a major depressive episode, evaluated by the MINI test (12) at the first visit and patients who have already been previously involved in relaxation training or in any migraine clinical trial.

Schultz relaxation technique

Training to Schultz relaxation technique was introduced individually in a one hour treatment session and was repeated once a week for 8 weeks. In all sessions, the therapist was the same headache specialist with extensive psychotherapy experience. AT is based on passive concentration on psychophysiological stimuli and bodily perceptions (e.g., heaviness and warmth of arms, legs, and abdomen; rhythm of breath; and heartbeat) (13). The aim of training is to develop voluntary mental control of specific physiological functions (reduction of heart rate, reduction of blood pressure, reduction of muscle tone etc.). There is an extensive literature about the effect of a specific relaxation technique on the body (3) and fMRI studies have shown that a parieto-premotor circuit becomes active during the processing of action-related sentences (14).

Multicenter study

Ten French pain clinics take part in this study. In each clinic, a medical doctor and a therapist specialised in Schultz relaxation technique take in charge the protocol. A clinical research assistant coordinates the study at national level, collects the diaries, monitors the data obtained in the pain clinics, with phone calls, e-mail backups, and on site visits.

Study

At the first visit (V1), the patients are given a clear explanation of the purpose of the trial and their role in it. They do a MINI test in order to exclude depressive patients. Obligations with which the subjects are expected to comply upon entry into the trial at the second visit V2 (daily completion of the headache diary, of the intensity of the migraine, of the treatment), are explained to the patients. Participants are told they should meet all predefined protocol inclusion and non-inclusion criteria. After the first visit to the Pain Clinic, a prospective baseline observation period of one month is started and includes the use of a headache diary by the patient.

At V2, patients are enrolled in the protocol if they meet the eligibility criteria, and are randomised to the relaxation or non-relaxation control group following the randomisation list. Prophylactic anti-migraine treatment with a beta blocker or oxyteron (left to the choice of the clinician, depending on the patient's past treatment and experience), is prescribed to the patient. Patients are informed about the mechanisms of migraine attacks, the possible adverse effects of drugs, and receive education tips for monitoring headache activity using headache diary, coping strategies, ways to change life style and advice to avoid triggers. Acute headache medication is allowed during the trial and patients are allowed to add any medication in an unrestricted manner but must write down any self administered medication in their diary.

Between V2 and V3 (2 months period), patients in the relaxation training group have a total of 8 sessions of relaxation, once a week. A quicker rhythm is however allowed (to a maximum of two sessions a week), to fit in with bank holidays. They are given a relaxation compact disc to reinforce the relaxation training at home. They come back two months later for the last visit (V4). At each visit patients bring back the headache diary they filled in at home since the last visit and fill in the questionnaires.

Randomization

Subjects are randomized after the run-in period (at V2) in small blocks in each pain clinic, to ensure balanced randomization across clinics, including 6 participants per centre (4 Relaxation and 4 Controls). A sealed envelope containing a prescription or non prescription of relaxation is opened by the practitioner at each new inclusion. It was calculated from literature data that 60 patients (30 per group) were required initially to detect a difference of 3 days of headache per month between the Relaxation and the waiting list group, with a power of 95%, a a risk of 5 %, assuming a drop-out rate of 30%.

Placebo control

Placebo control is impossible in studies involving relaxation techniques. The non-relaxation group was assigned to a waiting list, with the common agreement that relaxation would be started with these patients once the present trial would be completed.

Evaluation of results

The evaluation of the efficacy of the relaxation is based on headache diary information. Primary end points are 1- The percentages of change in the number of headache and in the headache score between visits (Vn+1-Vn)*100/Vn were grouped in two classes (=33% and =50%), and compared between groups, 2- the Number of Headache days per month ((NH) of any intensity)), 3- the Headache Score (HS) that takes account of the number and of the intensity of each headache (1=mild, 3=moderate, 5= severe) and is obtained by the following (number of headache of mild intensity *1 + number of headache of moderate intensity *3 + number of headache of sever intensity *5).

Secondary end-points are 1- Daily analgesics consumption according to the WHO classification (15): step 1 (paracetamol, non steroidal anti-inflammatory drugs), step 2 (tramadol, codeine, dextropropoxyphen, alone or in combination), step 3 (strong opiates); consumption of triptans and other antimigraine drugs, all in therapeutic units.

2- Healthcare outcomes and quality of life are studied by several questionnaires described below. Adverse events (AEs) if any, are noted in the diary and reported to local regulatory authority.

Questionnaires

At each visit the patients had a number of questionnaires to fill out:

Quality of life questionnaire. The SF36 (MOS 36-Item Short Form Survey Instrument) is the most widely used generic instrument for measuring health-related quality of life, and is frequently used in studies on headache (16).

Headache Impact Test (HIT). This tool measures the impact headaches have on a person's ability to function in everyday life (17). It covers six content categories represented in widely used surveys of headache impact and the highest the score obtained, the highest the impact of headache on the patient's quality of life.

Hospital anxiety and depression scale (HAD) is a self screening questionnaire (18) including 14 questions (7 for anxiety and 7 for depression) each rated from 0 to 3 with a total score of 21 each. Higher scores correspond to higher levels of anxiety and depression

Perceived stress scale (PSS). This scale (19) uses 4 items and is rated on a 5-point Likert scale ranging from 0 (never) to 4 (very frequently). Scores of items are reversed. Higher scores correspond to higher perceived stress.

Coping strategies questionnaire (CSQ). This questionnaire developed by Rosenstiel and Keefe 1983 (20), is composed of 48 items distributed in eight subscales each including six items: diverting attention, reinterpreting pain sensations, coping self-statements, ignoring pain sensations, praying and hoping, catastrophizing, increasing activity level, and increasing pain behaviour.

Multidimensional Health Locus of Control (MHLC) (21). There are three subscales of the MHLC: (1) Internal Health Locus of Control (IHLC), (2) Powerful Others Health Locus of Control (PHLC), and (3) Chance Health Locus of Control (CHLC). Each subscale comprises 6 items, resulting in a total of 18 items on the questionnaire. The scale was slightly adapted from the original scale. Patients are asked to rate, on a 4-point Likert scale, the degree to which they agree or disagree with each statement. Scores on each subscale can range from 6 to 36, with higher scores indicating a stronger belief in that type of control. The MHLC scale measures the extent to which an individual believes that external factors (i.e., other people and chance) and internal factors (i.e., one's own behaviour and thoughts) play important roles in determining his health.

Patient satisfaction remains in daily practice the gold standard of the efficacy of the treatment and is evaluated by the satisfaction of the patient with the treatment: very satisfied, satisfied, somewhat satisfied, no opinion.

Statistical analysis

Data analysis was done per protocol: we analysed only fully completed case report forms as regards headache and questionnaire results. Statistical analysis was done on SPSS statistical package (SPSS Inc Chicago, Illinois). Quantitative data, number and score of headaches have been analysed by ANOVA (significance <0.05) including group, visit and center effects. Intragroup data were compared by Student t test (significance <0.05). Qualitative data have been analysed with a Chi² test. All data are given as mean ± SD.

FINDINGS

42 out of the 60 included patients were analysed at V2, 21 AT and 21 ST patients, 21 AT and 21 ST at V3, 17AT and 19ST at V4. 3 patients withdrew, 6 stopped their treatment after V2, 4 were included erroneously by the clinician (2 with more than 15 days and 2 with less than 5 days of migraine per month), 3 did not attend all relaxation sessions, 8 had missing data in their diary (figure 1). We had more incomplete files than expected at the time we calculated the number of patients to include in order to give the study a satisfactory power, as the drop out was almost 50% instead of 30% we used for the calculation of the needed number of participants.

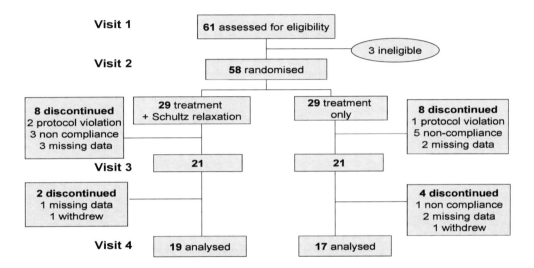

Figure 1. Flow Chart.

There were no significant differences between both groups concerning age ((43 ± 12 years (AT); 35 ± 14 years (ST)), weight (61 ± 12 kg (AT), 66 ± 13 (ST)), gender 19 (AT) and 16 (ST) female, and background treatment (11 betablockers and 12 oxytoron (AT) vs 12 and 11 (ST)). There were no differences between the pain centres. There were no differences between the groups as regards the number of headaches before starting relaxation, i.e between V1 and V2 (10 ± 3 vs 9 ± 3 (AT) and 9 ± 3 vs 9 ± 3 (ST)).

Primary end points

Response rate: when differences between visits are grouped in classes, the number of patients with a reduction of more than 33% of the headache score is significantly larger at V3 (p=0.050) and V4 (0.039) in the relaxation than in the standard treatment group. The number of patients with 50% of reduction of the headache score at V3 and V4 tends to be larger than with the standard treatment (p= 0. 1717 and 0.0969 respectively) (see figure 2).

Number of headache days per month (table 1) : Global analysis does not show pain centre nor group effect but a difference between the visits (p =0.0019). In the AT group, there are significant differences between visits V2 and V3 (-1,9 headaches) (p=0.0149), and V4 (-2.53

headaches) (p= 0.0008) while there is no significant difference in the ST group (-0.9 and -1.5 respectively).

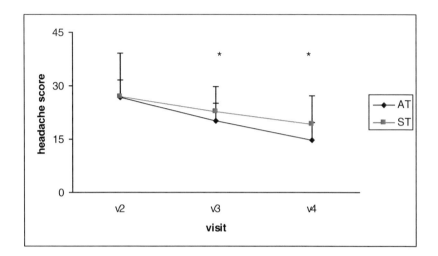

Figure 2. Improvement of migraine score with autogenic training (AT) (-33% (*=p<0.05)) at V3 and V4 compared to prophylactic treatment only (ST).

Table 1. Number of headaches and headache score (number of headache of mild intensity *1 + number of headache of moderate intensity *3 + number of headache of sever intensity *5) in the relaxation group (AT) and in the waiting list group (ST) at randomisation (V2), 2 months (V3) and 4 months (V4) later

group	visit	number of headaches (SD)	headache score (SD)
relaxation (AT)	v2	9.00 (3.19)	26.69 (12.25)
	v3	7.10 (2,98)	20.05 (6.82)
	v4	6.47 (3,24)	14.66 (8.08)
waiting list (ST)	v2	8.57 (2,38)	26.94 (14.03)
	v3	7.71 (3,13)	22.84 (11.28)
	v4	7.11 (4,31)	19.18 (11.92)

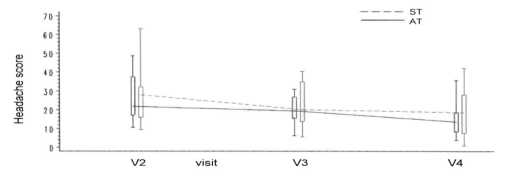

Figure 3. 75% of patients with relaxation and only 18% of patients with ST have a diminution of 50% of their migraine score when considering the median value of HS.

Headache Score (table 1): Global analysis does not show pain centre nor group effects but a difference between the visits (p <0.0001). In the AT group, there are significant differences between visits V2 and V3 (p=0.0115), and V4 (p< 0.0001), and between visits V2 and V4 (p=0.009) in the ST group. Interpreting from the median value and the fourth percentile (figure 3), 75% of patients with relaxation have a diminution of 50% of their migraine score and only of 18% in ST.

Secondary end-points

1- Paracetamol and non steroidal anti-inflammatory drugs (step 1), tramadol, codeine, dextropropoxyphen (step 2) and triptans have been taken by the patients during the protocol (table 2) with no consumption of strong opiates and other analgesics. NSAIDs is mainly ibuprofen, an over the counter drug. Global analysis shows that there is a significant difference between visits V2 and V4 for step I (p=0.0232), step II (0.0250) drugs, triptans (0.0166) and total consumption of analgesics (<0.0001). Intragroup analysis in AT shows a significant difference for step I (p=0.0199), triptans (p=0.0397) and total consumption of analgesics (p<0.0001). In ST, total consumption only is significantly diminished ((p=0.0048) (table2, figure 4).

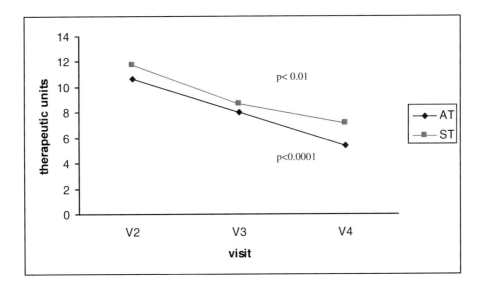

Figure 4. Total analgesics consumption.

2- Healthcare outcomes and quality of life have been studied by several questionnaires:

- SF36: There is no global difference between both groups. Intragroup analysis shows an improvement of the physical component in AT (0.031) and in ST (0.02) and in the vitality item only for AT at V4 (p<0.05).
- HAD: although our study was randomised there is a difference at V2, before randomisation, between the two groups concerning the anxious component of HAD

(p=0.0367) and this difference is maintained at V4 (p=0.0094). There are no global or intra-group differences for depression.

- HIT and PSS: no difference has been observed between the two groups.
- CSQ: There is no global difference between both groups. Both displayed less praying (p=0.024 (AT) and 0.034 (ST), more distantiation (p= 0.0017 (AT) and p=0.0043 (ST), less dramatisation (p=0.02 (AT) and p=0.0129 (ST)). Intra group analysis shows a significant difference for the items "reinterpretation" (p=0.01) for AT vs 0.994 for ST and ignorance (p=0.006 (AT) vs p=0.797 (ST)).
- MHLC: There is no global difference between both groups. Intragroup analysis shows in AT a significant difference between V2 and V4 for the Internal Health Locus of Control (p=0.002) and no difference for Powerful Others (p=0.1010), or Chance Health Locus of Control (p=0.2032). There is no significant difference for the ST group between the visits.

Table 2. Analgesics consumption (in therapeutic units per month) (step 1 = paracetamol and NSAIs) step 2 = weak opiates)

		step1			step2			Triptan		
		V2	V3	V4	V2	V3	V4	V2	V3	V4
AT	Mean	3.47	2.23	1.52	1.17	0.41	0.09	6.01	5.34	5.11
	SD	3.91	2.34	1.98	4.20	1.17	0.28	3.33	3.47	3.23
ST	Mean	2.66	2.42	2.20	3.73	1.50	1.68	5.13	4.75	3.97
	SD	3.61	3.52	3.59	7.07	3.59	3.59	4.07	3.48	2.46

No adverse events (AEs) were reported. The satisfaction in relaxation group reaches 90% very satisfied and 50% in the standard treatment group.

DISCUSSION

Our study was the first attempt to investigate the impact of autogenic training in a population of patients suffering from 5 to 14 days of headache per month and taking a prophylactic standard treatment (betablocker or oxyteron) in a controlled (versus waiting list) randomised clinical trial. The results showed a significant 33% reduction of the headache score when classes are considered, and a non-significant difference between the two groups when number of headaches and headache score are analysed.

Between V2 and V4, patients with AT have a significant diminution (-28%) in the number of headaches (-2,5 headaches) while the Headache score, that takes account of the headache intensity, diminishes by 45% : this underlines that the patients have either had less severe migraines or a milder intensity of each migraine when practising relaxation.

Both groups had a prophylactic treatment and the relief in ST is of -1,5 migraines/month at 4 months (non significant) and a decrease of the headache score (p<0.01), less significant however than for the AT group (p<0.0001). Prophylaxis is regarded as successful if frequency of attacks per month is decreased by at least 50% within 3 months (10): 75% of patients with relaxation have a diminution of 50% of their migraine score and of only 18% in ST when considering the median value of HS. Class intergroup comparison shows not only a significant 33% reduction of HS but also a tendency for a diminution of -50% (0.09) at V4.

Our study did not however demonstrate a significant intergroup difference in the number of migraines and the headache score: this is probably linked to the limited number of analysed patients that resulted from an unexpected number of missing data, leading to a lack of enough power to show significance; this may also be linked to the higher than expected inter-patient variability when we calculated the needed number for a resulting adequate power of the trial; this may also be linked to the fact the study has been performed in ten centres with different clinicians and therapists. Although the statistical analysis does not show significance for all the data, it is important to stress that having to face less episodes of headache every month (one less with AT than with ST) is clinically very pertinent for the patient. The results of this study converge to the conclusion that AT could act with time in synergy with the prophylactic treatment, potentiating its benefits and diminishing the number and the intensity of headaches. Although the study is underpowered, the findings are clinically pertinent for the patient.

This study was also interested in analysing the analgesics consumption of the patients who recorded in their diary all the drugs they took apart from the prescribed betablocker or oxyteron. No significant differences were shown between AT and SM, and both groups had a significant diminished consumption of drugs, but this diminution was however more marked for AT. All the more that in the AT group, we observed a significant diminution of paracetamol, NSAIDs and triptans, while no such significance is shown in the SM group. AT may therefore reinforce the impact of the prophylactic treatment on analgesics consumption. This finding is particularly interesting for health as well as for socio-economic reasons. Indeed, migraine is a chronic pathology and may last for a number of years. Although ibuprofen, used by the patients in this study, may have lower risks of gastro-intestinal complications than some other NSAIDs with higher antiCOX1/COX2 ratio like diclofenac or naproxen, the general long term deleterious impact of NSAIDs on renal function and potential nephropathy has been demonstrated (22).This is all the more important that the dose of NSAIDs, needs high dosing, e.g., 600 to 1200 mg for ibuprofen) to be fully effective in migraine. Likewise, paracetamol, considered as a safe drug even with a dosage of 4 grammes a day has potential hepatic side-effects (23).The other interesting result concerns triptans consumption as we observed a significant intra-group diminution of triptans consumption with AT. Although efficacious for migraine, triptans have still a high cost and have been described to have possible cardiovascular side-effects (24, 25). Hence, an even slightly decreased consumption of triptans, paracetamol and NSAIDs is always beneficial for the patient.

Another point this study was interested in was the impact of relaxation on a number of health related outcomes. The SF-36 which is a robust questionnaire shows that physical function is improved significantly in both groups, while mental function is not affected. Quite interestingly, vitality is significantly improved in the AT group: recent studies have showed that it is anxiety that mediates the effects of headache frequency on vitality (26) and plays an important role in the maintenance of chronic pain, (27). Unfortunately in our study the AT group happened to be more anxious than the ST group at V2 and we could not reproduce findings showing significant efficacy of relaxation training in reducing anxiety (28) or a link between anxiety and vitality. However, the improvement of vitality with relaxation in this pathology of chronic headache known to cause fatigue and to even lead to exhaustion of the patient, is a positive outcome that would need to be studied further.

Concerning the way patients coped with pain during the protocol, it is interesting to note that both treatments modified significantly a number of coping strategies, with more distantiation and less dramatisation, stressing that the prophylactic drug treatment has on its own a positive impact on the management of the pathology by the patient. Our study showed also that patients in the relaxation group develop adaptive strategies like reinterpretation and ignorance. Hence, the frequent inadequate or non-response to drug treatment of headache observed to be associated with low scores of positive reinterpretation (29) may find here a great help with the practise of relaxation to improve outcome.

Concerning health beliefs with the MHLC test, the internal locus of control is significantly improved in AT while a tendency is present for the external factors to diminish. Radat et al., 2008 (30), have identified a number of psychological variables that are associated with chronic headache and these include an externalized locus of control. In our study, AT patients not only tend to rely less on external persons or aspects, wishing to distance themselves from dependency to others, but focus more on their own personal control to regulate their health condition and manage their illness. We may interpret these findings as an impetus movement of the patients to gain more autonomy in the management of their pathology.

Finally, basic pain research has demonstrated that central sensitization can be generated by prolonged nociceptive inputs from the periphery (31), be secondary to chronic pain and may induce central neuroplastic changes that persist well after the initial trauma. Recent studies showed that headache frequency is related to sensitization (32). It is therefore crucial to combine all strategies, pharmacological and non pharmacological, to minimize, prevent and hopefully break the impact of central sensitization.

CONCLUSION

This randomised study has showed that the diminution of the headache frequency and the intensity of migraines was accompanied with positive changes of physical function and mental processes in both groups, although we lacked power to demonstrate a statistically significant difference between them because of a large drop-out of patients. The prophylactic drug treatment has indeed beneficial effects on headaches, drug consumption and on a number of domains of quality of life, health beliefs and coping strategies. The addition of autogenic training tends to enhance and potentiate these benefits, as regards headache score improvement of 33 %, lesser analgesics consumption, positive adaptive coping strategies and thoughts. The combination of pharmacological strategies and relaxation may be beneficial in a holistic approach of headache treatment and should be studied in a larger number of patients.

ACKNOWLEDGEMENTS

Financial support from the French Ministry of Health.

REFERENCES

[1] Rains JC, Penzien DB, McCrory AC, Gray RN. Behavioral headache treatment : history, revuiew of the empirical literature, and methodological critique. Headache 2005;45:S92-S109.

[2] Schultz JH, Luthe W. Autogenic methods. New York: Grune Stratton, 1969.

[3] Stetter F, Kupper S. Autogenic training: A meta-analysis of clinical outcome studies. Appl Psychophysiol Biofeedback 2002;27(1):45-54.

[4] Reich BA. Non-invasive treatment of vascular and muscle contraction headache: A comparative longitudinal study. Headache 1989;29:34–41.

[5] Zsombok T, Juhasz G, Budavari A, Vitrai J, Bagdy G. Effect of autogenic training on drug consumption in patients with primary headache: An 8-month follow-up study. Headache 2003;43:251-7.

[6] Silberstein S, Tfelt-Hansen P, Dodick DW, Limmroth V, Lipton RB, J Pascual J, et al. for the Task Force of the International Headache Society Clinical Trials Subcommittee. Guidelines for controlled trials of prophylactic treatment of chronic migraine in adults. Cephalalgia 2008;28:484–95.

[7] Bennett MI, Closs SJ. Methodological issues in nonpharmacological trials for chronic pain. Pain Clin Updates 2010;18(2).

[8] Linde D, Witt CM, Streng A, Weidenhammer W, Wagenpfell S, Brinkhaus B, et al. The impact of patients expectations on outcomes in four randomised controlled trials of acupuncture in patients with chronic pain. Pain 2007;128:264-71.

[9] Kanji N, White AR, Ernst E. Autogenic training for tension type headaches: A systematic review of controlled trials. Compl Ther Med 2006;14:144-50.

[10] Fumal A, Schoenen J. Current migraine management – patient acceptability and future approaches. Neuropsychiatr Dis Treat 2008;4(6) 1043–57.

[11] ICHD. Accessed 2013 Aug 01. URL: http://ihsclassification.org/

[12] Sheehan DV, Lecrubier Y, Sheehan KH, Amorim P, Janavs J, Weiller E, et al. The Mini-International Neuropsychiatric Interview (M.I.N.I.): the development and validation of a structured diagnostic psychiatric interview for DSM-IV and ICD-10. J Clin Psychiatry 1998;59(Suppl 20):22-33.

[13] Shapiro S, Lehrer P. Psychophysiological effects of autogenic training and progressive relaxation. Appl Psychophysiol Biofeedback 1980;5(2):249–255.

[14] Hauk O, Johnsrude I, Pulvermuller F. Somatotopic representation of action words in human motor and premotor cortex. Neuron 2004;41:301–7.

[15] Ventafridda V, Stjernsward J. Pain control and the World Health Organization analgesic ladder. JAMA 1995;274(23):1870-3.

[16] Brazier JE, Harper R, Jones NMB, OCathian A, Thomas KJ, Unsherwood T, Westlake L. Validating the SF-36 health survey questionnaire: new outcome measure for primary care. BMJ 1992;305:160-4.

[17] Kosinski M, Bayliss MS, Bjorner JB, Ware JE Jr, Garber WH, Batenhorst A, et al. A six-item short-form survey for measuring headache impact: the HIT-6. Qual Life Res 2003;12(8):963-74.

[18] Zigmond AS, Snaith RP. The hospital anxiety and depression scale. Acta Psychiatr Scand 1983;67(6):361-70.

[19] Cohen S, Kamarak T, Mermelstein R. A global measure of perceived stress. J Health Soc Behav 1983;24:385-96.

[20] Rosenstiel AK, Keefe FJ. The use of coping strategies in chronic low back pain patients: relationship to patient characteristics and current adjustment. Pain 1983;17(1):33-44.

[21] Wallston KA. The validity of the multidimensional health locus of control scales. J Health Psychol 2005;10(5):623-31.

[22] Kuo HW, Tsai SS, Tiao MM, Liu YC, Lee IM, Yang CY. Analgesic use and the risk for progression of chronic kidney disease. Pharmacoepidemiol Drug Saf 2010;19(7):745-51.

[23] Jalan R, Williams R, Bernuau J. Paracetamol: are therapeutic doses entirely safe? Lancet 2006;368(9554):2195-6

[24] Wammes-van der Heijden EA, Tijssen CC, Egberts AC. Treatment choices and patterns in migraine patients with and without a cardiovascular risk profile. Cephalalgia 2009;29(3):322-30.

[25] Barra S, Lanero S, Madrid A, Materazzi C, Vitagliano G, Ames PR et al. Sumatriptan therapy for headache and acute myocardial infarction. Expert Opin Pharmacother 2010;11(16):2727-37.

[26] Peñacoba-Puente C, Fernández-de-Las-Peñas C, González-Gutierrez JL, Miangolarra-Page JC, Pareja JA. Interaction between anxiety, depression, quality of life and clinical parameters in chronic tension-type headache. Eur J Pain 2008;12(7): 886-94

[27] Rollnik JD, Karst M, Fink M, Dengler R. Coping strategies in episodic and chronic tension-type headache. Headache 2001;41:297–302.

[28] Manzoni GM, Pagnini F, Castelnuovo G, Molinari E. Relaxation training for anxiety: a ten-years systematic review with meta-analysis. BMC Psychiatry 2008;8:41-5.

[29] Lucas C, Lantéri-Minet M, Massiou H, Nachit-Ouinekh F, Pradalier A, Mercier F, et al. The GRIM2005 study of migraine consultation in France II. Psychological factors associated with treatment response to acute headache therapy and satisfaction in migraine. Cephalalgia 2007;27(12):1398-407

[30] Radat F, Lantéri-Minet M, Nachit-Ouinekh F, Massiou H, Lucas C, Pradalier A et al. The GRIM 2005 study of migraine consultation in France. III: Psychological features of subjects with migraine. Cephalalgia 2009;29(3):338-50.

[31] Bendtsen L. Central sensitization in tension-type headache-possible pathophysiological mechanisms. Cephalalgia 2000;20:486-508.

[32] De Tommaso M, Sardaro M, Vecchio E, Serpino C, Stasi M, Ranieri M Central sensitisation phenomena in primary headaches: overview of a preventive therapeutic approach. CNS Neurol Disord Drug Targets 2008;7(6):524-35.

In: Disability and Chronic Disease
Editors: J. Merrick, S. Aspler and M. Morad

ISBN: 978-1-62948-288-0
© 2014 Nova Science Publishers, Inc.

Chapter 17

POSTURAL CONTROL AND CHANGES WITH AGEING AND EXERCISE

*Zachary Crowley, BHMS (Hons)[1], Pedro Bezerra, PhD[2] and Shi Zhou, PhD[*1]*

[1]School of Health and Human Science, Southern Cross University, Australia
[2]Instituto Politecnico Viana do Castelo, Portugal

ABSTRACT

Postural control is one of the functional capacities that are fundamental to an independent lifestyle. Ageing is frequently accompanied by a decrease of neuromuscular capacities which are associated with increased risk of falls and morbidity. Decreased muscle strength and power associated with ageing can cause adaptations in the strategies used by the nervous system in postural control. It has been reported that there is a change from an "ankle strategy" which relies on large moments at the ankle, to a "hip strategy" which relies on moments at the hip to rotate ankle and hip joints in opposite directions. The ability to control posture can be assessed using either traditional posturography or stabilogram diffusion analysis. The traditional postural control variables are most often characterised with the measures based on the displacement of the centre-of-pressure (COP), while the stabilogram diffusion analysis summarizes the mean square COP displacement as a function of the time interval between COP comparisons. Evidence in the literature indicates that appropriate exercise has a beneficial effect on the postural control. It appears that exercises that involve coordinative balance tasks, such as balance training and Tai Chi, are most effective in delaying the age-related decline in postural control. This review provides an analysis of the current literature on control of upright stance posture, with a focus on the effects of ageing on the factors that are essential for postural control and the effects of exercise interventions for improving postural control.

* Correspondance: Professor Shi Zhou, School of Health and Human Sciences, Southern Cross University, Lismore, NSW 2480, Australia. E-mail: shi.zhou@scu.edu.au.

INTRODUCTION

The ability in maintaining an upright standing position is of fundamental importance to daily life. The upright stance is a naturally unstable position that requires continuous adjustments of muscle contractions to maintain joint positions from the neck to the ankle. It requires maintenance of body's centre of gravity (COG) within the supporting base, ie. between the feet (1). The COG is usually located within the body at approximately the level of the second sacral segment. Despite this relatively large distance from the base of support (BOS) the body is able to provide suitable responses to changes in the location of the COG. The movement of the COG during an unconstrained standing can be measured by the trajectory of the Centre of Pressure (COP) when an individual stands on a force platform. The movements of COP are derived from the location of the vertical ground reaction forces on the surface of a force platform under the feet (2). These COP trajectories have, for many years, been used to infer biomechanical mechanisms of postural control (2) and some of the commonly used COP assessment methods are described in this review.

In the static erect posture the vertical projection of the COG is often termed the line of gravity (LOG) and this line has important implications in the maintenance of posture. Any shift in the location of the COG, e.g., anterior translation, will cause movement of the LOG in the same direction i.e., anteriorly. However, to maintain a static erect posture the LOG must fall within the border of the supporting feet to maintain equilibrium (3). When the LOG passes directly through the axis of rotation of a joint no net gravitational torque is produced. However, during quiet upright bipedal stance this optimal alignment of joints or "optimal posture" does not exist. Often when maintaining postural control the LOG passes either anteriorly or posteriorly to the axis of rotation of all joints involved which will cause gravitational torque around the joints. This torque will cause rotation around the joint which will consequently require a counterbalancing torque, through muscular contractions, to maintain the upright posture. Also the gravitational moment magnitude increases as the distance between the LOG and joint axis increases (3).

When analysing upright stance in the sagittal plane it can be seen that the LOG falls either anteriorly or posteriorly to the ankle, knee, and hip joint axes. For the ankle joint the LOG usually passes anteriorly to the lateral malleolus which is the ankle axis of rotation. This anterior LOG positioning causes a gravitational dorsiflexion moment. To counteract this dorsiflexion moment there is a need to activate posterior muscles such as the soleus and gastrocnemius (4). The activation of posterior lower limb muscles has been establish on several occasions (5) with some authors stating that the ankle muscles strength is the main modulator for ankle movement during postural control (6).

The knee joint is usually close to full extension during quiet stance, however the LOG passes just anterior to the knee joint axis which creates a gravitational moment causing extension at the knee joint. Posterior knee joint capsule tension and associated ligaments are usually sufficient to counterbalance the gravitational moment at the knee and therefore little muscle activity is needed. A small amount of activity, however, has been identified that a small amount of activation occurs in posterior thigh muscles which would help to counteract the extension moment due to gravity (3). It has also been hypothesised that activity of the soleus may augment the gravitational extension moment at the knee through its posterior pull on the tibia as it acts at the ankle joint (3). The LOG acting at the hip passes through the greater trochanter, which is slightly posterior to the axis of rotation. This posteriorly located gravitational line creates an extension moment at the hip which causes posterior rotation of the pelvis on the femoral head. This is supported by research that has shown activity within the hip flexors during standing.

While all the above examples were discussed in relation to a near optimal posture, in reality there is always movement of the body segments to counter the destabilization torque due to gravity. The LOG will often pass on the opposite side of the joint axis and would therefore require activation of the opposing muscles, compared to what was explained above. For example, if an individual adopted a flexed knee posture or the movement of the COG was posterior the LOG would pass posterior to the knee joint and create a flexion moment. To stabilise the knee and maintain erect posture, activation of the quadriceps muscles would then be required (3).

ASSESSMENT

Static posturography is a method in which the performance of the postural control system in a static position and environment is characterised. When an individual attempts to stand still, the COP under their feet moves relative to a global coordinate system. A plot of the time-varying coordinates of the COP is known as a stabilogram (7). Many researchers have measured the anterior-posterior (AP) and medial-lateral (ML) displacements of the COP in an attempt to evaluate and interpret the behaviour of the postural control system. The measurement of posture control is often conducted using either traditional posturography or stabilogram diffusion analysis, which are methods of computing the COP behaviours. Traditional postural control variables are most often characterised with the parameters based on the displacement of the COP measured with a force platform (also known as summary statistics) (2). The stabilogram diffusion analysis generates a stabilogram diffusion function that summarizes the mean square of the COP displacement as a function of the time interval between COP comparisons and is based on the assumption that erect posture is, in part, a stochastic process (8).

Stabilogram traditional parameters

The COP is the location of the vertical reaction vector on the surface of the force platform on which the subject stands. The COP reflects the orientation of the body segments (joint angels), as well as the movements of the body to keep the COP within the base of support. The anterior-posterior, medial-lateral displacement of the COP can be measured with the force platform. The COP parameters can be measured in 1) Time-Domain "distance" measures, 2) Time-Domain "area" measures, and 3) Time-Domain "hybrid" measures (2). Several authors in the literature have used combinations of these COP measurements to characterise the behaviour of the postural control system with a large majority of these parameters being drawn from the work of Prieto et al. (2).

The COP coordinate time series, AP and ML, are commonly used to compute measures of postural steadiness, and characterize the static performance of the postural control system.

These two time series also define the COP path relative to the origin of the force plate. The resultant distance (RD) time series is the vector distance from the mean COP to each pair of points in the AP and ML time series (2). The following procedures are for the composite measures computed using both the AP and ML time series, and those based on the AP time series. Every measurement defined for the AP time series is similarly defined for the ML time series (2).

Time-domain distance measures estimate a parameter associated with either the displacement of the COP from the central point of the stabilogram, or the velocity of the COP. The mean distance (Mdist) is the mean of the RD time series, and represents the average distance from the mean COP, while the mean distance-AP is the mean absolute value of the AP time series and represents the average AP distance from the mean COP (2). The root-mean-squared (RMS) distance from the mean COP is the RMS value of the RD time series and can also be calculated for just the RMS distance-AP and ML time series (2). The mean velocity (Mvel) is the average velocity of the COP and is also calculated for all three time series (RD, AP, and ML). In effect, this normalizes the total excursions to the analysis interval. The COP time series are filtered to the frequency range of interest to minimize the quantization noise that may inadvertently inflate measures such as mean velocity and total excursions (2).

Time-domain area measures and time-domain hybrid measures have also been used in the past but generally not to the same degree. These measures are methods that are statistically based estimates of the area enclosed by the stabilogram or are measures that model the stabilogram with a combination of distance measures respectively. Examples of Time-domain area measures include the 95% confidence circle area (Area-CC) and the 95% confidence ellipse area (Area-CE) while the sway-area (Area-SW) and mean frequency (MFreq) (2) are examples of time-domain hybrid measures. Although this is not an exhaustive list of the parameter used in traditional stabilogram analysis, there still is a need for future investigations to elucidate which measures best represent changes in the postural control system, e.g., due to ageing.

Stabilogram diffusion parameters

The statistical-biomechanics method of assessing the COP trajectories named stabilogram-diffusion analysis (SDA) was developed by Collins and De Luca (8). This analysis is based on the assumption that the movement of the COP represents the combined output of co-existing deterministic and stochastic mechanisms. The COP displacement analysis is calculated by computing the square of the displacements between all pairs of points separated by a specific time interval and averaged over the number of time intervals making up a COP time series. These analyses reveal that over short-term intervals of time during undisturbed stance the COP behaves as a positively correlated random walk whereby the COP tends to drift away from a relative equilibrium point. This is interpreted as an indication that the postural control system uses open-loop control mechanisms which operates without sensory feedback (descending commands which set the steady-state activity levels of the postural muscles) (1). In long-term intervals of time, it resembles a negatively correlated random walk whereby the COP tends to return to a relative equilibrium point, indicating that the postural control system now uses closed-loop control mechanisms. It is inferred that this period is one in which the postural control system operates with sensory feedback (from visual, vestibular and somatosensory systems) (1, 7, 8). This perspective has the advantage that it leads to the extraction of repeatable COP parameters which can be directly related to the steady-state behaviour and functional interaction of the neuromuscular mechanisms underlying the maintenance of upright stance (7).

Stabilogram-diffusion analysis involves the extraction of three sets of posturographic parameters: diffusion coefficients, scaling exponents, and critical point coordinates (7). The diffusion coefficient is an average measure of the stochastic activity of a random walker, i.e., it is directly related to its jump frequency and/or amplitude, and can be thought of as an indicator of the relative stability of the system. The short-term and long-term COP diffusion coefficients characterize the stochastic activity of the open-loop and closed-loop postural control mechanisms, respectively (7). Diffusion coefficients are calculated from the slopes of the resultant linear-linear plots of mean square COP displacement versus the change in time (7). The long-term and ML diffusion coefficients are usually lower than the respective short-term and AP diffusion coefficients which reflects the increased level of stochastic activity over the short-term time series and AP direction comparatively to long-term time series and ML direction, respectively (8).

Quantification of the correlation between the step increments that make up an experimental time series is the second posturographic parameter used in SDA and is termed "scaling exponents" (7). Scaling exponents are calculated from the slopes of the resultant log-log plots of mean square COP displacement versus the change in time. This measure can be thought of as providing an indication whether the motion of the COP is more or less likely to continue moving in the same direction that it is currently moving. Scaling exponents may assume a value in the range of 0 to 1. If the scaling exponents are equal to 0.5, then the increments in COP displacements are statistically independent. If the scaling exponent value is greater than 0.5, then past and future increments are positively correlated, i.e., future displacement increments tend to move in the same direction as the current displacement value (persistent behaviour). If scaling exponents are less than 0.5, then the stochastic activity is negatively correlated, i.e., increasing/decreasing trends in the past imply decreasing/increasing trends in the future (anti-persistent behaviour) (7). From a physiological standpoint, SDA scaling exponents quantify the correlated behaviour of the respective postural control mechanisms, i.e., short-term scaling exponents characterize the drift-like dynamics of the open-loop postural control mechanisms, whereas the long-term scaling exponents characterize the antidrift-like dynamics of the closed-loop postural control mechanisms (7).

The critical point coordinates approximate the transition region that separates the short-term and long-term regions. The estimation of the critical point coordinates is determined as the intersection point of the straight lines is fitted to the two regions of the linear-linear version of the resultant stabilogram-diffusion plot. The transition points occur at relatively small time intervals (0.33 s to 1.67 s) and small means square displacement (1.10 mm^2 to 29.37 mm^2) (7, 8). These coordinates approximate the temporal and spatial characteristics of the region over which the physiological postural control system switches from open-loop control to closed-loop control.

Several studies have utilised the SDA technique since the work of Collins & De Luca was first published with some authors using the technique to examine the age-related changes in postural control (1, 7). The SDA approach has the advantage that it can be directly related to the steady-state behaviour and functional interaction of the neuromuscular mechanisms underlying the maintenance of upright position. Thus, this statistical-biomechanics approach seems be useful to formulate and test hypothesis concerning the relative contribution of different sensorimotor subsystems (visual, vestibular and proprioceptive) and strategies to control posture (7, 8).

PHYSIOLOGY

Any detected angular deviation from upright stance applies neural strategies, at supraspinal and spinal levels, involving the interaction between the sensory and motor system to create continuous corrective torque to compensate for disturbances. Postural control involves integration of sensory information from the vestibular, visual and tactile-proprioceptive receptors which stimulate motor responses to maintain balance via several parts of the brain including the cerebellum, brainstem, basal ganglia and sensory-motor cortex (9). Once the postural system has integrated all sensory information the CNS sends out appropriate motor responses to effector muscles in an effort to maintain the posture. These corrective movements imply the ability to choose appropriate motor responses based on past experience, to modify these responses on the basis of the continuous sensory input and to produce the needed muscular contraction to stabilize posture (10).

Proprioception, vision, and vestibular inputs are the main sources of sensory information to guide and control posture and movement. This information is provided via kinaesthetic receptors located in the muscles, tendons, joints, skin, the eyes, and vestibular receptors and provides essential feedback for the maintenance of postural control. The peripheral sensations appear to be the most important sensory input in the maintenance of the postural control (10) and consists of two main sensory organs, the muscle spindle and the Golgi tendon organ. The vestibular and visual systems seem to contribute to the postural control system more when there is a reduced sensory feedback from proprioceptive inputs especially in some pathological conditions and ageing (10).

Muscle spindles are distributed throughout the belly of muscles and report the absolute amount of stretch and the rate of change of stretch in a particular muscle. The response to muscle length change, known as stretch reflex, plays an important role in counteracting the pull of gravity in upright posture. The tendon receptors, known as Golgi tendon organs, are sensitive to the amount of tension developed on a tendon and send the impulses to the spinal cord. This proprioceptive information is important in maintaining balance and adjusting posture during standing and has an increased role when both visual and vestibular information are poor or reduced (11). The vestibular apparatus is centrally involved in body balance and has close reflex connections with the visual system (6). A diminutive vestibular reflex has an impact on the maintenance of posture when both proprioceptive and visual information are unavailable or ambiguous (6).

In the motor system, the main factors associated with decreased postural control include the decline in muscle strength and power, and the reduced capacity to respond appropriately to disturbances in postural activity. The hip and lower limb muscle groups (knee extensors, knee flexors, ankle planarflexors and ankle dorsiflexors) should be examined closely because of their influence in controlling posture (1). The dynamic interaction between the agonists and antagonists in maintaining posture has received limited attention, however it has been suggested that an increase in strength of lower limb muscle groups may be a factor that could improve not only postural control but the stability of muscle contractions (1, 7). This could be especially important due to the contraction of hamstrings as a quadriceps' antagonist muscle and vice-versa in the thigh, while in the lower leg the same principle applies to the plantarflexors (e.g., gastrocnemius) and dorsiflexors (e.g., tibialis anterior) during postural control. Several studies have demonstrated that a reduced quadriceps and ankle dorsiflexion strength greatly increases body sway in a situation of reduced sensation and visual input (1), highlighting the importance of lower limb strength as a limiting factor in the control of upright stance.

Effects of ageing on postural control

Ageing is a natural process that brings with it many biological, physiological, and psychological changes. These changes often affect the individual's quality of living; nevertheless the fact remains that the ageing body can accomplish most, if not all, of the functions of its youth. However, these functions are often diminished with ageing, the main differences being that movements are less precise, take significantly longer time to produce, and require much more motivation (12). But as in youth, physiological function can be maintained to a degree through continued use and exercise (13).

In chronological terms, the older adult population is characteristically defined as individuals with age of 65 years and older. Still there is considerable heterogeneity among this age group and as a result older adults are often sub grouped into young-old (65 – 74 years), middle-old (75 – 84 years), and old-old (85+ years) categories. This further grouping of older individuals reflects more accurately the changes in physiological function (12).

Physiological changes often seen with ageing reflect a general decline in body system functions. These declines result in a diminution of various systems such as the muscular and neurologic systems resulting in a reduction of physical capabilities. The ageing muscular system experiences a decrease in muscular strength which is directly related to both a reduction in the size of existing muscle fibres (muscular atrophy) as well as a loss of muscle fibres. Accompanying this strength loss is a decline in reaction time which is often associated with type II muscle fibre loss while type I fibres are said to remain relatively stable throughout life (14). The progressive ageing-related decline in musculoskeletal strength cannot be stopped in entirety, however, it can be slowed with the introduction of appropriate exercise interventions (13). Neurological structural changes also occur with the ageing process that may interfere with day-to-day routines including a loss of neurons in both the brain and spinal cord. Another change in the nervous system with ageing is neuronal dendrite atrophy which results in impaired synaptic connections and diminished electrochemical reactions leading to the slowing of many neuronal processes (12). Sensorimotor changes with ageing include a decline in motor strength, slowed reaction time, diminished reflexes (especially in the ankles), and proprioceptive changes. These changes have functional consequences such as a compromised balance and postural control, and slowed and more deliberate movements (12).

Morphological and physiological alterations associated with ageing often cause degradation in the human's ability to maintain upright stance (15). It is often found that with ageing there is a decline in the capacity of postural control with an associated increase in the incidences of falls and a decrease in mobility. This ageing process often results in a decrease in stability of the open-loop postural control mechanisms (1) and also a greater delay in the closed-loop postural control (2, 16). Both the delay in the onset of the closed-loop postural control and the larger instability of the open-loop postural control causes an increase in the short-term postural sway through endorsing a higher level of stochastic activity (16, 17). It is possible that these age-related changes in the open-loop postural control mechanisms are due to a postural control strategy adopted by elderly individuals whereby they increase the level of muscle activity across their lower-limb joints (1). Moreover, compared with healthy young adults, older adults exhibit significantly increased levels of antagonist muscle co-activation in response to postural perturbations (16, 18). This co-activation of antagonistic muscles has been suggested to improve joint impedance and more specifically joint stiffness, which in turn contributes to the overall stability of the system (19).

It is also common to find in the postural control literature that, when using measures of COP traditional summary statistics, the elderly exhibit greater measured COP velocities, distances, and amplitude and/or frequencies. For example, Abrahamová & Hlavačka (15) found that under four sensory organisation test (SOT) conditions (combination of eyes open and closed on either hard or foam surface), the older group (60-82 years) exhibited significantly greater AP COP amplitude, velocity, and root mean square values when compared to a young group (20-40 years). In another study, Du Pasquier et al. (20) found that velocity measures were best at reflecting postural stability impairment with ageing. They also found that closure of the eyes increased sway but to a much greater degree in the older individuals compared to the younger group. All of the above authors attributed the decreased functionality of the postural control system to physiological changes in sensory and motor systems that are often seen with ageing.

Sensory inputs and ageing

Effective maintenance of postural control not only relies on appropriate application of muscle forces to maintain body position but also requires sensory inputs. These sensory inputs allow the nervous system to decide on the *when* and *how* the restorative forces are produced in an effort to maintain upright stance. When sensory inputs are altered or absent, as is the often experienced with natural ageing, the control system must interpret and respond to incomplete data. This partial reduction or complete lack of sensory feedback often causes alterations in a person's stability and postural control (20). These variations in sensory feedback can either be environmental, as in weightlessness, or physiological such as visual, vestibular, or proprioceptive abnormalities. All three of these physiological factors have been proven to diminish with ageing and have been implicated in alterations in postural control (20).

Vision
Visual inputs provide important information to the CNS regarding the motion and position of the head in relation to the surrounding environment. Visual inputs not only provide the postural system with motion information but it also provides a reference for verticality and further information such as colour, form, and depth which all contribute to sensory feedback and orientation with reference to the external environment (12). This visual information can

have significant effects on the maintenance of upright posture. For example, it has been found that sway increases when visual motion feedback is deprived or visual field is restricted and that visual environmental motion induces postural adjustments as well as illusions of self-motion (21).

In another study, Collins and De Luca (22) investigated the effects of eyes-open and eyes-closed on both open-loop and closed-loop postural control mechanisms in a group of healthy young adults. The authors interpreted the results as an indication that the visual system is integrated into the postural control system in one of two ways. Either visual input causes a decrease in the ML and AP stochastic activity of the open-loop control mechanism or it causes an increase in the stochastic activity and uncorrelated behaviour of the closed-loop control mechanism in the AP direction. It was hypothesised that in both schemes visual input serves to decrease the stiffness of the musculoskeletal system. However these alterations in postural control strategies in relation to visual inputs can differ when comparing young to older adults.

With ageing, there are multiple structural changes in the eye which cause functional constraints affecting the ability to maintain adequate postural control. There is typically a loss of visual field, a reduction in light transmission to the retina (causing an increase in visual threshold), a decline in visual acuity (caused by an increase in lens' stiffness, colour opacity, increased incidents of cataracts, and macular degeneration), and reduction in visual contrast sensitivity (which causes problems in contour and depth perception) (12). Many previous studies have demonstrated that age-related changes in visual information have undesirable effects on functional skills including postural control.

As humans age, the resulting reduction or alteration in the amount and quality of visual sensory information available to the motor cortex (2) is often associated with the deterioration in postural control . It is a common finding that the elderly exhibit significantly faster centre-of-pressure (COP) velocities, COP distances, and COP excursions in comparison with younger adults with the trend being exacerbated when eyes are closed (23). A study by Lord & Ward (23) found that under challenging conditions (standing on foam with eyes open or closed), vision, along with strength and reaction time, played a significant role in postural maintenance. It was concluded that up until age 65, balance control was significantly influenced by vision and that increasing sway areas in the oldest age groups (Over 65 years) were, in part, attributable to visual deficits effecting peripheral inputs.

Vestibular apparatus

Although we are not conscious of the vestibular sensation, as we are with other senses, vestibular inputs are important for the coordination of many motor functions. The vestibular organs are located in the inner ear and have a connection to the CNS. They contribute to the reflex activity necessary for effective posture and movement and provide information about the position and movement of the head with respect to gravity and inertial forces (24). In humans, our sense of equilibrium is facilitated by hair cells that line the vestibular apparatus of the inner ear. These hair cells are tonically active and synapse, via primary sensory neurons, to the vestibular nerve, in the vestibular nuclei of the medulla or run without synapsing to the cerebellum, which is the primary site of equilibrium processing (14). This vestibular sensory information has been shown on several occasions to be integral in the maintenance of upright posture.

Acute unilateral or bilateral loss of vestibular function has been shown to have devastating effects on postural control. This is particularly evident with ageing where there is a loss of 40% of the vestibular hair and nerve cells by 70 years of age which often leads to deteriorations in vestibular function. The extent of this disturbance, however, is often dependant on the ability of the nervous system to compensate for the loss of this important sensory input (24). This is due to the vestibular system functioning as a reference system for other sensory modalities (vision and somatosensory). Therefore vestibular sensory deficits can result in postural response alterations which give rise to a normal ankle strategy (24).

Although about one third of older adults suffer from disturbed vestibular reflexes, many studies have not found any effects on postural control (9, 23). The proposed reason for this lack of effect on postural control is that older people with adequate peripheral sensation and/or vision can compensate for reduced vestibular function. However, individuals with vestibular dysfunction experience conditions such as vertigo and nystagmus, suggesting that vestibular disorders influence postural control and that further research is required to better understand the vestibular contributions to the control of balance (25).

Proprioception

Proprioception is the afferent information that contributes to the sensation of muscle length and tension and segmental posture (joint stability). The sensory organs that are most commonly referred to as proprioceptors include muscle spindles, Golgi tendon organs, and joint receptors (14). Muscle spindles relay information about the muscles length and rate of stretch and are distributed throughout the belly of the muscle, while Golgi tendon organs are found in muscle tendons and transmit information regarding muscle tension or force. Muscle spindles provide sensory information by means of primary endings connected to the spinal cord via type Ia afferent fibres and secondary endings connected to the central nervous system via type II afferent fibres. The Golgi tendon organs send their impulses to the spinal cord via the Ib afferents fibres. Joint receptors are the third type of proprioceptor and are found in the capsules and ligaments around joints of the body. These receptors are stimulated by mechanical distortion that is experienced when the relative position of bones linked by flexible joints is changed (12, 14).

Proprioceptors provide the CNS with position and motion information with a reference to the supporting surface and is arguably the most important contributor to postural stability (25). Proprioceptive information from the ankle, regarding joint position in normal healthy individuals, has been said to be of principal importance in controlling standing balance (25).

Many previous studies have repeatedly found that with ageing, there are proprioceptive deficits including decreases in both cutaneous vibratory and joint sensation. These and other proprioceptive losses increase the threshold to movement detection and decrease postural stability (26). Age differences have been demonstrated when proprioceptive information was perturbed by means of tendon vibration of tibialis anterior and soleus muscles and were even greater when proprioceptive input needed to be reintegrated after the perturbation was removed (27). Doumas and Krampe (27) investigated adaptations and reintegration of proprioceptive information in young and older adults when undertaking postural tasks. Their results indicated that when inaccurate proprioception was introduced, AP sway path length increased. These increases were, however, comparable in both the young and older groups. What was different between the two age groups was the reintegration phase on restoration of a stable platform. In this stage, there was a sizable increase in AP path length which was greater in magnitude and duration for older adults. In another study, Kristinsdottir et al. (26) found that vibration sensation was the major determinant for postural control with those older adults that lacked intact vibration sensation exhibiting an increased high frequency sway compared with younger adults and those older with intact sensation. They concluded that the status of sensory receptors of the lower limbs were of the utmost importance for postural control in older people.

Motor outputs and ageing

The maintenance of upright postural control is not only reliant on effective sensory input but also the application of appropriate motor outputs. Both strength and power of lower limbs have been indicated as important factors in the control of balance, gait and preventions of falls and have traditionally been the focus of many papers in the ageing and postural control literature (4, 28). More recently however, there has been growing interest into the possible role that steady muscular contractions (usually termed steadiness) has on the control of posture (29).

Muscular strength
Muscular strength, or the amount of force a muscle produces, is a major contributor to the maintenance of posture. With ageing there is a decline in the strength of nearly all muscles of the body. However, in relation to lower limbs, strength declines at a steady rate of approximately 1–2% per year and it has been found that 20% to 40% of muscular strength is lost from the third to the eighth decade (30). Though, it is often seen that the major decrease in strength occurs after the fifth decade (31) which often results in modifications in functional tasks such as the control of posture.

It seems that muscle strength, as a musculoskeletal characteristic of postural control, is important in generating basic acceleration vectors to control posture. In both cross-sectional and longitudinal studies, lower extremity muscle weakness has been identified as a risk factor contributing to falls in the older populations (32). This has been shown to be especially true when considering muscles on the posterior side of the lower limbs. Kou & Zajac (33) conducted a biomechanical analysis of muscle strength based on a musculoskeletal model of the lower limb and reported that a 1% increase in knee flexors (KF) strength may result in approximately 0.9% increase in the maximum acceleration vector, while a similar increase in other muscles such as gluteus may have no such effect. It was also concluded that KF muscle strength is thought to have increased participation in both hip and ankle strategies to control posture. However, research has not examined whether the loss in KF' force has any impact on balance.

In a study by Lord et al. (32) it was shown that poor performance in two clinical measures of postural stability was associated with reduced quadriceps and ankle dorsiflexion strength. This suggests that in situations where there is a reduction in ankle proprioceptive inputs older subjects are more reliant on motor outputs such as muscular strength. In a similar study Daubney & Culham (34) it was found that the difference between fallers and non-fallers was muscular strength of the knee extensors and ankle dorsiflexors, which provides further evidence that the force generating capacity of lower limb muscles is important in the maintenance of postural control.

Power

Muscular power can be defined as the amount of force that is produced per unit of time and has been linked to the ability to control posture by many authors (4, 28). Generally, muscle power has been shown to decline at a faster rate than isometric muscle strength with age, at a rate of approximately 3.5% per annum, compared to the rate of strength decline of approximately 1.5% per annum (35). It has also been shown that power output can decrease by 50% or more from the third to the eighth decade (31).

Izquierdo et al. (4) examined the maximal and explosive force production capacity and balance performance in men of different ages. They found that the rate of force development was lower in older men compared with middle aged and was as much as 64% lower than young men. In both middle age and older groups the rate of force development (RFD) was significantly correlation with individual balance measures. It was concluded that ageing may lead to impaired postural control with a decrease in the speed of postural adjustments and that the decreased ability to develop force rapidly in older people seems to be associated with a lower capacity for neuromuscular responses in controlling posture.

Power output has also been implicated in the postural differences between fallers and non-fallers. Perry et al. (28) examined the difference between young and older people and between older fallers and non-fallers to assess if the history of falling is associated with strength and power output. Younger individuals were much stronger and more powerful compared to older people while there were significant differences between fallers and non-fallers. The fallers exhibited only 85% of the strength and 79% of the power of non-fallers. It was concluded by the authors that power output appears to be the most relevant measure of fall risk and its importance to postural control should be further studied.

Finally in a study by Bezerra et al. (36) in which they assessed RFD of the knee extensors and flexors in static knee extension and flexion and analysed the relationship with traditional COP and stabilogram parameters. Three groups of healthy volunteers, aged 18-30 (YG), 40-50 (MG) and 60-77 (OG) years, with 10 males and 10 females in each group, participated in the study. Results showed significantly lower RFD between OG compared with YG and MG in knee extensors and flexors. Both MG and YG were significantly better from OG in COP mean distance in AP direction and COP mean velocity in AP and ML directions. Moderate negative correlations were found between COP mean velocity in ML and the strength of the knee extensors and flexors in all posture testing conditions. It was concluded that higher RFD in the thigh musculature may contribute to better postural control performance. It was suggested that RFD be further examined for its validity as an indicator in postural control, particularly in the knee flexors.

Steadiness of force production

The ability to control force, termed steadiness (ST), can be understood as the magnitude of fluctuation in force when performing either isometric or anisometric (concentric and eccentric) steady contractions (37). Muscle steadiness has been examined in many different muscle groups and it has been reported that the upper limbs demonstrate a better control of force than do the muscle groups of the lower limbs. These findings have led to suggestions by some authors that individuals who experience an improved ST within lower limb muscle groups may also have difficulties in the performance of daily activities (29).

Available research has reported that the muscle steadiness is better maintained in young adults than older adults (37) and it has been suggested that both isometric and anisometric muscle steadiness may be limiting factors for older adults in performing daily tasks such as postural control (29). This line of thoughts seems logical because the maintenance of upright bipedal stance is another motor task requiring the capacity to control forces of the lower limb because of the continuous need to neutralize destabilizing forces. Despite this assumption, the potential association between the performance of daily activities and force fluctuations during isolated voluntary steady contractions has not been clearly shown.

Of the limited research that has been completed there have been some promising results. Kouzaki and Shinohara (29) investigated the functional significance of force fluctuations during voluntary contractions of the plantar flexors and postural sway during quiet stance. They found a positive correlation between the coefficient of variation (CV) of COP measures and CV of force during plantar flexion in both young and older adults. This correlation was only seen at contraction intensities of $\leq 5\%$ maximal voluntary contraction which corresponds to commonly seen muscle activity levels during quiet stance. In another study in our laboratory (38) it was found that in older adults moderate correlations existed between COP mean distance and root means square in anterior-posterior direction and steadiness at low contraction intensities of the plantar flexors, dorsiflexors, and knee extensors. Therefore further research should be conducted to verify whether ST of all four muscle groups of the lower limbs is important in postural control.

Strength ratio between agonists and antagonists

It has been emphasized in the literature that the Hamstring to Quadriceps Ratio (HQR) is of integral importance in the maintenance of knee joint stability and the prevention of knee injuries such as ACL ruptures or hamstring muscle tears (39). Previously it has been found that the HQR appears not to be affected by age in young individuals (12 to 17 years) and no differences in HQR have been reported across sport, gender or side of the body (39). However, very little investigation has been conducted on the age-related changes of the HQR in older populations and the possible complications that may cause in the everyday functioning of these individuals.

Just as the HQR has been proven to provide stability to the knee joint, the Dorisflexors to Plantarflexors Ratio (DPR) also has a potential functional role. It is common in the literature to highlight that strength of the lower limb musculature is a limiting factor in the maintenance of posture especially when considering the muscles acting at the ankle joint (34). Considering that there is a dynamic interaction between the ankle plantarflexors and dorsiflexors during functional task such as postural control, it is surprising that there has not been more in depth examination of the influence of these strength ratios in relation to posture and falls.

From the above information, it seems plausible that the balance between agonist/antagonist muscle strength may play a key role in knee and ankle stability and therefore functional tasks such as postural control. These roles seem to increase when the ankle joint is in the neutral position and when the knee joint angle approaches those angles commonly used in daily tasks such as posture. Therefore, the age-related decline in KF and plantarflexors (PF) strength may contribute to a lack of knee and ankle stability respectively, and eventually may compromise posture in an older population. To date, little research has investigated the HQR or DPR and their age-related changes in relation to postural stability. Whether the HQR and DPR are correlated with the ability to control posture, and whether and how this relationship is affected by ageing and/or training, has not been extensively examined.

However, of the few studies that have investigated the role of strength ratios of lower limb agonist/antagonist muscle pairs in postural control, there have been some interesting findings. In our laboratory it was found that there are significant age-related declines in quadriceps and hamstrings maximal voluntary contraction strength and HQR. An additional finding was that the HQR exhibited significant negative correlations with most stabilogram parameters. The authors concluded that a higher HQR may be associated with better postural control performance and suggested that the HQR should be further examined for its validity as a meaningful indicator in postural control, particularly in relation to ageing (40).

Postural control strategies and ageing

When standing in an upright position the COG is continuously repositioned via a flexible inverted pendulum about the ankles and is dependent on the effective control of the torques at the ankle, knee and hip joints (16). This COG fluctuation causes a COP drift away from the relative equilibrium point during the maintenance of stance (7). Such slow movements of the body are detected by the sensory system and integrated by the CNS and reflex pathways. These signals generate the commands necessary to drive the muscles involved around the lower limb joint, so that these muscles restore body balance (41). These postural control movements are often categorized into two discrete control strategies: either "ankle strategy" or "hip strategy" (41). However, other strategies have been hypothesised that highlight the role of knee joint dynamics and also the use of muscle coactivation around the joints of the lower limb (18). The strategy selected by individuals is based on sensory information, area of support, musculoskeletal characteristics, degree of freedom, task constraints, and particularly the age of the individual.

Ankle strategy
The ankle strategy was defined first by Nashner and McCollum in 1985 who characterised the human postural control system as a single-segment inverted pendulum (17). This strategy was said to occur when there was early activation of ankle joint muscles and then activation radiated in sequence to the thigh and then trunk muscles. Therefore, it is thought that the nervous system controls postural movement through activation of the ankle joint muscle groups, while keeping the knee and hip joints in a fixed position (17, 41). Keeping the knee fixed is not equivalent to keeping the knee muscles inactivated as torque is still needed from both the agonists and antagonists to maintain the constraint (17). Under this strategy, the aim is to keep the trunk parallel to the legs without changing the angle of the hip and knee joints, while at the same time the hip moment is regulated approximately proportional to the ankle moment (41). This strategy is mainly used in situations in which the perturbations to equilibrium are small, when the inclination angle is small, the area of support is large, and the support surface is firm (17, 41). The ankle strategy is also most commonly seen in young adults in comparison with older adults, who generally adopt a postural strategy termed hip strategy (42).

Hip strategy

The hip strategy has been categorised as the early activation of ventral trunk and thigh muscles, i.e., top down activation, and is related with the motion of the body as a double-segment inverted pendulum with counterphase motions at the hip and ankle joints (5). This strategy is more complex than the ankle strategy because the moments around the two joints are not simply proportional and require at least two independent sensory inputs. When a large disturbing force is applied to body segments, or the area of support is not wide enough to receive a sufficient amount of the ankle moment, the inclination angles of the body become so large that the ankle strategy may not be able to restore body balance. Therefore, near the body limits of stability, the nervous system regulates the joint moments using the hip strategy (5, 17, 41). This strategy has been reported to be highly effective in the maintenance of postural control and an efficient means of stabilizing body posture especially in older individuals (16).

The hip strategy is most often associated with older adults in comparison with young adults who utilize the ankle strategy more regularly (42). This over-reliance on hip strategy in older adults has been linked to degeneration in neural, muscular, and skeletal mechanisms leading to increased susceptibility to falls (16). Possible explanations for the greater hip strategy dependence seen in the elderly include inadequate torque production by ankle muscles and insufficient proprioceptive contribution from the distal lower limb and foot as a result of peripheral neuropathies (16).

Agonist/antagonist coactivation

The concept of coactivation (also known as co-contraction) of agonist/antagonist pairs around the joint of the lower extremity has only recently gained much attention. It has been found in past investigations that coactivation level is dependent on several factors. These factors include age, joint angle, and the muscle groups being investigated of which all may have an influence on the postural control strategy adopted (18).

Ageing may also have an influence on the coactivation level. Healthy young individuals produce the net torque at a joint by optimally scaling the activation of the prime movers and the concurrent activity of the antagonist muscles. In contrast, old adults generate the desired torque with a different neural strategy that involves a near complete activation of the agonist combined with a disproportionately heightened coactivation of the antagonist muscles. Changes in spinal reflex circuitry are the traditionally accepted mechanism that influences coactivation. However, recent imaging, EEG, microstimulation, and magnetic brain stimulation studies make the hypothesis tenable that, in conjunction with modulations of spinal circuits, cortical and possibly subcortical mechanisms are also responsible for the age associated changes in coactivation (43). It has been shown that during postural task and tasks that involve stepping the level of coactivation at the ankle joint is significantly increased in the elderly (19). This association is further enhanced when older adults have restricted visual feedback, narrow base of support, or are required to undertake dual cognitive tasks while maintaining posture (18, 19). It has previously been speculated that the elderly adopt this coactivation strategy in an effort to stiffen the ankle joint which helps to reduce excessive movements thus decreasing postural sway (19). Due to this adopted strategy it may be hypothesised that the relative strength ratios of these agonist/antagonist muscles may play a role in the degree of coactivation during postural tasks.

EFFECTS OF EXERCISE

The regression of the physiological process and functional performance with ageing has evident impacts on the quality of life of older individuals. Loss of strength, decreasing aerobic capacity and increased risk of falls are well-known consequences associated with the ageing process (23). As the aged population continues to grow, the development and implementation of cost-efficient and effective exercise interventions for the improvement of postural control and prevention of falls is of utmost importance. Research concerning exercise habits and lifestyle choices in older adults has produced strong evidence that exercise and other forms of physical activity can produce health benefits. Also, training studies involving resistance exercises (44), Tai Chi (45), electromyostimulation (46), and balance exercises (47) have shown that older adults respond positively to exercise and often produce enhancements in functional abilities and health variables.

Resistance exercise

A decline in muscular strength occurs with ageing and is often associated with the observable decline in functional performance. This lack of capacity by the muscle effectors to respond appropriately to disturbances is frequently linked to impaired postural control (9). It has been shown that systematic strength training can lead to considerable increases in lower limb strength and improvement in postural stability (44, 48). Ryushi et al. (48) conducted a 10 week resistance training schedule that was focused on strength development of the quadriceps muscle group. It was found that the quadriceps strength and the percentage limits-of-stability to the rear were increased, and the percentage change in the path length was decreased significantly with strength training. The authors concluded that strength gains in the quadriceps is thought to possibly enable accurate movement of the COG farther towards the rear, suggesting that strength gains have a positive influence on a person's perception of their postural control. Similar findings were shown by Hess & Woollacott (44) when they also conducted 10 weeks of high intensity strength training of the quadriceps, hamstrings, tibialis anterior, and triceps surae. After training, there were considerable improvements in strength, Berg Balance Scale, Timed Up and Go, and the Activities-Specific Balance Confidence Scale in the experimental group. These findings showed that strength training can effectively strengthen lower extremity muscles in balance-impaired older individuals which, in turn, results in significant improvements in functional balance ability and decrease falls risk.

Tai Chi exercise

Postural equilibrium requires proprioceptive acuity. It is well established in the literature that proprioception is impaired with age (42) and it has previously been postulated that this decrement in proprioceptive acuity makes it difficult for older individuals to detect changes in body position (49). Indeed, some studies have shown that diminished proprioception is a major contributing factor to falls in older populations (9). Exercise has been shown to have beneficial effects on improving a number of sensorimotor systems that contribute to stability

(9). Of the exercise modes available, it appears that proprioceptive exercises such as Tai Chi (TC) have a more beneficial effect on the proprioceptive capacity post training compared with bioenergetic activities such as resistance exercise or walking (49).

Tai Chi is a traditional Chinese exercise and has been used for centuries. It was originally developed as a form of martial arts, however now it has become popular among many older populations as a form of exercise to improve health and physical wellbeing. The basic exercise involved in TC is a series of individual movements that are linked together in a continuous manner and that flow smoothly from one movement to another. These elements incorporate the elements of postural muscle strengthening, balance, and postural alignment. The simple, soft, and fluid movements of TC are ideal for older people regardless of previous exercise experience. TC is performed in a semi-squat posture that can place a large load on the muscles of the lower extremities. The movements demand guided motions of the hip, knee, and ankle joints in various directions, requiring concentric, eccentric, and isometric contractions of the hip, knee, and ankle muscles (50). Tai Chi has been demonstrated to cause significant improvements in the neuromuscular and somatosensory systems which have particular importance in the performance of postural control and hence has become important in the areas of falls prevention and healthy ageing (51).

Several studies have examined the effects of TC interventions on balance control and the prevention of falls. In one such study, Voukelatos et al. (52) examined the effectiveness of a 16 week TC program with the aim of improving balance and reducing falls in a group of adults with age 60 years and older. It was concluded in that study that participation in TC for one hour per week over 16 weeks can prevent falls and improve balance in relatively healthy community-dwelling older populations. In other studies, there have been shown significant improvements in postural control and falls risks when undertaking shorter TC interventions such as 4 to 8 weeks (53) or 12 weeks (45). The positive effect of TC on postural control and falls prevention has also been studied for older practitioners of TC who have practiced for one or more years. In a majority of these studies, positive health outcomes directly or indirectly related to improved posture and falls prevention have been establish. For example, long term TC practice (minimum of 1.5 hours per week for at least 3 years) was found to improve knee muscle strength, body sway in perturbed one-legged stance, and balance confidence (51). In other studies that investigated the long term effects of TC practice in older adult population, it has been found that TC improves standing balance under reduced or conflicting sensory conditions (54), improves isokinetic knee extensor strength and reduces postural sway (55), and improves balance control, flexibility, and cardiovascular fitness (56).

Other types of exercise and interventions

Several other exercise modes have been examined in the past in relation to their effect on postural control in older populations. Of these exercise modes, most are easily implemented, cost effective, and simple enough to be conducted at home.

Electromyostimulation
Electromyostimulation (EMS) is a mode of training that induces a muscular contraction by the application of an external electrical stimulus on the muscle. The artificial stimulus evokes an action potential independent and different from normal voluntary contractions. Research

has suggested that EMS recruits different types of muscular fibres in a reverse order relative to normal voluntary contractions (57).

EMS has been considered an important tool in physiotherapy and rehabilitation and is increasingly used by post-injury and post-operation individuals. However, EMS has only recently been considered as a training methodology to improve strength and postural control in older adults (46, 57). Little is known about whether EMS training is effective in improving postural control. Of the little research that has been conducted, it was found by Amiridis et al. (46) that after 4 weeks of EMS training (40 mins per session, 4 sessions per week) there was a decrease in postural sway, greater ankle muscle EMG activity, greater stability of the ankle joint, and significant changes in the mean position of all three joints of the lower limb. Therefore further research should be conducted to clarify whether lower limb EMS training has a beneficial impact on postural control in older adults.

Balance training

Balance training is another coordinative exercise that has previously been utilised as a possible exercise intervention for the improvement of postural control. The inclusion of balance training in exercise programs appears to be important for older age groups and tailored balance training has been shown to improve postural stability (13). These exercise programmes, including low intensity strength and balance training, have improved the balance and reduced the fall rates compared with the controls. These finding are similar to that of Nagy et al. (47) who found that 8 weeks of balance training produced a significant improvement in postural control.

Inclusion of balance training has previously shown to be effective in substantially reducing fall rates and improving postural control in older persons. In a systematic review and meta-analysis of effective exercise for the prevention of falls (13), it was found that exercise could prevent falls and improve balance in older individuals and that greater relative effects were seen in programs that included exercises that challenged balance. The effect of exercise on postural control has been further highlighted in the publication, Frailty and Injuries: Co-operative Studies of Intervention Techniques (58) which, on prospective meta-analysis of individual participant data from eight trials, found a pooled estimate of a 17% lower falls risk from exercise programs that included balance training.

CONCLUSIONS

The human's ability to maintain upright posture is of the utmost importance and essential to everyday functioning of most people. To maintain this upright position the human body has to integrate several sensory modalities and produce appropriate motor responses to counteract internal and external perturbations. With ageing, however, there are many physiological degenerative processes that take place which reduce the effective control of posture. An effect of this diminished ability to maintain posture is often associated with falls and injuries. In an effort to reduce the incidents of falls and uncover those most at risk of postural control abnormalities, it is important to continue to develop appropriate postural control assessment techniques and optimal interventions for improving balance control. The evidence in the current literature indicates that appropriate exercise has a beneficial effect on the postural control. Amongst the training modalities that have been examined it appears that exercises that involve coordinative balance tasks, such as balance training and Tai Chi, are the most effective in delaying the age-related decline in postural control.

REFERENCES

[1]   Laughton CA, Slavin M, Katdare K, Nolan L, Bean JF, Kerrigan DC, et al. Aging, muscle activity, and balance control: physiologic changes associated with balance impairment. Gait Posture 2003;18(2):101-8.

[2]   Prieto TE, Myklebust JB, Hoffmann RG, Lovett EG, Myklebust BM. Measures of postural steadiness: differences between healthy young and elderly adults. IEEE Trans Biomed Eng 1996;43(9):956-66.

[3]   Levangie PK, Norkin CC. Joint structure and function: A comprehensive analysis. 3rd ed. Sydney: MacLennan Petty, 2001.

[4]   Izquierdo M, Aguado X, Gonzalez R, Lopez JL, Hakkinen K. Maximal and explosive force production capacity and balance performance in men of different ages. Eur J Appl Physiol 1999;79(3):260-7.

[5]   Runge CF, Shupert CL, Horak FB, Zajac FE. Ankle and hip postural strategies defined by joint torques. Gait Posture 1999;10:161-70.

[6]   Horak FB, Earhart GM, Dietz V. Postural responses to combinations of head and body displacements: vestibular-somatosensory interactions. Exp Brain Res 2001;141(3):410-4.

[7]   Collins JJ, De Luca CJ, Burrows A, Lipsitz LA. Age-related changes in open-loop and closed-loop postural control mechanisms. Exp Brain Res 1995;104(3):480-92.

[8]   Collins JJ, De Luca CJ. Open-loop and closed-loop control of posture: a random-walk analysis of center-of-pressure trajectories. Exp Brain Res 1993;95(2):308-18.

[9]   Lord SR, Ward JA, Williams P, Anstey KJ. Physiological factors associated with falls in older community-dwelling women. J Am Geriatr Soc 1994;42(10):1110-7.

[10]   Era P, Schroll M, Ytting H, Gause-Nilsson I, Heikkinen E, Steen B. Postural balance and its sensory-motor correlates in 75-year-old men and women: a cross-national comparative study. J Gerontol A Biol Sci Med Sci 1996;51(2):M53-63.

[11]   Winter J, Allen TJ, Proske U. Muscle spindle signals combine with the sense of effort to indicate limb position. J Physiol 2005;568(Pt 3):1035-46.

[12]   Porth CM, Matfin G. Pathophysiology - concepts of altered health sates. 8th ed: Lippincott Williams &Wilkins, 2009.

[13]   Sherrington C, Whitney JC, Lord SR, Herbert RD, Cumming RG, Close JCT. Effective exercise for the prevention of falls: a systematic review and meta-analysis. J Am Geriatr Soc 2008;56(12):2234-43.

[14]   Silverthorn DU. Human Physiology: An intergrated approach. 5th ed. Sydney: Pearsons, 2010.

[15]   Abrahamová D, Hlavačka F. Age-related changes of human balance during quiet stance. Physiol Res 2008;57(6):957-64.

[16]   Amiridis IG, Hatzitaki V, Arabatzi F. Age-induced modifications of static postural control in humans. Neurosci Lett 2003;350(3):137-40.

[17]   Kuo AD, Zajac FE. Human standing posture: multi-joint movement strategies based on biomechanical constraints. Prog Brain Res 1993;97:349-58.

[18]   Benjuya N, Melzer I, Kaplanski J. Aging-induced shifts from a reliance on sensory input to muscle cocontraction during balanced standing. J Gerontol A Biol Sci Med Sci 2004;59(2):166-71.

[19]   Melzer I, Benjuya N, Kaplanski J. Age-related changes of postural control: effect of cognitive tasks. Gerontology 2001;47(4):189-94.

[20]   Du Pasquier RA, Blanc Y, Sinnreich M, Landis T, Burkhard P, Vingerhoets FJG. The effect of aging on postural stability: a cross sectional and longitudinal study. Neurophysiol Clin 2003;33(5):213-8.

[21]   Guerraz M, Bronstein AM. Mechanisms underlying visually induced body sway. Neurosci Lett 2008;443(1):12-6.

[22]   Collins JJ, De Luca CJ. The effects of visual input on open-loop and closed-loop postural control mechanisms. Exp Brain Res 1995;103(1):151-63.

[23] Lord SR, Ward JA. Age-associated differences in sensori-motor function and balance in community dwelling women. Age Ageing 1994;23(6):452-60.

[24] Horak FB. Postural compensation for vestibular loss and implications for rehabilitation. Restorative Neurol Neurosci 2010;28(1):57-68.

[25] Lord SR, Sturnieks DL. The physiology of falling: assessment and prevention strategies for older people. J Sci Med Sport 2005;8(1):35-42.

[26] Kristinsdottir EK, Fransson PA, Magnusson M. Changes in postural control in healthy elderly subjects are related to vibration sensation, vision and vestibular asymmetry. Acta Oto-Laryngologica 2001;121(6):700-6.

[27] Doumas M, Krampe RT. Adaptation and reintegration of proprioceptive information in young and older adults' postural control. J Neurophysiol 2010;104(4):1969-77.

[28] Perry MC, Carville SF, Smith CH, Rutherford OM, Newham DJ. Strength, power output and symmetry of leg muscles: effect of age and history of falling. Eur J Appl Physiol 2007;100:553-61.

[29] Kouzaki M, Shinohara M. Steadiness in plantar flexor muscles and its relation to postural sway in young and elderly adults. Muscle Nerve 2010;42(1):78-87.

[30] Doherty TJ. Invited review: Aging and sarcopenia. J Appl Physiol 2003;95(4):1717-27.

[31] Izquierdo M, Ibanez J, Gorostiaga E, Garrues M, Zuniga A, Anton A, et al. Maximal strength and power characteristics in isometric and dynamic actions of the upper and lower extremities in middle-aged and older men. Acta Physiol Scand 1999;167(1):57-68.

[32] Lord SR, Clark RD, Webster IW. Postural stability and associated physiological factors in a population of aged persons. J Gerontol 1991;46(3):M69-76.

[33] Kuo AD, Zajac FE. A biomechanical analysis of muscle strength as a limiting factor in standing posture. J Biomech 1993;26(Suppl 1):137-50.

[34] Daubney ME, Culham EG. Lower-extremity muscle force and balance performance in adults aged 65 years and older. Phys Ther 1999;79(12):1177-85.

[35] Thomas GN, Tomlinson B, Hong AWL, Hui SSC. Age-related anthropometric remodelling resulting in increased and redistributed adiposity is associated with increases in the prevalence of cardiovascular risk factors in Chinese subjects. Diabetes Metab Res Rev 2006;22(1):72-8.

[36] Bezerra P, Zhou S, Crowley Z, Baglin R. Age-related changes in knee extensors and flexors rate of force development and its relation to postural stability. Paper preseted at the 14th Congress of the European College of Sport Science, Oslo, Norway, 2009.

[37] Laidlaw DH, Bilodeau M, Enoka RM. Steadiness is reduced and motor unit discharge is more variable in old adults. Muscle Nerve 2000;23(4):600-12.

[38] Bezerra P, Zhou S, Crowley Z, Baglin R. The relationship between lower limbs muscles steadiness and posture maintenance in older adults. Paper presented at the15th Annual Congress of European College of Sport Science, Antalya, Turkey, 2010.

[39] Gabbe BJ, Finch CF, Bennell KL, Wajswelner H. Risk factors for hamstring injuries in community level Australian football. Br J Sports Med 2005;39(2):106-10.

[40] Bezerra P, Zhou S, Crowley Z. Age-related changes in quadriceps to hamstrings strength ratio and its relation to postural stability. Paper presented at the Australian Association for Exercise and Sports Science Conference, Melbourne, Australia, 2008.

[41] Fujisawa N, Masuda T, Inaoka Y, Fukuoka H, Ishida A, Minamitani H. Human standing posture control system depending on adopted strategies. Med Biol Eng Comput 2005;43(1):107-14.

[42] Xu D, Hong Y, Li J, Chan K. Effect of tai chi exercise on proprioception of ankle and knee joints in old people. Br J Sports Med 2004;38(1):50-4.

[43] Hortobagyi T, Devita P. Mechanisms responsible for the age-associated increase in coactivation of antagonist muscles. Exerc Sport Sci Rev 2006;34(1):29-35.

[44] Hess JA, Woollacott M. Effect of high-intensity strength-training on functional measures of balance ability in balance-impaired older adults. J Manipulative Physiol Ther 2005;28(8):582-90.

[45] Choi JH, Moon J-S, Song R. Effects of Sun-style Tai Chi exercise on physical fitness and fall prevention in fall-prone older adults. J Adv Nurs 2005;51(2):150-7.

[46] Amiridis IG, Arabatzi F, Violaris P, Stavropoulos E, Hatzitaki V. Static balance improvement in elderly after dorsiflexors electrostimulation training. Eur J Appl Physiol 2005;94(4):424-33.

[47] Nagy E, Feher-Kiss A, Barnai M, Domján-Preszner A, Angyan L, Horvath G. Postural control in elderly subjects participating in balance training. Eur J Appl Physiol 2007;100(1):97-104.

[48] Ryushi T, Kumagai K, Hayase H, Abe T, Shibuya K, Ono A. Effect of resistive knee extension training on postural control measures in middle aged and elderly persons. J Physiol Anthropol Appl Human Sci 2000;19(3):143-9.

[49] Gauchard GC, Jeandel C, Tessier A, Perrin PP. Beneficial effect of proprioceptive physical activities on balance control in elderly human subjects. Neurosci Lett 1999;273:81-4.

[50] Xu D, Hong Y, Li J. Tai Chi exercise and muscle strength and endurance in older people. Med Sport Sci 2008;52:20-9.

[51] Tsang WWN, Hui-Chan CWY. Comparison of muscle torque, balance, and confidence in older tai chi and healthy adults. Med Sci Sports Exerc 2005;37(2):280-9.

[52] Voukelatos A, Cumming RG, Lord SR, Rissel C. A randomized, controlled trial of tai chi for the prevention of falls: the Central Sydney tai chi trial. J Am Geriatr Soc 2007;55(8):1185-91.

[53] Tsang WWN, Hui-Chan CWY. Effect of 4- and 8-wk intensive Tai Chi Training on balance control in the elderly. Med Sci Sports Exerc 2004;36(4):648-57.

[54] Tsang WWN, Wong VS, Fu SN, Hui-Chan CW. Tai Chi improves standing balance control under reduced or conflicting sensory conditions. Arch Phys Med Rehabil 2004;85(1):129-37.

[55] Wu G, Zhao F, Zhou X, Wei L. Improvement of isokinetic knee extensor strength and reduction of postural sway in the elderly from long-term Tai Chi exercise. Arch Phys Med Rehabil 2002;83:1364-9.

[56] Hong Y, Li JX, Robinson PD. Balance control, flexibility, and cardiorespiratory fitness among older Tai Chi practitioners. Br J Sports Med 2000;34(1):29-34.

[57] Bezerra P, Zhou S, Crowley Z, Brooks L, Hooper A. Effects of unilateral electromyostimulation superimposed on voluntary training on strength and cross-sectional area. Muscle Nerve 2009;40(3):430-7.

[58] Province MA, Hadley EC, Hornbrook MC, Lipsitz LA, Miller JP, Mulrow CD, et al. The effects of exercise on falls in elderly patients. A preplanned meta-analysis of the FICSIT Trials. Frailty and Injuries: Cooperative Studies of Intervention Techniques. JAMA 1995;273(17):1341-7.

In: Disability and Chronic Disease
Editors: J. Merrick, S. Aspler and M. Morad

ISBN: 978-1-62948-288-0
© 2014 Nova Science Publishers, Inc.

Chapter 18

UPDATES IN SELF-CONCEPT, SELF-ESTEEM AND SELF-WORTH IN CHILDREN WITH HEALTH CONDITIONS

Betty V DeBoer, PhD, MPE and Greta von der Luft, PT, MEd, PhD*
Department of Psychology, University of Wisconsin-La Crosse, La Crosse,
Wisconsin and Physical Therapy Program, MCPHS University, Worcester,
Massachusetts, US

The overall health and wellbeing of children is linked to their self-concept, self-esteem and self worth. There is a renewed interest in self-concept, self-esteem, and self-worth in children with different health conditions, which seems related to the World Health Organization launching the International Classification of Functioning, Disability, and Health (ICF). It is important to use a comprehensive approach when investigating self-concept, self-esteem, and self-worth in children with health conditions. First, it is critical to clearly define the terms self-concept, self-esteem and self-worth. Second, it is important to use an outcome measure that has been validated for use with the target population with health conditions. This creates a challenge when many measures are not fully validated on even their target population of children without health conditions. Third, it is important to consider the impact of personal and environmental factors on the development of self-concept, self-esteem and self-worth in children without health conditions to understand the development of these characteristics in typically developing children. In children with health conditions, body functions and structures, activity limitations and participation restrictions, as well as other personal and environmental factors will need to be considered to best understand how self-concept develops in this population. Once we establish factors that impact a child's self-concept, self-esteem and self-worth, we can better structure their environments and opportunities to help them develop healthy characteristics.

---

* Correspondence: Betty V DeBoer, Psychology Department, University of Wisconsin-La Crosse, La Crosse, Wisconsin, 54601, United States. E-mail: bdeboer@uwlax.edu.

INTRODUCTION

There is an increasing interest in self-concept, self-esteem, and self-worth in children with different health conditions (1-3). There are a couple factors related to assessment that could improve future research on self-concept, self-esteem and self-worth in children with health conditions. First, it is critical to define our terminology clearly (4-6). Second, it is important to consider the psychometrics of tools that assess these concepts when used on children without health conditions (4-6). Once the psychometric merits of the tools are established for children without health conditions, we can validate those tools for use with children with health conditions (7-9). With appropriate terminology and validated tools in place, future researchers can make more solid determinations of how children with health conditions may feel about themselves. These future findings can be made even more powerful if personal and environmental factors impacting children with health conditions are also evaluated (10-12).

Researchers, clinicians and educators are encouraged to review the self-concept, self-esteem, and self-worth literature involving children to further understand how these may be impacted by the child's personal and environmental characteristics (10-14).

This increased interest in self-concept, self-esteem, and self-worth seems related to the World Health Organization launching the International Classification of Functioning, Disability, and Health (ICF) (15). This model encourages using a holistic viewpoint to assess people with health conditions and to determine how these conditions may affect a person contexually by looking at both personal and environmental factors. Due to this push, many researchers are now more comprehensively investigating how health conditions affect people's views of themselves (16). The purpose of this chapter is to review the relevant terminology, the psychometrics of the most commonly used standardized paper-and-pencil measures as well as new measures, and what is already known about self-concept, self-esteem and self-worth in people with health conditions.

DEFINITIONS

There are no universal definitions of self-concept, self-esteem, or self-worth; however there are universal themes surrounding these terms. Self-concept is generally thought of as a global description of oneself. Self-esteem is widely viewed as how one evaluates oneself (4). Lastly, self-worth is frequently used interchangeably with self-esteem (17).

There are many concepts that are embedded within the term "self-concept." Self-concept is an organized collection of the thoughts and feelings concerning oneself that can govern behavior and adjustment (18). When considering one's own self-concept, one may or may not necessarily make comparisons between one's self and others (19).

Although related to self-concept, self-esteem differs in that it is how someone evaluates their own self-concept (4). That is, self-esteem is a summation of how good or bad one feels about oneself using one's characteristics and capabilities (20). This evaluation of self-concept is based upon the discrepancy between the actual and the ideal self as well as the attitudes of others (21). Thus, self-esteem refers to how people feel about their perceived worth as individuals and when compared with others (22).

Self-worth is the same as self-esteem and thus these terms can be used interchangeably without causing a change in meaning or definition (17). The authors will use the terms self-worth and self-esteem together for the remainder of this chapter.

MEASUREMENTS IN CHILDREN WITHOUT HEALTH CONDITIONS

In choosing a measure to assess self-concept, self-esteem, or self-worth in children without health conditions, the measure's definition of the construct as well as the measure's psychometric properties should be considered (18). The authors will review the most commonly used measures in the field. These are the Piers-Harris Children's Self-Concept Scale: Second Edition, the Coopersmith Measure of Self-Esteem Inventory, the Tennessee Self-Concept Scale: Second Edition, the Self Perception Profile for Children, and the Self Description Questionnaire-I.

The Piers-Harris Children's Self Concept Scale: Second Edition, (The Way I Feel About Myself) is a 60-item scale that asks whether children and adolescents agree or disagree with statements about themselves. Using these statements, the test developers created a six factor structure supporting the six domains which include freedom from anxiety, behavioral adjustment, intellectual and school status, physical appearance and attributes, popularity, and happiness and satisfaction. The Piers Harris scales have internal consistency scores that range from 0.60-0.93 and the construct validity is quite variable with almost half of the items loading on two different factors (23). Thus, it is unclear whether the Pier-Harris is actually assessing what it purports to measure.

The Coopersmith Measure of Self Esteem Inventories are three self-report questionnaires that measure how children, adolescents and adults view themselves. There are four domains including peers, parents, school, and personal interests (24). The internal consistency scores range from 0.87-0.92. The construct validity of this measure is not substantiated through factor analysis and concurrent validity (25). Thus, it may be questioned whether the Coopersmith Measure of Self Esteem Inventories examines the four domains that it states it is measuring.

The Tennessee Self-Concept Scales: Second Edition provides a 'self-picture' (4), of 'who am I,' and 'how do I feel about myself.' There are six scales including the physical, moral, personal, family, social, and academic/work scales with internal consistency scores ranging from 0.73-0.93 (26, 27). The test developers do not address the variable factor structure or update the construct validity information in the current version (27). These limitations decrease the psychometric support for use of the Tennessee Self-Concept Scales: Second Edition.

The Self Perception Profile for Children measures competence, self-adequacy, and self-perception in six scales including scholastic competence, social acceptance, athletic competence, physical appearance, behavioral conduct, and global self-worth with the internal consistency scores of the subscales ranging from 0.71-0.86. There are overlapping factor structures with variable factor loadings ranging from 0.33-0.82 (28). The low and overlapping factor loadings may indicate that the Self Perception Profile for Children is measuring factors other than those the test developer intended.

The Self Description Questionnaire-I measures self-concept with the understanding that self-concept is descriptive, evaluative, and multidimensional. There are eight scales including peer relations, parent relations, physical appearance, physical abilities, general school, reading, math, and general self with the internal consistency scores ranging from 0.80-0.90 (29). The test developers have done extensive research finding a stable and expected factor structure with low factor intercorrelations (6, 29). In summary, the Self Description Questionnaire-I appears to have better internal consistency and a more reproducible factor structure (6, 29) when compared to the Tennessee Self-Concept Scale (26, 27), Coopersmith Self Esteem Inventory (24, 25), and the Self Perception Profile for Children (28). The Self-Description Questionnaire-I demonstrates the greatest promise for use with children with health conditions; however additional research still needs to be conducted to validate this measure with various populations.

A new way of examining emotional, social and mental health is through the use of computer adapted testing (CAT) that relies on item response theory (IRT). The NIH Toolbox for the Assessment of Neurological and Behavioral Function (NIH Toolbox) and the Patient Reported Outcomes Measurement Information System (PROMIS) each have different tests that measure personal wellbeing. The NIH Toolbox measures emotion and cognition. The emotion domain consists of psychological well-being, social relationships, stress and self-efficacy, and negative affect. The domains for the PROMIS are under construction and will include mental and social health. There have been substantial psychometric studies on the PROMIS and the NIH Toolbox. While neither the NIH Toolbox or PROMIS are measures of self-concept, self-esteem or self-worth, both have promising psychometrics that could be helpful in studying aspects off children's wellbeing. For more information on the NIH toolbox, please refer to: http://www.nihtoolbox.org/Pages/default.aspx and for more information on the PROMIS, please refer to www.nihpromis.org

MEASUREMENTS IN CHILDREN WITH HEALTH CONDITIONS

Before a measure is used to assess self-concept, self-esteem, or self-worth in a different population than the one for which it was developed, it should be validated for use in that new target population (5). There have been a few studies which attempted to do this including a precursor to the Self Perception Profile for Children (7), the Self Perception Profile for Children (30) and the Self Description Questionnaire-I (8, 9).

There were two different attempts to validate the Self Perception Profile for Children for use with children with mild intellectual impairment (MID) (7) and with children with cerebral palsy (30). When the Self Perception Profile for Children was validated for use with children with MID, a different factor structure emerged than when it was used with children without health conditions and its internal reliability also changed (7). When the Self Perception Profile for Children was used with children with cerebral palsy, the test-retest reliability ranged from 0.56-0.75 for the different subscales (30).

There were two different attempts to validate the Self Description Questionnaire-I for use with children with MID (8) and with children with cerebral palsy (9). Both of these studies found good internal consistency for the different scales and the same expected factor structure found in children without health conditions (8, 9).

The Quality of Life in Neurological Disorders (Neuro- QOL) is a newer self-report measure that assesses the health related quality of life of children with neurological disorders (31). This outcome measure is evolving and utilizes CAT and IRT, similar to the PROMIS and NIH Toolbox. The domains for the Neuro-QOL include pediatric social relations and interactions with peers, and pediatric stigma. These domains have strong psychometrics and are still being expanded. The participants in the most current pediatric normative sample seem to only have the health conditions of epilepsy and muscular dystrophy; however, there are plans to increase the normative sample to include more health conditions. Although not a specific self-concept, self-esteem or self-worth measure, the Neuro-QOL promises to have application in studies looking to assess well being in children with many health conditions. For more information on the Neuro-QOL please refer to: http://www.neuroqol.org/WhatandWhy/Pages/default.aspx

In summary, the paper-and-pencil Self Description Questionnaire-I seems to have better psychometric properties when used with children with health conditions (8, 9) in comparison with the Self Perception Profile for Children (7, 30). Additionally, newer techology using CAT and IRT has resulted in the development of promising measures such as the Neuro-QOL, the PROMIS, and the NIH Toolbox which have substantially improved psychometrics over all former paper-and-pencil measures that assess self-concept, self-esteem, and self-worth. Although the NIH Toolbox, PROMIS and Neuro-QOL are not measures of self-concept, self-esteem or self-worth, they are promising measures that may be useful in studying the wellbeing of children. It should be noted that the majority of the articles references later in this article did not necessarily use self-concept, self-esteem or self-worth tools that were standardized on the populations they assessed. The findings, although interesting and often consistent with expectations, should be interpreted cautiously.

ICF MODEL

The ICF model provides a clear framework for research considering individuals with health conditions. Generally, health conditions are defined in terms of the specific impariment of body functions and structures, and concomitant limitations in functioning. These impairments may lead to activity limitations that then affect activities that the person would like to complete. The activity limitations, when combined together, may affect a person's life situation. All of these may be affected by personal factors and environmental factors. The personal factors may include gender and age while the environmental factors may include social attitudes and architectural environment (15).

Limitations in a child's body structures and functions are important in understanding a child (15) as these may impact the child's ability to care for their own personal needs and participate in greater society. Children who have health conditions that negatively impact their body structures and functions can be psychologically impacted by these differences (32). Some authors argued that researchers should assess functional independence in daily living tasks when assessing people with physical disabilities (33). The child's physical capabilities and performance are fundamental to the formation of physical self-concept, global self-concept (32), self-esteem and self-worth. Furthermore, the severity of physical disability affects how a child is treated by peers and society. For example, in cerebral palsy, if the physical disability is highly visible, the general population often assumes that the individual also has an intellectual disability and often treats the individual with cerebral palsy non-equitably (34).

Studies on children with health conditions should include control of, or information on, additional factors that may be relevant to that population. This review will highlight some of the more salient factors that may be helpful to consider in future research on the development of self-concept, self-esteem and self-worth in children without and with health conditions.

BODY FUNCTIONS AND STRUCTURES

The main hypothesis in a number of investigations was that the self-concept of children with cerebral palsy would be different from the self-concept in children without health conditions (1, 21, 35). Findings were variable with some researchers reporting differences in self-concept and others reporting none. Many studies have documented ways in which having impairments in body functions and anatomical structures negatively impacted children's self-esteem. For example, one study reported that children with hemiplegic cerebral palsy demonstrated lower self-esteem and self-concepts than did age and sex-matched peers (36). The authors of a meta analysis concluded that children with spina bifida reported lower self-worth, physical appearance, athletic competence, social acceptance, scholastic competence and self-concept than did children without health conditions (37). In another study, children in 3rd, 6th and 9th grades with minimal sensorineural hearing loss exhibited lower self-esteem than did children with normal hearing (38).

An important related factor to consider is the severity of impairment in body functions and anatomical structures in children. For example, severity of impairment was found to be important in boys with Developmental Coordination Disorder (DCD) (39). Boys with DCD reported lower self-concepts in physical abilities and in peer relations compared to the norms provided on the Self Description Questionnaire. Boys with more severe DCD rated their self-concept even lower for physical abilities. Further, boys with ADHD in addition to DCD reported lower self-concepts compared to boys with just DCD (39).

Not all studies noted differences in self-concept, self-esteem or self-worth based on severity of impairment. However, until we can articulate when severity is important and when it is not, future studies should control for, or at a minimum clearly report, each child's impairment in body functions and structures (12) as well as the severity of that impairment.

Actual performance of tasks or perception of performance can also impact how a child with a health condition develops self-esteem. For example, teachers of children with DCD and a learning disability estimated that these students had significantly lower academic self-esteem and lower self-reported physical and cognitive competence than did children without health conditions (40).

Intellectual functioning is an important aspect of human development. Children with health conditions vary in their intellectual functioning (41). As stated earlier, self-concept is generally thought of as a global description of oneself, self-esteem is generally viewed as how one evaluates oneself (4) and self-worth is often used interchangeably with self-esteem (17). All of these require that the child is able to reflect and, at times, make a judgment on the self. The formation of self-concept, self-esteem, and self-worth therefore rely heavily on the child's ability to understand and process the information that is available from social interactions (18, 42). Children with mild intellectual disabilities (MID) may not be able to reflect on how they perceive themselves in as sophisticated of a manner as do typically developing children (7). Intellectual deficits may also limit how well a child can report social comparisons, as required by most scales assessing self-concept (43), self-esteem and self-worth, thus affecting the construct validity of current tools (7). A final concern is that children with MID may not develop differentiated self-concepts at the same rate as do typically developing children (7). The authors found no studies on self-concept, self-esteem or self-worth in persons with greater intellectual impairment (e.g., moderate, severe, profound) perhaps due to the difficulty in assessing these characteristics appropriately in these populations (5, 7, 8, 44). Based on this summary, it is important to report on or control for intellectual ability when assessing self-concept, self-esteem and self-worth. Miyahara and Piek (19) also noted that it is important to identify additional co-morbid conditions such as learning disabilities, Attention Deficit Hyperactivity Disorder, Asperger's Syndrome, behavior problems and Autism in participants.

ACTIVITY LIMITATIONS AND PARTICIPATION RESTRICTIONS

Recent research on activity limitations and participation restrictions has highlighted the need to document these areas as they may impact a person's psychological well being (45). Studies have demonstrated that many children with health conditions have limitations in self-care, mobility, socialization (46) and activities of daily living (47) that may impact the child's psychological adjustment (45). Some studies reported that children with health conditions, such as cerebral palsy, report being involved in a range of leisure activities that they enjoy (48), however, there are frequently associated participation restrictions.

Children with health conditions may have participation restrictions in a variety of domains and for an array of reasons. Students with chronic physical health conditions are less able to attend school regularly (49). This restricts the child's ability to comprehensively fulfill the role of "student". The extracurricular and non school activities that children with health conditions participate in tend to be less structured and less intensive than the activities that children without chronic health conditions participate in (48, 50). Also, the activities are often more informal, require less skill, and are less community-based (48). Children with health conditions are therefore restricted in the variety of extracurricular and non school opportunities that are available to them and therefore have fewer opportunities to fulfill the variety of "social" roles available to children without health conditions. Even with fewer opportunities to engage in intensive activities, children with chronic health conditions sustain more injuries than do children without health conditions (51). When children sustain injuries, this further restricts their participation in activities. Additionally, these same children are more likely to live in poverty and receive fewer health care services (52). Injuries and poor health care access may further limit the child's ability to fulfill the "student" and "social" roles by limiting the child's access to school and friends. Cognitive and behavioral challenges, and parental stress serve as additional barriers to participation (48). In children with health conditions that do not present cognitive and behavioral challenges, motor requirements may be a barrier to participation with the most limited students having most barriers (53). Other barriers that were found to impact participation include low familial financial resources, single parenthood, lower parental education (54), negative social attitudes, unsupportive physical environments (50) as well as lower mastery motivation and less involvement with rehabilitation (48).

Assessment of a child's activity limitations and participation restrictions allows for a better understanding of the opportunities a child has to fulfill "student" and "social" roles and to develop positive self-concept, self-esteem and self-worth. Since participation in activities is related to positive self-concept, self-esteem, and self-worth in children without health conditions, it is reasonable to hypothesize that activity limitations and participation restrictions may be related to self-concept, self-esteem and self-worth in children with health conditions. Some children with health conditions have significant activity limitations and participation restrictions that may prevent them from fulfilling their social roles as "student" or "friend" in the same ways that children without health conditions are fulfilling such roles. Thus, their inability to fulfill their role as "student" or "friend" may negatively impact their self-concept.

PERSONAL FACTORS

Personal factors are within child variables that are important to consider when studying the development of self-concept, self-esteem or self-worth. Two personal factors, age and gender, have been found to be important in the formation of these aspects of growth. For example, self-concept evolves as the child progresses through childhood and adolescence. This process begins early in childhood (age 5 years) where the child's self-concept is often overly positive. The strong self-concept is perhaps due to their limited ability to evaluate actual competence and to accurately compare their abilities with those of peers (11). It is also possible that their strong self-concept may be due to their focus being on how much they have grown in that skill area rather than how they rank relative to other children. In middle childhood (age 8 years) their self-concept declines to more realistic levels. When children transition to middle school, their self-concepts initially decline but then start to increase into a more balanced representation of their capabilities in late childhood (age 12 years). As children enter adolescence and transition into high school, their self-concepts change again, becoming imbalanced with inconsistent assessments of their competencies (11). Self-esteem and self-worth follow similar patterns (17).

Gender is an important variable to consider when studying self-concept, self-esteem and self-worth as there are noted gender differences in these in children without health conditions. Gender differences among children without health conditions fluctuate according to age and school class type (co-ed or same sex) with the differences becoming less noticeable in same sex classes (55). Gender differences in global self-concepts have been studied heavily. In a metaanalysis and literature summary, the authors concluded that boys report a small but consistent advantage in self-esteem over girls. The effect size is similar to that reported in boys' math performance over girls'. Girls and boys have the largest discrepancy between the ages of 15 and 18 years. The authors noted that 92% of males and females overlapped in scores and concluded that the genders are still more similar than different (56). Less research has been conducted looking at all the domains in self-concept, self-esteem and self-worth. In kindergarten through second grades, girls report significantly lower self-concepts in physical ability, and higher self-concepts in physical appearance, reading and parent relations. The girls' physical ability self-concept domain difference increases with age during this period (42). In adolescence, females report lower physical abilities and physical appearance self-concepts compared to boys (13). Sahlstein and Allen (57) concluded based on their meta-analysis, that the impact of sex differences in cognitive, social and physical self-esteem development need to be studied further to explain the differences observed across time. Thus, from this brief synopsis, it appears that age and gender should be clearly reported and controlled for when investigating the development of self-concept, self-esteem and self-worth.

PERSONAL FACTORS IN CHILDREN WITH HEALTH CONDITIONS

The development of self-concept, self-esteem and self-worth in children with health conditions may be impacted by personal variables such as age, gender, intellectual impairment, body structures and functions and activity limitations and participation restrictions (3, 32). At this point in time, it is unclear if children with health conditions go through similar stages of development in these areas as do children without health conditions. It is possible that children with health conditions vary in how they develop self-concept, self-esteem and self-worth based on the severity of their impairment and subsequent restriction of participation. Studies on self-concept must clearly report and control for age to provide meaningful results.

It is also not clear whether or how gender affects self-esteem, self-concept (3) and self-worth in children with health conditions compared to children without health conditions. There is evidence that some differences do exist. For example, researchers provided initial evidence that there are gender differences in the development of self-concept in children with cerebral palsy when compared to their peers without physical impairment (3). Girls and boys with cerebral palsy were compared to matched peers (average age 11 years 8 months) without health conditions to see if there are differences within genders. Girls with cerebral palsy demonstrated lower social acceptance than girls without health conditions. Boys with cerebral palsy demonstrated lower scholastic competence than boys without health conditions. Both girls and boys reported lower athletic competence than did their counterparts without health conditions. Interestingly, neither boys nor girls with health conditions demonstrated lower global self-worth (3). Future studies would ideally report outcomes in global as well as specific areas of self-concept, self-esteem and self-worth to better illustrate the development of these characteristics.

ENVIRONMENTAL FACTORS

There are many environmental factors that have been investigated and that have shown promise to contributing to a child's development of self-esteem, self-worth or self-concept. The quality of the parent-child attachment relationship predicts many important behavioral aspects including aggression, social stress and self-esteem (58). Children with secure attachments to their caregiver demonstrate higher self-esteem than do those without secure attachments (59). Many researchers have demonstrated that child maltreatment is related to later low self-esteem in the victim (39). Other areas related to home environment are also being proposed or being investigated. For example, there is very preliminary research exploring the dynamics of siblings and birth order with some research stating that first born children have higher self-esteem (60) and some international studies not finding a difference between first and latter born children (60). Researchers have studied self-concept, self, esteem and self-worth in children dealing with parental divorce (62). Another interesting study (63) noted that self-reported parenting stress when their child was age 10 years, predicted the adolescent's self-concept at age 14 years. Goodman and colleagues (64) noted that maternal depression and paternal psychiatric status are risk factors that explain much variability in children's social and emotional competence. Researchers concluded from a meta-analysis that parenting impacts children's self-esteem (65). Multiple research studies support the idea that family environment plays an important role in the development of one's self-concept, self-esteem and self-worth (63, 65).

ENVIRONMENTAL FACTORS AND CHILDREN WITH HEALTH CONDITIONS

When investigating self-concept, self-esteem and self-worth, it is critical that the ecology of human development be considered (16). A child's developing self-concept, self-esteem and self-worth can be considered using Bronfenbrenner's Systems Model of Human Behavior. Each system influences the formation of the child's self-concept, self-esteem and self-worth either directly or indirectly. Moreover, these different systems provide a framework from which a phenomenological perspective can be established by assessing the different settings, people, relationships, and cultural and societal demands which occur to help form the developing self-concept of the growing child (10). We have reason to believe that many of the factors discussed above that impact children without health conditions would also impact children with health conditions. Unfortunately, little research has been conducted in those areas using children and adolescents with health conditions.

One salient environmental factor that has been discussed regarding children with disabilities is that of educational placement. Educational placement appears to play an important role in the development of self-concept in the lives of children with health conditions such as cerebral palsy (66).

Children with cerebral palsy and other health conditions may develop their self-concepts differently in a microsystem which includes attending a special segregated school for children with health conditions as opposed to attending an integrated school setting with exposure to children without health conditions (66). Children with cerebral palsy who attend a special school may initially develop a "big fish little pond affect" (14).When they reach adolescence and compare themselves to typically developing peers using their more honed abstract reasoning skills, however, their exaggerated self-concepts may plummet to levels lower than those in children with health conditions who attended an inclusive school all along (8, 14).

Unfortunately, if children with cerebral palsy attend an inclusive school they may develop lower self-concepts earlier in childhood. These lower self-concept levels may evolve as their concrete self-comparisons may be made to peers without health conditions who seem to be excelling in sports, academics, and social relationships (68). These lower self-concept levels may become resistant to changes as the child becomes older (11).

Far less in known about the impact of environmental factors such as attachment, parental mental health, maltreatment, sibling, birth order, urban vs. rural residence, divorce, and family environment specific to children with health impairments. It is likely that these, as well as personal variables known to impact children without health conditions, should also be given consideration.

In sum, the self-concept, self-esteem and self-worth levels of children with health conditions may be at risk simply because of their health condition and the resulting implications. Moreover, these differences may be heightened or diminished depending on the different systems and their respective processes and linkages such as home setting, presence of family members, school setting, and cultural influences (10). It is therefore important to report on and control for what is reliably measurable, and known to have an impact. The educational environment is one of those important environmental variables to report on when studying children with health conditions (12).

CONCLUSION

Parents, health care professionals, researchers, lay persons and educators strive to understand how to best develop positive mental well-being in children. The onus is on researchers to use current tools and knowledge to comprehensively investigate self-concept, self-esteem, and self-worth in children with health conditions to assist in this process. Several points are important to keep in mind. First, it is critical to clearly define the terms self-concept, self-esteem and self-worth. Second, it is important to use an outcome measure that has been validated for use with the target population with health conditions. This creates a challenge when many measures are not fully validated on even their target population of children without health conditions.

Luckily, the recent use of CAT has allowed for significant improvements in measurement. Measures such as the NIH Toolbox, the PROMIS, and the Neuro-QOL allow researchers, educators and clinicians to more accurately and comprehensively assess important characteristics in children.

Third, it is important to consider the impact of personal and environmental factors on the development of self-concept, self-esteem and self-worth in children without health conditions to understand the development of these characteristics in typically developing children. In children with health conditions, body functions and structures, activity limitations and participation restrictions, as well as other personal and environmental factors will need to be considered to best understand how self-concept develops in this population. Once we establish factors that impact a child's self-concept, self-esteem and self-worth, we can better structure their environments and opportunities to help them develop healthy characteristics.

ACKNOWLEDGMENTS

This work was partially supported by a University of Wisconsin – La Crosse Faculty Research Grant, a semester Sabbatical and a small grant for Dr. Betty DeBoer.

REFERENCES

[1]   Harvey D, Greenway A. The self-concept of physically handicapped children and their non-handicapped siblings: An empirical investigation. J Child Psychol Psychiatr Allied Disciplines 1984;25:273-84.

[2]   Schuengel C, Voorman J, Stolk J, Dallmeijer A, Vermeer A, Becher J. Self-worth, perceived competence, and behaviour problems in children with cerebral palsy. Disabil Rehabil 2006;28(20):1251-8.

[3]   Shields N, Yijun L, Murdoch A, Taylor N, Dodd K. Self-concept of children with cerebral palsy compared with that of children without impairment. Dev Med Child Neurol2007;49:350-4.

[4]   Butler B, Gasson S. Self-esteem/self-concept scales for children and adolescents: A review. Child Adolesc Ment Health 2005;10(4):190-201.

[5]   Byrne B. Measuring self-concept across the life-span: Issues and instrumentation. Washington, DC: Am Psychol Assoc, 1996.

[6]   Marsh H, Hattie J. Theoretical perspectives on the structure of self-concept. In: Bracken B, ed. Handbook of self-concept: Developmental, social, and clinical considerations. Oxford: John Wiley, 1996:38-90.

[7]   Silon E, Harter S. Assessment of perceived competence, motivational orientation and anxiety in segregated and mainstreamed educable mentally retarded children. J Educ Psychol 1985;77:217-30.

[8]   Tracey D, Craven R, Marsh H. Multidimensional self-concept structure for preadolescents with mild intellectual disabilities. Educ Psycholl Measurement 2006;66(5):795-818.

[9]   von der Luft G, Harman L, Koenig K, Nixon-Cave K, Gaughan J. Cross validation of a self-concept tool for use with children with cerebral palsy. J Dev Phys Disabil 2008;20:561-72.

[10]   Bronfenbrenner U. Ecology of childhood. Sch Psychol Rev 1980;9:294-7.

[11]   Harter S. The development of self-representations. In: Eisenberg N, ed. Handbook of child psychology. New York: John Wiley, 1998:553-617.

[12]   von der Luft G, DeBoer B, Harman L, Koenig K, Nixon-Cave K. Improving the quality of studies on self concept in children with cerebral palsy. J Dev Phys Disabil 2008;20(6):581-94.

[13]   Harter S. The self. In: Eisenberg N, Damon W, Lerner R, eds. Handbook of child psychology, 6 ed. Hoboken, NJ: John Wiley, 2006:505-70.

[14]   Marsh H. The big fish little pond effect on academic self concept. J Educ Psychol1987;79(3):280-95.

[15]   WHO. Towards a common language for functioning, disability and health. ICF: The international classification of functioning, disability and health. Geneva: WHO, 2002.

[16]   Llewellyn A, Cheung-Chung M. The self-esteem of children with physical disabilities-Problems and dilemmas of research. J Dev Phys Disabil 1997;9:265-75.

[17]   Harter S, Whitesell N. Beyond the debate: Why some adolescents report stable self-worth over time and situation, whereas others report changes in self-worth. J Personal 2003;71:1027-58.

[18]   Hughes H. Measures of self-concept and self-esteem for children ages 3-12 years; A review and recommendations. ClinPsychol Rev 1984;4:657-92.

[19]   Miyahara M, Piek J. Self-esteem of children and adolescents with physical disabilities: quantitative evidence from meta-analysis. J Dev Phys Disabil 2006;18(3):219-34.

[20]   Jambunathan S, Hurlburt N. Gender comparisons in the perception of self-competence among four-year-old children. J Genetic Psychol2000;161:469-77.

[21]   Arnold P, Chapman M. Self-esteem, aspirations, and expectations of adolescents with physical disability. Dev Med Child Neurol 1992;34:97-102.

[22]   Davis-Kean P, Sandler H. A meta-analysis of measures of self esteem for young children: A framework for future measures. Child Dev 2001;72:887-906.

[23]   Oswald D. Review of the Piers-Harris Children's Self-Concept Scale, Second ed (The Way I Feel About Myself). MentMeasurements Yearbook Database, 2004.

[24]   Peterson C, Austin J. Review of the Coopersmith Self-Esteem Inventories. Ment Measurements Yearbook Database, 2004.

[25]   Sewell T. Review of the Coopersmith Self-Esteem Inventories. Ment Measurements Yearbook Database, 2004.

[26]   Brown R. Review of the Tennessee Self-Concept Scale, Second ed. Ment Measurements Yearbook Database, 2004.

[27]   27,   Hattie J. Review of the Tennessee Self-Concept Scale, Second ed. Ment Measurements Yearbook Database, 2004.

[28]   Harter S. Manual for the self-perception profile for children. Denver, CO: Univ Denver, 1985.

[29]   Marsh H. Self-description questionnaire-I: Manual. Sydney, Australia: Self-concept enhancement learning facilitation, 1990.

[30]   Dodd K, Taylor N, Graham H. Strength training can have unexpected effects on the self-concept of children with cerebral palsy. Pediatr Phys Ther 2004;16:99-105.

[31]   Lai J, Nowinski C, Victorson D, Bode R, Podrabsky T, McKinney N, et al. Quality-of-life measures in children with neurological conditions: Pediatric neuro-QOL. Neurorehabil Neural Repair 2012;26:36-47.

[32]   Stein R. Physical self-concept. In: Bracken BA, ed. Handbook of self concept. New York: John Wiley, 1996:374-94.

[33]   Tam A, Watkins D. Towards a hierarchical model of self-concept for Hong Kong Chinese adults with physical disabilities. Int J Psychol 1995;30(1):1-17.

[34]   Hebl M, Kleck R. The social consequences of physical disability. In: Heatherton T, Kleck R, Hebl M, Hull J, eds. The social psychology of stigma. New York: Guilford, 2000:419-39.

[35]   Scholtes V, Vermeer A, Meek G. Measuring perceived competence and social acceptance in children with cerebral palsy. Eur J Spec Needs Educ 2002;17:77-87.

[36]   Russo R, Goodwin E, Miller M, Haan E, Connell T, Crotty M. Self-esteem, self-concept, and quality of life in children with hemiplegic cerebral palsy. J Pediatrics 2008;153(4):473-7.

[37]   Shields N, Taylor N, Dodd K. Self-concept in children with spina bifida compared with typically developing children. Dev MedChild Neurol 2008;50(10):733-43.

[38]   Bess F, Dodd-Murphy J, Parker R. Children with minimal sensorineural hearing loss: prevalence, educational performance, and functional status. Ear Hearing 1998;19(5):339-54.

[39]   Stern A, Lynch D, Oates K, O'Toole B, Cooney G. Self esteem, depression, behaviour and family functioning in sexually abused children. J Child Psychol Psychiatr Allied Disciplines 1995;36(6):1077-89.

[40]   Willoughby C, Polakajko H, Wilson B. The elf-esteem and motor performance of young learning disabled children. Phys Occupat Ther Pediatr 1995;14(3/4):1-30.

[41]   Odding E, Roebroeck M, Stam H. The epidemiology of cerebral palsy: incidence, impairments and risk factors. Disabil Rehabil 2006;28(4):183-91.

[42]   Marsh H, Craven R, Debus R. Structure, stability, and development of young children's self-concepts: A multicohort-multioccasion study. Child Dev 1998;69:1030-53.

[43]   Finlay W, Lyons E. Methodological Issues in interviewing and using self-report questionnaires with people with mental retardation. Psychol Assessment 2001;13(3):319-35.

[44]   Harter S. Special groups of children. The construction of the self. New York: Guilford, 1999:137-40.

[45]   Witt W, Riley A, Coiro M. Childhood function status, family stressors, and psychosocial adjustmet among school-aged children with disabilities in the United States. Arch Pediatr Adolesc Med 2003;157(7):687-95.

[46]   McDowell B, McDonough S, Kerr C. The relationship between gross motor function and participation restriction in children with cerebral palsy: An exploratory analysis. Child CareHealth Dev 2007;33(1):22-7.

[47] Msall M, Tremont M, Avery R, Lima J, Rogers M, Hogan D. Functional disability and school activity limitations in 41, 300 school-age children: Relationship to medical impairments. Pediatrics 2003;111(3).

[48] Majnemer A, Shevell M, Law M, Birnbaum R, Chilingaryan G, Rosenbaum P, et al. Participation and enjoyment of leisure activities in school-aged children with cerebral palsy. Dev Med Child Neurol 2008;50(10):751-8.

[49] McDougall J, King G, de Wit D, Miller L, Hong S, Offord D, et al. Chronic physical health conditions and disability among Canadian school-aged children: a national profile. Disabil Rehabil 2004;26(1):35-45.

[50] Imms C. Children with cerebral palsy participate: A review of the literature. Disabil Rehabil 2008;30(24):1867-84.

[51] Sinclair S, Xiang H. Injuries among US children with different types of disabilities. Am J Public Health 2008;98(8):1510-6.

[52] Porterfield S, McBride T. The effect of poverty and caregiver education on perceived need and access to health services amond children with special health care needs. Am J Public Health 2007;97(2):323-9.

[53] Donkervoort M, Roebroeck M, Wiegerink D, van der Heijden-Maessen H, Stam H. Determinants of functioning of adolescents and young adults with cerebral palsy. Disabil Rehabil 2007;29(6):453-63.

[54] Law M, King G, King S, Kerstoy M, Hurley P, Rosenbaum P, et al. Patterns of participation in recreational and leisure activities among children with complex physical disabilities. Dev MedChild Neurol 2006;48(5):337-42.

[55] Marsh H, Relich J, Smith I. Self-Concept: The construct validity of interpretations based upon the SDQ. J Personal Soc Psychol 1983;45:173-87.

[56] Kling K, Hyde J, Showers C, Buswell B. Gender differences in self-esteem: A meta-analysis. Psychol Bull 1999;125(4):470-500.

[57] Sahlstein E, Allen M. Sex differences in self-esteem: a meta-analytic assessment. In: Allen M, Preiss RW, Gayle BM, Burrell NA, eds. Interpersonal communication research: advances through meta-analysis. Mahwah, NJ: Lawrence Erlbaum, 2002:59-72.

[58] Yoon P, Ang R, Fung D, Wong G, Yiming C. The impact of parent-child attachment on aggression, social, stress, and self-esteem. Sch Psychol Int. 2006;27(5):552-66.

[59] Laible D, Carlo G, Roesch S. Pathways to self-eteem in late adolescence: The role of parent and peer attachment, empathy, and social behaviours. JAdolesc 2004;27(6):703-16.

[60] Gates L, Lineberger M, Crockett J, Hubbard J. Birth order and its relationship to depression, anxiety, and self-concept test scores in children. J Genetic Psychol 2001;149(1):29-34.

[61] Watkins D, Astilla E. Birth order, family size, and self-esteem: a filipino study. J Genetic Psychol 1980;137:297-8.

[62] Reifman A, Villa L, Amans J, Rethinam V, Telesca T. Children of divorce in the 1990s: a meta analysis. J Divorce Remarriage 2001;36(1-2):27-36.

[63] Putnick D, Bornstein M, Hendricks C, Painter K, Suwalsky J, Collins W. Parenting stress, perceived parenting behaviors, and adolescent self-concept in european american families. J Fam Psychol 2008;22(5):752-62.

[64] Goodman S, Brogan D, Lynch M, Fielding B. Social and emotional competence in children of depressed mothers. Child Dev 1993;64:516-31.

[65] Cedar B, Levant R. A meta-analysis of the effects of parent effectiveness training. Am J Fam Ther1990;18(4):373-84.

[66] Nadeau L, Tessier R. Social adjustment of children with cerebral palsy in mainstream classes: peer perception. Dev Med Child Neurol 2006;48:331-6.

[67] von der Luft G. Self concept in children with cerebral palsy. Dissertation. Philadelphia, PA: Temple Univ, 2006.

[68] Marsh H, Hau K. Big-fish-little-pond effect on academic self-concept: A cross cultural (26-country) Test of the negative effects of the academically selective schools. Am Psychol 2003;58(5):364-76.

In: Disability and Chronic Disease
Editors: J. Merrick, S. Aspler and M. Morad

ISBN: 978-1-62948-288-0
© 2014 Nova Science Publishers, Inc.

Chapter 19

DIGNITY AND WAR DISABLED VETERANS

Zdravka Leutar[*], PhD and Tihana Jašarevic, MA

Department of Social Work, Faculty of Law, University in Zagreb, Zagreb, Croatia

ABSTRACT

This chapter deals with an analysis of the concepts of dignity in disabled veterans of the homeland war. In the introduction we try to clarify dignity, defining the term on the basis of earlier research. Then we present an invalid of the homeland war, and finally we discuss the choice of qualitative methodology for doing research in this field. The aim of this study was to gain insights into disabled veterans' personal experiences and attitudes about dignity. An interview was conducted with 17 ex-soldiers during 2007, invalids of the homeland war and members of five different associations of war veterans in Zagreb and Varaždin. All interviewed persons had the status of war invalids with degrees of invalidity from 30 to 90%. On the basis of qualitative analysis of the interview results, six categories were formed: 1) social equality; 2) valorization of past experiences and personal contribution to the common good; 3) preservation of tradition and remembrance of the Homeland war; 4) social participation; 5) protective role of the State; 6) respect of basic human rights. Accordingly, a schematic model of relationships between these categories was made, showing how important involvement in society is for the disabled war veterans, since universal human dignity (Menschenwuerde) stems from social involvement.

INTRODUCTION

Human rights and human dignity are concepts that are inseparable and we can hardly consider them being two separate concepts. Human rights enter the domain of dignity assuming its existence, and vice versa – dignity is considered to be the domain of human rights, since in most cases the dignity of a person represents a group of rights that belong to that person; that is - when we respect some person's dignity, we respect the rights that belong to that same

---

[*] Correspondence: Prof. dr. sc. Zdravka Leutar, Law Faculty, Department of Social Work, University in Zagreb, Nazorova 51, HR- Zagreb, Croatia. E-mail: zleutar@inet.hr.

person. Accordingly, it is right to interpret dignity as a key category of human rights; as the basic human right.

Historically, the concept of dignity appeared in Ancient Greece when an attempt was made to differentiate a man from an animal according to man's ability to think (1). In Ancient Rome dignity was also discussed. It was connected to social ideas and considered to be based on social roles (2). In the Middle ages this concept was linked to personality (1). During the Renaissance period the concept of dignity was linked to the concepts of human identity, creative ability and a person's ability to influence his/her own life in the sense of doing good or bad (3). In the 17th century the concept of dignity was connected with the changes in relation to vulnerable social groups and was not linked to any particular social position, which was especially emphasized in the works of artists (4). According to European tradition, personality and individuality make one person unique and singularly (1).

In international law we find the appeals to human dignity, especially in its preambles. In the Charter of the United Nations from 26 June 1945 it is stated that "We the peoples of the United Nations determined ... to reaffirm faith in fundamental human rights, in the dignity and worth of the human person ... " Article 1 of the programmatic Universal Declaration of Human Rights adopted by the UN General Assembly on 10 December 1948 states (5): "All human beings are born free and equal in dignity and rights. They are endowed with reason and conscience and should act towards one another in a spirit of brotherhood." The preamble of The International Covenant on Civil and Political Rights (19 December 1966) (5) states that "... recognition of the inherent dignity and of the equal and inalienable rights of all members of the human family is the foundation of freedom, justice and peace in the world, recognizing that these rights derive from the inherent dignity of the human person ... " In the opening pages of the Constitution of UNESCO signed on 16 November 1945 we find this paragraph: "The Governments of the States Parties to this Constitution on behalf of their peoples declare ... That the great and terrible war which has now ended was a war made possible by the denial of the democratic principles of the dignity, equality and mutual respect of men ..." That the emphasis on human dignity was a "reaction" to the horrors and crimes of World War II is palpable in these texts. At the same time it is a decree (fiat) for the future to be modeled as deserving of man (6).

In Croatian language there has been one widely accepted definition of dignity given by professor Anic, which says: "dignity is an abstract noun that signifies totality of virtues which rouse respect" (7). Although correct, such a definition of dignity implies that the respect of a person simply means that we have a good opinion about that person, and we realize his/her qualities. Numerous studies of this "abstract noun" have made a step further from such an unilateral and incomplete definition.

Nordenfelt (8-10) conducted a research project on the dignity of older Europeans. He investigated a group of concepts of human dignity and, on the basis of that research, he presented four forms of human dignity and the differences between them.

The first form of dignity he calls "dignity according to credits". Here we find a concept of dignity that depends on a social rank and position, in other words, a particular hierarchy in the society. Because of the dependency on the social hierarchy, this form of dignity appears in different degrees and many varieties, being very unevenly distributed between human beings. Generally, we distinguish two varieties of this type of dignity: so-called formal and informal forms. The formal form of dignity can be inherited or gained through profession or social status; we may say that this is the variety from which certain rights originate - namely, the rights closely connected to that particular social position, which should be respected by other members of society. Somewhat different, the informal form of dignity represents the concept where people gain respect according to their personal accomplishments, in other words, their deeds.

The second form of dignity is called "dignity of moral or existential greatness" and is the result of a person's moral deeds, the deeds that do not bring any private profit or personal rights to that person. In that sense, this form of dignity can be reduced or lost through immoral deeds of an individual. This variety is similar to the first one in the sense of being unevenly distributed between human beings and in different degrees. It is closely connected to the ideas of dignified character and dignity as a virtue. To have dignity in this sense means to have specific moral standards.

The third form of dignity is called "dignity of identity" and is closely connected with the integrity of the body and mind of a person and often, although not always, depends on the picture that a person has about himself/herself as a human being. This is a dignity that people possess as complete and independent persons, persons with their past and future and their personal relationships with other people. This form of dignity can occur, but also disappear, as a result of changes in a person's body and mind. The main characteristic of this form of dignity is that it can be taken away from a person by various external events such as accidents, other people's treatment, diseases and the process of aging. A person with a disability is a person with reduced and limited independence and autonomy and, often, a drastically changed identity and sense of dignity. And, although the majority of people have some basic respect of their own identity in spite of possibly negative moral or foreign standpoints, this form of dignity can be easily destroyed by cruel or dishonest behaviour of other people.

Although each is different, those three forms of dignity have two characteristics in common: they belong to people in different degrees; and they may be won, received or appear but they may also be lost and disappear.

The fourth form of dignity is the one that is completely different from the first three. It is called "universal human dignity" or "Menschenwürde". This is the form of dignity belonging to all human beings and cannot be lost during their lives. This dignity is possessed by everyone, or at least assumed to be so, as the result of simply being humans. This form of dignity is a specific human value and belongs to everyone in the same proportion and with the same respect. A characteristic is that it cannot be taken away from a person while he/she lives. It is this form of dignity that is the one referred to as "birthright" in the Universal Declaration of Human Rights.

Although defined as something "abstract", dignity is more than an everyday phenomenon, state or feeling. In transactional models of stress, according to which both an individual and his/her environment have equal influence on the stress, we observe dignity as a phenomenon that is affected by the environment (external valuation), the variables connected to an individual (internal valuation), and the interactivity between an individual and the environment (interactive valuation).

Consequently, dignity depends on how others see us and treat us and on the way we see ourselves. This implies that human dignity can be supported and respected in two ways – internally and externally. All of this also makes dignity dependent on the interactivity of individuals with the environment. According to this view, persons will experience the feeling of inner value only when they see themselves and treat themselves with dignity and self-respect. But if only inner valuation of inner values exists, others would not be able to recognize dignity. And vice versa: if only external valuation existed, it would be difficult to evaluate how persons see themselves, internal valuation. Thus the importance of all three types of valuation - all three being necessary and vital for understanding the concept of dignity (11).

Subsequently, it is justifiable to conclude that dignity is more than a part of everyday social life, equally influenced by everyday external, relational and internal influences and events that are constantly going on around every individual. A too narrow view of influences may be the reason why the concept of dignity is so frequently used in too simplified a manner, and with no true perception of its real meaning and influence on human lives. Although the influences that support or, on the contrary, reduce dignity are different according to particular categories and populations of people, the majority of qualitative research on dignity is unanimous about the effects that respect or lack of respect have on persons.

Miller and Keys (11), in their research on the dignity of homeless people, presented results that show how showing respect for one's dignity, treating one another with dignity, and being in an environment that generally supports dignity results in better self-respect among the people who live there, better motivation for taking control of one's life, and feelings of satisfaction and happiness. And the opposite is also documented - showing no respect for another's dignity results in anger, depression and feelings of unworthiness. Anderberg and associates (1) analyse the concept of dignity in the context of care for the aged and state five essential dimensions: individual care, respect, support, advocacy, sensitive listening.

Other research conducted on other types of populations similarly showed that the results of showing or not showing respect for one's dignity are a common denominator for almost all categories of people (12-16). To recognise someone's dignity means to recognise his or her value as a human being, regardless of his or her social status or social role. Dignity is a key aspect of humanity; it is a part of the wholeness of who we are, not of what we have or own (11). Social stigmas, stereotypes and prejudice against any individual or social group create one form of degradation and inhuman conditions of life that may threaten the dignity of these persons or social groups and, at the same time, reduce and destroy the possibility for them to be seen or to see themselves as worthy human beings (17).

Research connected with the dignity of war veterans from the Home Defense Regiments is rare, and approaches to the databases about them usually result in finding numerous studies connected with PTSP syndrome. This is why we, in this study, are going to approach this specific population of the defenders in the Croatian Homeland War from another aspect to analyse the concept of their dignity.

In the Legislation about the rights of Croatian veterans from the Homeland war and the members of their families (Article 5), we find a legal definition of this population: "Croatian war invalid from the Homeland war is a Croatian soldier-defender from the Croatian Homeland war whose organism is damaged at least 20% due to a wound or injury that was caused during the defending of sovereignty of the Republic of Croatia, or during imprisonment, as being imprisoned either in a prison or in the enemy's camp during the Homeland war. Croatian war invalid is also a Croatian soldier-defender from the Homeland war whose organism is damaged at least 20% due to a disease, and that disease, its occurrence or its progression must be the direct consequence of participation in the defence of sovereignty of the Republic of Croatia during the Homeland war" (18).

Invalids of the Homeland war represent a specific population in the sense that they really are invalids, persons with disabilities because of being in the military and war, not because of birth or civil accidents. These characteristics of "war" and "military" are the ones that differentiate them from other persons with disabilities, and that carries numerous implications for almost all aspects of their lives. The causes of their invalidity are different because of the fact that they, soldiers and warriors, were seriously wounded and became disabled almost overnight.

Every person is a unique integration of biophysical and psychological characteristics, consisting of personal identity, individuality and personality. Thus it is logical that every injury of the physical integrity of a person necessarily results in the injury of psychological integrity as well (19). We have to accentuate that most of these persons, even before their wounding, had passed through numerous stressful and traumatic events; the wounding itself was only the last in a series of traumatic events. Due to such circumstances these individuals, apart from their physical/corporal injuries, have many psychic/mental injuries caused by the traumatic events of the war - they had to fight for their own lives and/or the lives of their war companions/fellow soldiers (20).

Thus far, the research about the population of the invalids of the Homeland war has been mostly conducted to define their number, their structural and demographic characteristics, their rights, and the finances spent for their cause. In most cases these research projects are quantitative, e.g., statistics, percentages and other figures. With this emphasis, the inner life of these invalid persons is ignored as is the way they see the society in which they live. The whole field of their personal experiences is neglected including the way they perceive themselves and evaluate how their environment treats them.

One of the basic characteristics of a qualitative approach is that it is conducted in natural life situations, while effort is made to gain complete insight into the investigated surroundings. The aim of such an approach is to make a detailed study of the perception of the people who participate in the research and, from their patterns, to give preference to the intentional ones,

e. g., informed persons. Qualitative methods are based on the analysis of textual material obtained on the basis of personal experiences, life stories, individual and group interviews, observance and other documents that equally describe both everyday and exceptional moments relevant to the life of an individual (21).

These kinds of qualitative studies of the population of the invalids of the Homeland war are a completely neglected field of scientific research although the numeric growth of persons with disabilities continued during the post-war period. Qualitative studies that take into consideration the personal experiences of war invalids are necessary for enlightening their real state of being, their status, and their degree of content or discontent. The concept of dignity as the key human right is mentioned in our society only declaratively, because no relevant studies in that field exist. Research on stigma and discrimination most often studies the general attitudes of the public and neglects the personal and subjective experiences of the very people who face stigma from others in their everyday lives.

The aim of this research was to get an insight into the personal experiences and attitudes about dignity of veterans who are invalids. According to that aim, the following problem was stated: to define what the dignity means to the invalids of the Homeland war.

OUR STUDY

The research was conducted during November 2007, using the method of a half-structured interview. Seventeen defenders from the Homeland war with the status of Croatian war military invalids were questioned. The research started in the Association of Vukovar Defenders from Zagreb and with their help and agency, we continued the research with other five associations: the Association of Croatian Volunteers and Veterans of Homeland war, the Association of Homeland war Participants, the Members of 150th brigade, the Association of Croatian Volunteers of Homeland war, the Association of the Defenders – Camp Imprisoners from the City of Zagreb and its surroundings, and a branch of HVIDR- (Croatian Homeland War Veterans Association) in Varaždin.

The defenders were ready and willing to participate in this research. Before the interview started, the research topic and aim had been explained, in detail, to all participants and, after confidentiality and anonymity were guaranteed, all the participants agreed to having the interview recorded.

The interview was conducted on the basis of a previously prepared set of questions, which were modified according to the course of an interview. Every interview lasted, on average, for 15 minutes. Interviews were taped and, afterwards, literally copied into a textual form.

Participants in the research

Seventeen defenders from the Homeland war with the status of Croatian war military invalids participated in the research. The degree of their invalidity/disability ranged from 30% to 90%: two participants had 30% invalidity/disability, two 40%, four 50%, five 60%, three 70%, and one participant with 90%.

The average age of the participants was 47 years. Their age ranged from 37 to 65 years. Eleven participants finished secondary school; all had worked actively before the war at different working places (four policemen, one bank account officer, one computing technician, one craftsman, a couple of qualified workers and one manager). Six of them had graduated at the university and they also had different professional profiles: one participant had finished two college programs and was studying for a master's degree at the time of the interview; one had a master of sciences; also among them was one academic painter, a lawyer, an economist and a policeman. Sixteen participants were pensioned; only one was actively working.

Fifteen participants were married, one was divorced, and one single. One participant had no children; the other 16 have children as follows: 10 with two children, five with one, and one with three children. Fourteen participants have their own place for living, three still have a housing problem (one lives as a subtenant at his friend's place, one in a municipal flat and one is on the waiting list for a flat for veterans). Among the 17 participants, nine stated that they were satisfied with their financial income, five were not completely satisfied, and three felt completely unsatisfied.

Data analysis

For the data analysis we used a method of open coding that consisted of the following steps (22):

1. Applying terminology to empiric material;
2. Grouping similar terms into categories;
3. Analysing the meaning of terms and categories.

We now provide an example of the way the collected data were organised according to the above mentioned steps. The numbers in the brackets represent the participants in the interview who made the statement.

Table 1. Applying terminology to empiric material and grouping similar terms into categories according to the level of abstraction

Participants' statements about personal perception of the concept of dignity	LEVEL II	LEVEL III
Normal way of life... all those factors that make normal functioning in every day life possible for a man... one normal contact man-to-man... (1) ...to treat me like a person (4) ...to let us alone, everybody... I want them to let us live our life... let finally things flow their way (5) That I can work and live normally... normal relations (6) ...live and work normally... (16) ...normal relationship... (17) ...that incongruous relations would not exist... equality with all other citizens (9) Normal human relationship... fair man-to-man relation (11) To be respected as a man, without privileges and priority status... normal relationship (12)	- normal way of life - equality	- social equality
Means that no one offends his personality, his person, does not underestimate him... behaviour with owing respect in the sense of pure respect of personality and individuality of every person (1) ...that no one devaluates me and tells what is not true about who I am and what I have been through... (11) ...that somebody respects me... situations where one respects the other... situations where there exists mutual respect of attitudes, acts, opinions, jobs and activities done (4) ...just respect and mutual esteem as for any other person (17) ...not to be humiliated... I want just to be respected as a human being, receive the recognition for what I had passed through, and that will bring me dignity and moral satisfaction (16)	- respect - recognition	- valorisation of past experiences and contributions

Table 2. Applying terminology to empiric material and grouping similar terms into categories according to the level of abstraction

Participants' statements about personal perception of the concept of dignity	LEVEL II	LEVEL III
Normal way of life… all those factors that enable man to function normally in every day life… one normal contact man-to-man… (1) …to treat me like a person (4) …to let us alone, everybody… I want them to let us live our life… let finally things flow their way (5) That I can work and live normally… normal relations (6) …live and work normally… (16) …normal relationship… (17) …that incongruous relations would not exist… equality with all other citizens (9) Normal human relationship… fair man-to-man relation (11) To be respected as a man, without privileges and priority status… normal relationship (12)	- normal way of life - equality	- social equality
Means that no one offends his personality, his person, does not underestimate him… behaviour with owing respect in the sense of pure respect of personality and individuality of every person (1) …that no one devaluates me and tells what is not true about who I am and what I have been through… (11) …that somebody respects me… situations where one respects the other… situations where there exists mutual respect of attitudes, acts, opinions, jobs and activities done (4) …just respect and mutual esteem as for any other person (17) …not to be humiliated… I want just to be respected as a human being, receive the recognition for what I had passed through, and that will bring me dignity and moral satisfaction (16) Respect and recognition of what I had passed through all together with the others … respect, not to be insulted (15) Paying respect… that people respect you due to the fact that you are an invalid as a result of what you had done for our people, for the country, for all of them (2) Recognition of all my deeds and decisions … what we had done for this society should be revered (3) That my environment respects me in a way… to take into consideration a bit more everything I had been through… to treat my war experience with more reverence… that people respect and appreciate us just a little (5) …the fact that if it had not been for us, this state would not exist should be respected… to acknowledge that my invalidity is due to the war, the fight for the establishment of this country (6) …to acknowledge just one thing – that we, at a given moment, helped everybody to live better yesterday and today (13) …that the state and the rest of society thank us for our courage (10) …valorisation of what I had done… to show gratitude to the defenders and appreciate their contribution, and that way, valorisating them… society should treat us well and appreciate our deeds (8) …some moral satisfaction… that people do not speak about the contribution I made in creation of this country in a sneering manner, underestimating me (9) …our status should be recognized, and we claim the right on it as moral satisfaction (13) …how the others behave is important to me, it is important for my personal moral satisfaction (15) …I want only to be respected as a man, I want recognition of what I had been through, and that will bring me dignity and moral satisfaction (16) …dignity of us, war invalids, we can observe from material and spiritual, moral side (17)	- respect - recognition	- valorisation of past experiences and given contributions

Participants' statements about personal perception of the concept of dignity	LEVEL II	LEVEL III
	- gratitude - moral satisfaction	
...we should not let some things that happened in the Homeland war become forgotten... by preserving tradition and remembrance on what happened (2) ...we have to be active, working on keeping remembrance on those who gave their lives, were wounded and left their health in war (3) ...the past should not be forgotten... preserving tradition and remembrance on those who gave their lives (8)	- preserving tradition - keeping remembrance	- preserving tradition and remembrance of the Homeland war
That participation in socialization and in society in general would be as easy and as accessible as possible... so that a man could be a real participant and member of that society (2) ...help the defenders to get more easily integrated into today's society (13) ...not to ignore us... not to take us into their settings and install us as representatives of something... to have our place in society (7) ...to acknowledge us as a part of society, namely its vital part (11) ...we should stay active as long as possible, keep working activity... to feel we are socially efficient (9) ...that people get their place within society... to have something to do in your life... to be given an opportunity and satisfaction to be activated within society... (10) ...not only material rights of a man are important... here is a wish to work, to feel useful, to feel that he contributes to the society and family (16)	- position in society - working activity - social efficiency	- social participation
...to provide real care to real invalids... that society makes attempt to re-socialize us... that the society helps us to try to function best we can [4] ...State institutions that should protect us from all that... local administration should take care about their defenders and help them... all those people, who came out of an extremely difficult situation, should be taken care of (8) ...procedures of the State... to give help to those who can survive and work... to assist us in finding job (10) The State should give instructions to those who do not know where to go and what to do... that the State helps us in a realisation of our rights and alleviates our suffering while gaining or verification of those rights (12)	- help and support of the society - help and support of the State	- protective role of the State
The right to health... the right to work... the right to all Constitutional categories contained in the Constitution (2) ...to respect the rights of every person no matter of age, sex, religious or national determination (9) ...is the most important part of a person (11) ...not to be maltreated... not to be proscribed... to think freely, to work and act, and that your deeds (if their motto is right) are not convicted (13) ...something that belongs to every person and what every man should have if he wants to feel as a human being... there is no bigger right (15) ...something that man carries in his soul... something that makes man a man... all man's emotions, honesty, education... the wholeness of existence... (17)	- legal and Constitutional rights - a part of person that cannot be taken away	- respect of basic human rights

DISCUSSION

By qualitative analysis of the conducted interviews we have data that provide insight into personal concepts of dignity from these Homeland war veterans themselves and their experiences and thoughts about their own position and status in society. From these data we also extracted discoveries about protective factors that help the Homeland war invalids in every day life and their vision of the future.

The meaning of dignity for invalids of homeland war

To get a better insight into the personal comprehension of the concept of dignity from the Homeland war invalids themselves, we asked them the following question: "What does the concept of dignity mean for you personally?". By analysing the participants' answers, we name six different categories.

Social equality

What is primary to the Homeland war invalids for experiencing dignity and feeling that they are the persons whose dignity is respected, is social equality. Although included in numerous international documents and national programs of the Republic of Croatia, the category of social equality is usually defined as equality in the rights of different kinds. This is essentially different from the Homeland war invalids' personal attitudes. For them, social equality primarily includes a normal way of life ("…Normal way of life… all those factors that enable man to function normally in every day life… one normal contact man-to-man… (1)"; That I can work and live normally… normal relationship (6)"; "…to live and work normally… (16)"; "…normal relations… (17) "and, after that, equality in sense of proper relationships and human conduct from the side of the others ("…that incongruous relations do not exist… equality like for all other citizens (9)"; "…Normal human relationship… fair relations like man-to-man (11)"; "To be respected as a man, without privileges and priority status… normal relationship" (12).

Valorisation of past experience and given contributions

Literally, valorisation means to increase or hold someone's value, to respect or positively estimate somebody or something. In that sense, invalids of the Homeland war claim the valorisation of traumatic war experience and the contributions they gave as defenders for their country to be the crucial category of dignity. That valorisation is expressed through respect people show to them in their environment ("…that somebody respects me… situations where one respects the other… situations where there exists mutual respect of attitudes, acts, opinions, jobs and activities done (4)."; "… just respect and mutual esteem as for any other person (17)"; " not to be humiliated… I want just to be respected as a human being, receive the recognition for what I had passed through, and that will bring me dignity and moral satisfaction" (16)), recognition of the past experiences ("...Respect and recognition of what I had passed through all together with the others ... (15)"; " Recognition of all my deeds and decisions (1)"; "... to acknowledge just one thing – that we, at a given moment, helped everybody to live better yesterday and today (13)") and showing due respect for courage and deeds that were done during the war ("...that the state and the rest of society thank them for courage (10)"; "...valorisation of what I had done... to show gratitude to the defenders and appreciate their contribution, and that way, valorisating them... society should treat us well and appreciate our deeds (8)"). Apart from respect, recognition and gratitude, through which valorisation is being expressed, another important part of that valorisation is the moral satisfaction of war invalids ("...how the others behave is important to me, it is important for my personal moral satisfaction (15)"; "...I want only to be respected as a man, I want recognition of what I had been through, and that will bring me dignity and moral satisfaction (16)"; "...some moral satisfaction... that people do not speak about the contribution I made in creation of this country in a sneering manner, underestimating me (9)").

Similar to the data collected by analysing the Homeland war invalids' answers are data that had been collected by research with Vietnam veterans. The soldiers who came back from the war in Vietnam are always very sensitive to the level of support they get from society, especially immediately after their return (23-26). All the research has shown how important it is for all war veterans to find and get some kind of public recognition, both in the form of a moral attitude of the community and in the form of evidence that what they had done and passed through during their participation in war was meaningful. The thing that war veterans, after they come back from war, want to understand is how they are accepted by their community and society. Accordingly, their basic need appeared to be a wish to know whether society perceived them in a positive or negative way.

The research has shown that the attitude of the community towards veterans who returned from war played a very important role in their re-entry into civil society. The atmosphere of acceptance of veterans from the community made their integration into a peaceful life easier; an atmosphere of rejection from the public increased their isolation (27). Using the data for social support and public recognition from the Vietnam veterans, the valorisation of their past experience and given contributions and the data we gathered from the Homeland war veterans, we may conclude that all war veterans have similar attitudes about the reactions they expect from their environment. No matter what the time the war was fought, the causes which led to it, or what kind of society veterans have come back to, what is most essential is for them to feel respected and maintain their sense of dignity.

Preserving tradition and remembrance of the Homeland war

The majority of the Homeland war invalids attach remarkable importance to preserving tradition and keeping remembrance of the Homeland war and the people who participated in it. They consider those things essential for their moral satisfaction ("...we should not let some things that happened in the Homeland war become forgotten... by preserving tradition and remembrance on what had happened (2)"; "...we have to be active, working on keeping remembrance on those who gave their lives, were wounded and left their health in war (3)"; "...the past should not be forgotten... preserving tradition and remembrance on those who gave their lives (8)").

Previous studies that dealt with the return of Vietnam veterans to civil society (23-26) have demonstrated that the Vietnam soldiers were faced with the criticism of the public and a rejection of the war in which they had participated. After their return from the war, they were traumatized for the second time. But the public confession of society that it felt sorry for their loss was the means of reducing this secondary victimization of Vietnam veterans. However, the results of similar qualitative research about veterans after every war shows that the soldiers are annoyed by the general lack of public awareness and the lack of interest and attention from the public.

The primary fear that soldiers who survive a war feel is that their sacrifices soon will be forgotten. This is the reason why Vietnam veterans were establishing veteran associations after they came back from war. Their primary purpose was to make sure that the public would not forget their war trauma and experiences. Therefore, they insisted on medals and monuments, memorial days, parades and public commemorations and on personal compensations for their wounds as well (24). The general aspiration for preservation of traditions and remembrances of war and the persons who participated in it is a common characteristic of both Vietnam veterans and the Homeland war veterans-invalids. Their common fear, expressed in the possibility of social oblivion of everything they had passed through during war, is what connects them in forming different associations and organisations that try to prevent such a possibility. Non-oblivion, as one aspect of social relation towards the Homeland war veterans-invalids, becomes the foundation of their dignity and makes a contribution to their feeling of moral satisfaction.

Social participation

Most participants, when their sense of dignity was in question, put a special emphasis on the category of social participation as a possibility for equal participation in the life of both society in general and the community that surrounded them. Thus, social participation for them primarily means to have their own place in society ("...That participation in socialization and in society in general would be as easy and as accessible as possible... so that a man could be a real participant and member of that society (2)"; "... not to ignore us...not to take us into their settings and install us as representatives of something... to have our place in society (7); "...to acknowledge us as a part of society, namely its vital part (11).

Apart from a place in society, as a major part of social participation, the Homeland war invalids emphasize working activity and the sense of being socially efficient – a feeling of usefulness (...we should stay active as long as possible, keep working activity... to feel we are socially efficient (9)...that people get their place within society... to have something to do in your life... to be given an opportunity and satisfaction to be activated within society...(10)...not only material rights of a man are important... here is a wish to work, to feel useful, to feel that he contributes to the society and family (16).

Similar to those experiences are the experiences of Vietnam veterans. The research has shown that, after their return home, the wounded Vietnam veterans expressed the feeling of isolation (24). The war was a traumatic event that had destroyed the feeling of a mutual connection between the soldiers and the community to which they had belonged before it. Upon their return, their involvement in the wider community appeared to be crucial and necessary for them to regain the feeling that life makes sense. The research results showed that it is of major importance to find a place in society for the war veterans after they come back from war as a kind of protective bond (27).

Social participation is extremely important for war veterans and invalids because it offers them a chance to regain a place in society they had strived to reach before the war. This is the place they could have reached before the war and that was suddenly taken from them because of the war and their contribution to it. Aspirations for being an active worker and socially efficient do not differentiate the veterans from other persons in community except for the fact that these are expressed more strongly due to their war experiences. The war has changed the way they participate in society in two aspects: First, the position they had had in society until the war was completely lost and abruptly changed by a new, unplanned role that transformed them in many different ways and made them unable to come back to the place in society they had had before the war. Second, this new disability is compensated by a new ability they acquired by their participation in war. The fact that they participated in the war presumes their strength and their possession of many skills. Many defenders and invalids of the Homeland war think that these are the basis by which they should be characterised as persons capable of social participation, as persons who can give their contributions to social life as they were giving it during the war.

Protective role of the state

Modeled on the experiences of other countries that had experienced war and, therefore, all the issues that appear after a war, the Republic of Croatia adopted the National program of protection and promotion of human rights in 2004 in which the protective role of the State towards veterans is emphasized as being primary (28). That protective role is defined as the sole responsibility and duty of the State for providing adequate protection and care for those persons who defended the country and ensured its sovereignty and independence, and for all other victims and participants of the war.

Thus, the Homeland war invalids see their dignity, among other things, as reflected in the protective role of the State. What is primary to the Homeland war invalids in the State's expressing of that protective role is to provide help and support, most of all, in the process and for the purpose of their resocialization and integration into a peaceful community. This represents the way of establishing new social connections that were abruptly broken when going to the war ("...to provide real care to real invalids... that society makes attempt to resocialise us... that the society helps us to try to function best we can (4)). Apart from society, the Homeland war invalids attribute an important place and protective role in preservation of their dignity and moral satisfaction to the State and its institutions. This role is mostly in providing assistance and support to those war invalids who have difficult existential situations and also providing assistance to those who do not know how to exercise their rights ("The State should give instructions to those who do not know where to go and what to do... that State helps us in realisation of our rights and alleviates our suffering while gaining or verification of those rights (12)"; "...procedures of the State... to give help to those who can survive and work... to assist us in finding job (10)"; "...State institutions that should protect us from all that... local administration should take care about their defenders and help them... all those people, who came out of an extremely difficult situation, should be taken care of (8)". The Homeland war invalids do not speak about help from the State and society from the position of helpless members of that society who need continuous help, but from the standpoint of those who need the «hand» of society and the State as a short-term help and a necessary impulse and initiative for further functioning.

Respect of basic human rights

Dignity is a key category of human rights. Human rights and dignity are closely linked together in the sense that respect of human rights is a premise for the existence of dignity and vice versa. Such very close connections between those two categories were found by analysing the participants' answers because dignity, for them, primarily means the respect of the rights provided by the Constitution, laws, and numerous international documents: ("...The right to health... the right to work... the right to all Constitutional categories contained in the Constitution (2); ...to respect the rights of every person no matter of age, sex, religious or national determination (9)"). Respect of basic human rights determines personal, inner feelings of dignity in the Homeland war invalids and, in that sense, they consider that dignity is the part of a human being that cannot be taken away from anybody ("...is the most important part of a person (11)"; "...something that belongs to every person and what every man should have if he wants to feel as a human being... there is no bigger right (15)"; "...something that man carries in his soul... something that makes man a man... all man's emotions, honesty, education... the wholeness of existence... (17)").

CONCLUSION

This study presents the results of the research, the aim of which was to get an insight into the sense of dignity of the Homeland war invalids on the basis of their personal experiences and reflections. The data were collected by interviewing 17 veterans, invalids of the Homeland war and members of five different associations of war veterans in Zagreb and Varaždin during 2007.

On the basis of a qualitative analysis of the interview results, six categories were identified: 1) social equality; 2) valorisation of past experiences and personal contributions to the common good; 3) preservation of tradition and remembrance of the Homeland war; 4) social participation; 5) protective role of the State; 6) respect of basic human rights.

Accordingly, a schematic model of the relationships between the categories was made. (see table 2) The relationships of the six categories important for the dignity of the invalids of the Homeland war can be related to the previously presented four forms of human dignity (8-10).

Dignity on the merits includes our second category: Valorisation of past experiences and personal contributions to the common good; Dignity of existential and moral greatness includes our third category: preservation of tradition and remembrance of the Homeland war. The third form, the dignity of identity, includes our three categories that are related to identity in social context, e.g., social equality, social participation and protective role of the State. The fourth form, universal human dignity, is our sixth category: respect of basic human rights.

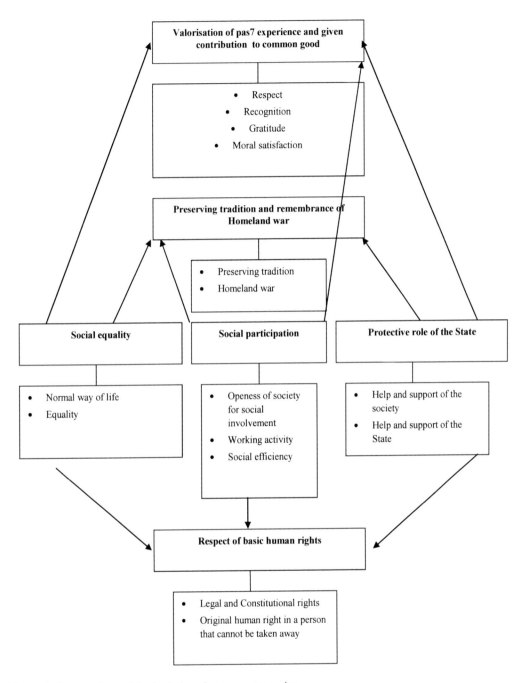

Figure 1. Schematic model of relations between categories.

In this study data and conclusions from other research, made with other groups of people but focused on the concept of dignity, are analysed including some that researched war veterans. From this other research we found some common characteristics in our war invalids related to dignity, but also some peculiarities characteristic for our Homeland war invalids only. Specifically, for them the concept of dignity of identity contains a very clearly emphasized social context - found remarkably important during our research. Thus we may define the concept of dignity of the Homeland war invalids as their social involvement, where their dignity is expressed in the forms of acquired merits for their deeds done for the common good, valorisation of the Homeland war and universal human dignity.

Particularly important for their sense of dignity and moral satisfaction is their participation in the social life of the community in which they live. The Homeland war invalids, being equal to other members of society, find their place in their community primarily through a particular form of working activity, which in them creates a feeling of being useful through making contributions to society and family. This working activity means that they do not demand any material rights from the State or society, but only protection in the form of better care for themselves and help with the processes of integration and resocialization, processes that have not been completely implemented as of now.

To improve their position, based on equality and social involvement, the legal norms must be changed to harmonize with the real life situations of the Homeland war invalids. It is important to involve persons and professionals who were direct participants in war activities into the social services that help with the issues of the defenders because they can observe those issues from the standpoint of the Homeland war invalids themselves. Activities of social involvement and equal social position are, actually, direct contributions to the dignity of the Homeland war veterans-invalids.

REFERENCES

[1]   Anderberg T, Lepp M, Berglund AL, Segesten K. Preserving dignity in caring for older adults: a concept analysis. J Adv Nurs 2007; 5(6):635-43.
[2]   Moody HR. Why dignity in old age matters. In: Disch R, Dobrof R, Moody HR. Dignity and old age. New York: Haworth Press, 1998:13–37.
[3]   Baker, H. The image of man: A study of the idea of human dignity in classical antiquity, the middle ages, and the renaissance. New York: Harper Torchbooks, 1961.
[4]   Edgar A. Vela´zquez and the representation of dignity. Med Health Care Philosophy 2003;6:111–21.
[5]   Opca deklaracija o ljudskim pravima (Universal Declaration of Human Rights) http://www.amnesty.hr/stranica.php?sifra_str=opca_deklaracija, 1948.
[6]   Haeberle P. Ljudsko dostojanstvo i pluralisticka demokracija (Human dignity and pluralistic democracy). Politicka misao 2006;43(2):3–41.
[7]   Anic, V. Rjecnik hrvatskog jezika (Dictionary of Croatian language), Novi Liber, Zagreb, 2007.
[8]   Nordenfelt L. Dignity of the elderly. Med Health Care Philosophy 2003;6:99–101.
[9]   Nordenfelt L. Dignity and the care of the elderly. Med Health Care Philosophy 2003;6:103–10.
[10]   Nordenfelt L. The varieties od dignity, Health Care Analysis 2004;12(2):69-81.
[11]   Miller AB, Keys CB. Understanding dignity in the lives of homeless persons. Am J Comm Psychol 2001;29(2):331-4.
[12]   Mairis ED. Concept clarification in professional practice – dignity. J Adv Nurs 1994;19:947–53.
[13]   Disch R. Dignity, cultural power and narrative redemption: aging male writers confront the medical system. J Gerontol Soc Work 1998;29:93–109.
[14]   Kane RA. Long-term care and good quality of life: bring them closer together. Gerontologist 2001;41:293–304.
[15]   Chochinov HM, Hack T, McClement S, Kristjanson L, Harlos M. Dignity in the terminally ill: a developing empirical model. Soc Sci Med 2002;54:433–43.
[16]   Cynthia S, Jacelon TW, Connelly RB, Proulx K, Vo T. A concept analysis of dignity for older adults. J Adv Nurs 2004;48(1):76-83.
[17]   Manzo JF. On the sociology and social organization of stigma: some etnomethodological insights, Hum Stud 2004;27:401-16.

[18] Zakon o pravima hrvatskih branitelja iz domovinskog rata i clanova njihovih obitelji (The Law about the Rights of Croatian Homeland war Defenders and their families), Narodne novine 174/04, 92/05, 2/07

[19] Jašarevic T, Leutar, Z. Samopercepcija društvenog položaja invalida Domovinskog rata (Self-perception of social position of Homeland war invalids), Društvena istraživanja, (being printed), 2009.

[20] Frigelj D. Vojna psihologija (Military psychology), MORH, Zagreb, 2003.

[21] Milas G. Istraživacke metode u psihologiji i drugim društvenim znanostima (Research methods in psychology and other social sciences). Jastrebarsko: Naklada Slap, 2005.

[22] Deklaracija o Domovinskom ratu (Declaration on Homeland war) Narodne novine 2000:2000/102 .

[23] Ustav Republike Hrvatske (Constitution of the Republic of Croatia), Narodne novine, 56/1990., 135/1997., 8/1998. – procišceni text, 113/2000., 124/2000. – procišceni text, 28/2001., 41/2001. – procišceni text, 55/2001. – corrected

[24] Mesec, B. uvod v kvalitativno raziskovanje v socialnem delu (Introducion to qualitative method in social studies). Visoka šola za socialno delo, Ljubljana, 1998.

[25] Lifton RJ. Home from the war: Vietnam veterans: Neither victims nor executioners, New York: Simon Schuster, 1973.

[26] Shatan C. The grief of soldiers: Vietnam combat veterans self-help movement. Am J Orthopsychiatry 1973;43:640-53.

[27] Lifton RJ. The concept of the survivor. In: Dimsdale JE. Survivors, victims, and perpetrators: Essays on the Nazi Holocaust. New York: Hemisphere 1980:113-26.

[28] Charles RF, Leventman S. Strangers at home: Vietnam veterans since the war. New York: Prager, 1980.

[29] Herman JL. Trauma i oporavak (Trauma and recovery), Druga, Zagreb, 1996.

[30] Nacionalni program psihosocijalne i zdravstvene pomoci sudionicima i stradalnicima iz Domovinskog rata (National program of psycho-social and medical help for participants and sufferers from Homeland war) http://vlada.hr/hr/content/download/6613/50485/file/64-02.apdf (24.10.2007.)

[31] Nacionalni program zaštite i promicanja ljudskih prava u Republici Hrvatskoj od 2005. do 2008. godine (National program of protection and reinforcement of human rights in the Republic of Croatia from 2005 to 2008), (2004) http://www.vlada.hr/hr/content/download/6514/49952/file/56-02.pdf (17.10.2007)

SECTION THREE: TRANSITION TO ADULT CARE

In: Disability and Chronic Disease
Editors: J. Merrick, S. Aspler and M. Morad

ISBN: 978-1-62948-288-0
© 2014 Nova Science Publishers, Inc.

Chapter 20

THE SELF-MANAGEMENT AND TRANSITION TO ADULTHOOD PROGRAM "UNC STAR$_x$"

Maria E Ferris[*]*, MD, MPH, PhD*[1]*, Michael T Ferris, BA*[2]*,*
Carolyn Viall, RN, PhD[3]*, Heather D Stewart, MD*[1]*,*
Nicole Fenton, MS[1]*, Cara Haberman, MD*[4]*, Edward A Iglesia, BA*[5]*,*
Lauren E Hancock, PNP[4]*, Donna H Harward*[1]*,*
Donna Gilleskie, PhD[6]*, James O'Neill*[7]*, Robert Imperial*[7]*,*
Zion Ko[1]*, Mary H Benton*[1]*, May Doan, BA*[1]*, Kristi Bickford*[1]*, BA,*
Randy Detwiler, MD[1]*, Kenneth Andreoni, MD*[8]*,*
John D Mahan, MD[8]*, Zachary Smith, MD,*[1]
Keisha Gibson, MD, MPH[1] *and Steve Hooper*[9]

[1]University of North Carolina Kidney Center, Chapel Hill, North Carolina, [2]Script-a-wish and Simione Health Care Consultants, Cincinnati, Ohio, [3]The North Carolina Children's Hospital, Chapel Hill, North Carolina, [4]Victory Junction Camp and Wake Forrest University, Winston-Salem, North Carolina, [5]Robert Wood Johnson Medical School, Piscataway, New Jersey, [6]University of North Carolina School of Economics, Chapel Hill, North Carolina, [7]University of North Carolina Department of Internal Medicine, Chapel Hill, North Carolina and [8]University of Florida, US [9]UNC Carolina Institute for Developmental Disabilities

ABSTRACT

The University of North Carolina's Self-management and Transition to Adulthood with R$_x$=therapies Program (UNC STAR$_x$) was created in 2006. This manuscript describes the

---

[*] Correspondence: Maria E Ferris, MD, MPH, PhD, Associate Professor of Pediatrics and Medicine, The University of North Carolina at Chapel Hill, Founder and Director, the UNC TR$_x$ANSITION and Self-management Program, Director, Pediatric Dialysis and Kidney Transplant Programs, Chapel Hill, NC 27599-7155, United States. E-mail: maria_ferris@med.unc.edu.

program's evolution from a nephrology-centric intervention to addressing multiple-conditions in an institution-wide interdisciplinary program. We illustrate the lessons and insight informed by youth with chronic conditions/disabilities, their parents, health provider and community partners across the continuum of health care transition (HCT). Specifically, we describe lessons relate to program sustainability, including the importance of a dedicated program coordinator, inter and intra-institutional collaboration to validate tools that promote and assess patient self-management skills and HCT, strategies to improve youth, provider (pediatric and adult-focused) and parent communication, and the important role for peer volunteers (in person or through social media) addressed. The UNC STAR$_x$ Program's collaboration has produced IRB-approved tools that promote communication between youth with chronic conditions and providers, while outlining customized interventions based on patient's level of knowledge and mastery of HCT skills. Two private foundations provided initial funding and it now has become an institution-wide collaborative funded primarily by the North Carolina Children's Hospital. The UNC STARx partners include youth with chronic conditions and disabilities, families and researchers from several disciplines and institutions in our state, nation and the world. Our innovative program holds great promise and it already appears to improve health outcomes and quality of life for youth and their families (based on participation rate and user satisfaction both at >95%). Our lessons from the field may assist other institutions as they strive to improve adolescents'/young adults' health outcomes through evidence-based and cost-effective interventions.

INTRODUCTION

Health care transition (HCT) is a dynamic, patient- and family-centered process that involves the purposeful, planned movement of adolescents and young adults with chronic physical and medical conditions from child-centered to adult-oriented healthcare systems (1-3). The consensus goal of HCT is for adolescents and young adults (youth) to successfully engage the adult healthcare system in order to receive high-quality, developmentally-appropriate health care services, thus maximizing their lifelong functioning, potential, and quality of life (3, 4). Toward this end, the HCT process is deliberate and focused, meets the needs of an individual, and prepares an adolescent or young adult with a chronic illness to assume progressive increasing responsibility for the management of their health (3, 5-7).

HCT preparation ensures a smooth, uninterrupted, and coordinated transfer from pediatric to adult health care providers and services. Ideally, the HCT process is flexible, responsive, continuous, comprehensive, and well-coordinated, that is championed by a transition program and/or care providers that ensure appropriate HCT planning and support are provided (3, 4, 6, 7). The recommended key components of an effective HCT program are: 1) a designated professional responsible for HCT coordination, 2) development of written HCT plans at the onset of adolescence and 3) formulation of a written portable medical summary ready at the time of transfer to adult providers (3, 5-7).

Despite consensus recommendations that youth with chronic conditions benefit from HCT programs (3-7), barriers to the establishment of effective HCT programs still persist. Firstly, there is lack of agreement regarding a theoretical model to support transition, despite a few proposals of interest (8, 9). By extension, there is lack of agreement about the identified targets of intervention and clinical outcomes to measure transition (10). Secondly, there is no consensus about which individual should serve as the HCT coordinator, the coordinator's level of training, or the coordinator's function. Thirdly, health provider compensation to carry out HCT services also remains a barrier. Lastly, HCT program funding is a critical barrier as most HCT programs are not supported by institutional budgets and thus must rely on external sources of funding.

In this paper, we describe our experience in launching our institution-wide HCT program: called the UNC STAR$_x$ (Self-management and Transition to Adulthood with Rx=treatment). We share the lessons we have learned and the insight we have gained from working with youth, parents, and community partners. We also briefly describe the tools that we have developed, currently utilize, and continue to validate in order to guide youth with chronic medical conditions/disabilities, their families, and the health providers who serve them in the HCT process.

PROGRAM ORGANIZATION AND SUSTAINABILITY

In 2006, with the enthusiastic support of adolescent/young adults with chronic conditions and their parents, the need for the interdisciplinary self-management and transition program was acknowledged and addressed. The initial impetus for this collaborative effort was triggered by anecdotal experience with survivors of pediatric-onset chronic kidney disease who had poor outcomes (loss of transplant, lost to follow up, or death) subsequent to their transfer to adult-focused health. In preparation for establishing a formal program at UNC, the founder and program director visited the transition programs of Dr. Alan Watson (Nottingham, UK) and Dr, Janet McDonagh (Birmingham, UK) and conducted semi-structured interviews with published experts in the field of transition (see acknowledgments). The purpose of these initial discussions was to explore organizational models, ascertain how programs were funded, determine how multidisciplinary, intra-institutional partners were identified/ recruited, and identify available tools for assessing young adults' progression in achieving readiness for (see acknowledgments). Two distinct lessons derived from these exploratory visits informed our programmatic plans: 1) no validated tools were available for dissemination, and 2) funds to support a targeted transition program were difficult to secure.

It was clear that a distinct organizational advantage at UNC was that pediatric nephrology resides within the internal medicine nephrology group. This embedded model provides pediatric nephrology with greater fiscal stability and shared clinic space, promoting collaboration between child and adult-focused providers. In addition, increased communication between UNC pediatric and adult nephrology providers engendered improved communication between external providers who either referred or received adolescent/young adult patients.

Initial funding for the STAR$_x$ Program was through a three-year award from the K.B. Reynolds Charitable Trust, and following HCT consensus guidelines a full-time transition coordinator position was established. This position proved critical to achieving timely execution of readiness assessments and was instrumental in providing patient-centered education and in promoting communication between community partners (teachers, support agencies), the health care providers, the patient and the parent(s). Ms. Kristi Bickford has a BA degree in Psychology and extensive experience working with children and adolescents in the judicial, social service, and mental health fields. Until the last two years, Ms. Bickford had been the sole transition coordinator.

Following the expiration of the initial grant support, bridge funding was secured from the UNC Departments of Internal Medicine and Pathology. A grant from the Agency for Healthcare Research and Quality through the UNC Center for Education Research and Therapeutics, partly supported the development one of our tools, the $STAR_x$ Survey; a self-administered questionnaire to assess transition readiness and disease management skills (11). The UNC Kidney Center and the Department of Pediatrics partially funded the development of our second tool, the $TR_xANSITION$ Scale™ It is a provider-administered survey to measure the adolescent/young adult's self-management skills and disease specific knowledge. The development of a parallel $TR_xANSITION$ Scale-Parent Version™ was partly funded by the Renal Research Institute. Dr. Maria Ferris had previously developed and used a medical passport, which was adapted to be used in the $STAR_x$ Program started, and it is now known as the $TR_xANSITION$ Medical Passport.™

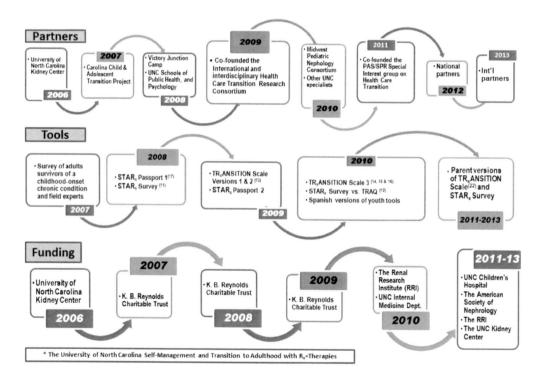

Figure 1. Transition and Self-Management UNCSTARx* Program Timeline.

Since 2011, the University of North Carolina Children's Hospital Administration has funded for the program's full time transition coordinator, providing important stability. This substantial financial support has facilitated the expansion of services to receiving care in other pediatric subspecialties, including: Gastroenterology, Rheumatology, Endocrinology, Hematology, and Pulmonology. Additional research manpower, in the form of a psychology graduate student, two medical students and a coordinator, has been achieved with awards from the Renal Research Institute and the American Society of Nephrology, supporting two one-year funding for two medical students and 20% of Dr. Ferris' salary. In-kind donations from the UNC Kidney Center and the UNC Schools of Arts and Science, Public Health, and Nursing, as well as the Carolina Institute for Developmental Disabilities, the Center for Faculty Development and the Odum Institute are essential sources in our continued effort (administrative support, office space and research program). With a dedicated HCT coordinator and additional research personnel, over 500 adolescents and young adults with chronic conditions are being followed longitudinally, including post-transfer to adult focused health care. For further detail on the program timeline, partners, tools and funding, please see Figure 1.

PATIENTS SERVED AND STAFF/VOLUNTEERS

Patients

Our program enrolls patients between the ages of 12-24 years who have been diagnosed with a chronic health condition for at least 6 months. Additional inclusion criteria are: taking at least one medication daily for the diagnosed chronic condition and the cognitive ability (as deemed by their medical provider) to understand and answer questions about their medical condition(s) and treatment. All patients that accept our invitation to participate in our program sign an IRB-approved consent permitting access to their medical and pharmacy records for longitudinal data collection. Patients and their parents are enrolled in person during a routinely scheduled clinic visit. During the clinic visit the majority of the tool administration and assessments are completed, followed by phone or online administered surveys when necessary. We currently have a 95% program enrolment rate with an equally high proportion of reported participant satisfaction in the program at 95%). Our program is primarily focused on clinical services, but our patients/parents are invited to participate in research projects as applicable.

Program staff and volunteers

By in large, our most influential team members are the youth with chronic medical conditions and their parents who volunteer their time, knowledge, and suggestions, guiding the advancement in our work. The STAR$_x$ team is multi-disciplinary and composed of paid staff, grant funded researchers, and volunteers. The medical director receives 20% salary support via grant funding and a fulltime transition coordinator whose salary is 100% supported by the UNC Children's Hospital. We collaborate with professionals amongst various disciplines including: nursing (nurses and nurse practitioners), pharmacy, clinical psychology, developmental disabilities, education, social work, public rehabilitation health and recreational therapy. Furthermore, the UNC STAR$_x$ Program is aided by the work of five diligent student researchers (two medical and one psychology graduate student whose positions are funded by research grants provided by the American Society of Nephrology; and two part-time pre-medical students funded by the Renal Research Institute). Our team is also composed of diverse student researchers volunteering their time during summer breaks.

TOOLS TO MEASURE TRANSITION READINESS

The STAR$_x$ Transition-Readiness Survey

This questionnaire was result of collaborative work utilizing valuable input from adolescents and emerging adults with various chronic medical conditions. The 18-question survey was developed through the use of patient focus groups, focused interviews, and cognitive interviews, including the "concurrent think-aloud" technique in which responses are probed extensively. This tool was created with supplemental input acquired from patient-graduates and existing patients of our pediatric renal program; information obtained from published transition checklists; and interdisciplinary collaboration between students of the UNC School of Public Health (Sarah Massie, Victoria Pham, Department of Health Behavior/Health Education) and Sue Tolleson-Rinehart, PhD of the UNC Schools of Medicine and Public Health. Using the Stages of Change Model, the STARx survey was designed to longitudinally measure self-reported health care transition readiness and disease self-management skills. The STARx Transition-Readiness Survey includes self-reported knowledge of 1) disease diagnosis, 2) medications/treatment, 3) health insurance, 4) ability to make medical appointments, 5) ability to use health resources and 6) disease self-management. This web-based tool is administered every 6-12 months and is undergoing validation in clinical and therapeutic camp settings (11). Most recently, we are comparing the performance of this survey among adolescents with chronic conditions to another self-administered tool (12) (see figure 1).

The TR$_x$ANSITION Scale

The TR$_x$ANSITION Scale™ (trademark 2006, University of North Carolina) is a tool used to assess and monitor the HCT process longitudinally; and is readily accessible (web-based) and reproducible in clinical practice (Ferris et al., Renal Failure). This scale produces a collective score using the following 10 transition related domains: **T**ype of illness, **R**x (medications), **A**dherence, **N**utrition, **S**elf-management, **I**ssues of reproduction, **T**rade/school, **I**nsurance, **O**ngoing support, and **N**ew health providers. The scale has been revised thrice to support and reflect the current structured interview format. It should be noted that administration of the scale is not limited to health providers. Our program is an example of how people with limited to no medical knowledge or backgrounds can be trained to effectively administer this tool (reproducibility kappa score 0.76). The scale collects information through both, confirmation of attained knowledge and skill mastery claimed (i.e., the patient has to name his/her medication(s) to get credit for the answer) and patient self-report (13-16). This allows the health provider to commend the youth on their attained knowledge/skills and helps them provide developmentally-appropriate patient-education activities in the areas of low competency. The scale is administered every 6-12 months, monitoring progress in a de-identified web-based format.

Preliminary analysis of a cross-sectional pilot study revealed adolescents younger than 17 years had a significantly lower score than older teens and young adults, with those younger than 14 years having the lowest scores (13, 14, 16). This may reflect life experiences and time-varying development as the adolescent matures. Validation studies are underway to assess the instruments' effectiveness in a longitudinal study design. Internal medicine and combined internal medicine-pediatrics fellows assume the care of transitioned patients when the youth achieve a TR$_x$ANSITION Scale™ score of > 80%.

The TR$_x$ANSITION medical passport™

This tool helps teach youth with chronic medical conditions about their disease and facilitates communication between health care providers in emergency rooms and clinic settings. This laminated, wallet-sized document contains the following patient-specific health information: medical diagnosis, current medication list (type, dosage, frequency, and purpose), drug allergies, and medical provider contact information. The TR$_x$ANSITION Medical Passport™ also includes the patient's name, photograph (if they wish), emergency contacts, and their unique patient ID number. The medical passport is updated every 6-12 months to reflect their most current health and personal information. In an effort to evaluate retention and usability, patients are contacted and asked if they have their medical passport in their possession (17). To confirm that they do in fact have it through telephone conversations, they are asked to read their ID number located in the upper right-hand corner of the card. User satisfaction and feedback from providers (in emergency departments and clinics throughout the state) has been enlightening and rewarding.

Peer-support and on-line Facebook™

Our transition coordinator is the administrator of a Facebook™ page for some of the young adults who participate in our STAR$_x$ program. She monitors communication between the invited members and proposes relevant, age-appropriate topics of discussion. This expansion into a social media forum has led the participants to discuss their challenges to self- manage their conditions, and finding the appropriate support systems. This platform encourages active communication among members and provides a non-threatening, non-judgmental environment. Youth share stories, coach one another, ask questions, and seek support. There have been several instances when a group member has been hospitalized and other members coordinate a visit to the hospital. Many of the young adult members of this group have said that they don't feel comfortable posting status updates about their health on their personal Facebook™ pages. In contrast, our HCT Facebook™ page monitored by our transition coordinator provides is an environment where they feel comfortable to post about their feelings (e.g., being different from "healthy" peers, sadness about having a health condition, frustration with taking medications daily), struggles (e.g., medication side effects, special diets, wheel-chair dependence), and triumphs (e.g., hospital discharge, receiving a transplant, medication removed, etc.) related to their health. Table 1 depicts recommendations for health providers that the youth in our program have given us. Table 2 summarizes the recommendations parents of our patients have proposed. Recurring themes youth have taught us through personal and on-line conversations include:

- The importance that health providers have in their lives and sense of well-being.

- Providers can inspire trust particularly if they express confidence in the youth's ability to manage their condition and lives. On the other hand, providers can also inspire distrust if the youth are treated without respect or their opinions are discounted.
- Youth...
  - like to be included in all conversations that affect their lives
  - actually hear what the health providers advise, but don't necessarily agree at times
  - worry about the burden their diagnosis brings to their parents/siblings and family
  - like to have peer support and the ability to share "war stories" and advice from peers who are experiencing the same struggles they encounter (18)
  - would like having more relaxed communications with their providers as conversations expand to survival and life goals
  - want to be affirmed of their growing autonomy

Table 1. UNC STAR$_x$ Program Youth Recommendations to Health Providers

[1] Customer service
In the outpatient setting:
a. Everyone should have a smile to show they are happy to see you
b. Good bed-side manners by providers
c. All signage should be clear and visible (as in an airport) to navigate the system.
d. Clean environment in the clinic but not smelling like a hospital
e. A waiting room that is the "Apple™ stores of clinic", airy, nicely designed, not cluttered
f. Magazines that are up to date and today's news-paper,
g. Relaxing music in the background at low volume/having a fish tank
h. Health message in posters, computer screens or TV monitors with nicely designed graphics with colors that are great to look at, almost artistic; surprising the consumer that they are actually health education messages
i. Email system for staggered appointments with times that are respected.
j. Paying co-pays up-front to stand in line at the check-in/out counter once
k. Patient portal to access medical record
In the in-patient setting:
l. Hospital gowns are not cool, they are demeaning and revealing
m. Children's wards prevents the youth from getting sleep (crying babies next door)
n. Adult wards is also not appropriate and they would prefer an adolescent and young adult unit that caters to their unique needs and morbidities
o. Being able to eat or drink on a timely basis if a potential procedure is cancelled

[2] Health care providers that
a. Direct the conversation to the adolescent and young adult
b. Ask for the youth's opinion
c. Ask the parents to leave the room
d. Reassure the youth that all conversations are private
e. Inspire confidence and trustworthiness, as a friend. Youth patients often "don't know what we don't know" until they are faced with a question or having to explain it to someone else.
f. Listen to the youth's concerns
g. Relates to young-adults interests by being up-to-date in music, movies, sports
h. Encourage questions by the youth and help navigate the system
i. Teach how to explain their condition to their peers
j. Showing the awards the clinic or providers have received or the results of the research

[3] Continuous Quality Improvement
a. Individualized patient and parent education, re-education and re-training, particularly those patient who were diagnosed early in life
b. Counseling about how to successfully self-manage their condition
c. Meeting older patients serving as mentor/coaches or even examples of what not to do with tangible consequences (i.e. Somebody who lost a transplant due to no-compliance)

[4] Creating a patient health ambassador program: Using the principle " You see something, you do something ,you teach something"

[5] Getting a Health Care Transition Graduation Certificate

[6] Ecological Aspects of Health
1. Secure individualized education plans and assistance with 504 Educational plans
2. Participation in therapeutic camp
3. Involvement in peer-support group

Table 2. UNC STAR_x Program Parent Recommendations to Health Providers

1. Customer service: Similar to the youth recommendations plus...
   In the outpatient setting:
      a. Have a care coordinator, particularly if multiple consultants are involved
      b. Psychological services should be offered as soon as the chronic diagnosis is made and presented to the family as an expected referral <u>for all</u> patients
      c. Schedule 2-4 appointments in one day to avoid losing work days
      d. Identify parent and patient support groups
   In the inpatient setting
      a. As much as possible be consistent with the rounding time, so that they can rest and are able to talk with the provider every day
      b. Have a multidisciplinary family meeting once per week to improve communication with all involved
      c. Having the same nurse care for their child to allow continuity
      d. Participate in holiday-related decorations or floor activities to be considered part of the team, improve the environment and get respite
      e. Getting blood work at 4:00 AM is not friendly, especially when it has been a rough night
      f. Try to do blood work from peripheral IV when possible to decrease veni-punctures
      g. Admission to the same floor whenever possible
      h. Minimize radiation exposure
      i. Have laundry-related services available for long-term admissions
      j. Being able to have your child use regular clothes and not the hospital gowns
      k. Have a parent tray of food
2. Their fears
      a. That their child will not be able to survive
      b. Who will assist their child manage their health conditions and their lives as they age
      c. Financial burden
      d. Strain in their marriage
      e. Losing their jobs
      f. Having enough time for their other children and themselves
      g. Keeping their sanity and optimism

3. Their need for continuous education on
      a. Their child's diagnosis, especially if the diagnosis is early in life.
      b. Education material that is literacy- and culturally-appropriate
      c. Guidance on how to find community resources

LESSONS FROM THE PARENTS OF YOUTH WITH CHRONIC MEDICAL CONDITIONS

For youth with chronic medical conditions, parents assume a variety of roles that include care coordinator, medical expert, and patient advocate (19). Additionally, as their child develops through adolescence and acquires self-management skills, the role of a parent ideally transitions from that of a manager, to a supervisor, and then finally a consultant (20). Through their monitoring, supervision, coaching, and support of skill-development, parents play a significant role in HCT (8, 9, 21)

Initially, the UNC TR$_x$ANSITION Scale™ was administered to patients in private, without their parent(s) present. About two years ago, our transition coordinator began to administer the scale to the youth in the presence of their family members, as long as the family members remain silent during the assessment. Due to time constraints and limited clinic space, she recognized that a parent's non-participatory presence during assessment served as an excellent learning and teaching opportunity to both, the youth and the parent. By doing this, our HCT coordinator discovered that many parents did not know the level of skills their children possessed, or, worse yet; parents would mention that they themselves did not know the answer to many of the questions related to their child's medical condition(s) and management. This was a very concerning finding, since parents are important facilitators of their children's acquisition of medical knowledge and disease self-management. We considered this as one of the most valuable lessons from the field as this experience reinforced the need for a targeted educational intervention that is both patient- and family-centered.

As a direct result of this experience, the complement to the UNC TR$_x$ANSITION Scale™ for Adolescents and Young Adults was expanded to include a parent version (22). This parent version serves as an assessment of a parent's disease and medication knowledge of their child's condition and as an additional proxy report for the youths' self-management, medication adherence and other HCT-related skills mastery (23). In table 2 we have summarized the UNC TR$_x$ANSITION Program parent recommendations for health providers.

COMMUNITY PARTNERS AND VOLUNTEERS

We have partnered with Victory Junction, a camp located in Randleman, NC, providing year-round programming for children with chronic and life-threatening conditions and their families. Victory Junction has allowed the UNC STAR$_x$ Program to conduct summer research programs that include the deployment of web-based surveys to children and adolescents with a variety of chronic medical conditions (18, 23). In-kind donations by Victory Junction have allowed an expansion of services to organize the annual Young Adult Weekend, serving adolescent and emerging adult patients with chronic medical conditions. During this annual weekend, 16-24 year-old participants are able to engage in camp activities and teambuilding sessions, while learning about health care transition and disease self-management.

The UNC STAR$_x$ Program has attracted the assistance of undergraduate, graduate and medical students from several institutions. Two of our students have received "abstract of the year awards" in international conferences (22, 23) and summer students have secured funding from the NIH and private foundations. This year, two of our participating medical students each received a 12-month grant from the American Society of Nephrology to conduct research in the area of health care transition (14, 22).

Partnering with other HCT programs

The UNC STAR$_x$ Program collaborated with the North Carolina Health and Transition Project, a grant by the Agency of Healthcare Research in Quality to the North Carolina Department of Health. Following the conclusion of the grant, we continued our state-wide collaboration by contacting other HCT programs and researchers outside of North Carolina. As a result, we co-founded what is now known as the *International and Interdisciplinary Health Care Transition Research Consortium* with the following website: https://sites.google.com/site/healthcaretransition/. This consortium holds monthly telecommunication conferences and has bi-annual face to face meetings, with the purpose of advancing the evidence in the field of HCT (22). This has allowed for formal research collaboration of our proprietary tools with Nationwide Children's Hospital/The Ohio State University (pediatric and adult transplant programs), Carolinas Medical Center, the University of Michigan, Hospital Infantil de Mexico, and Universidad de Puerto Rico.

The (long) road ahead

Our program will continue to provide needed services while collecting longitudinal data and evidence on health care transition readiness and disease self-management. Innovation and program development will continue, driven by our patients' experiences and what they teach us. Generalizability of these innovative tools and applications will come from collaborative studies with our committed present and future partners. Understanding and appreciation of the efforts of other practitioners and investigators in this field will continue to inform and help us all develop the science of HCT. Of paramount importance will be defining cost-effectiveness of our efforts – the costs of failed transplants and unnecessary medical complications is all too evident to many - We need to systematically assess this program's costs to determine both, cost-effectives and evidence for best practices.

   We will continue to recognize and honor the essential input of youth and their families who ultimately define how we can best serve their needs. Interdisciplinary collaboration among pediatric patients, their families, team members and practitioners will further assist in tool refinement to assure general application. Our commitment to collaboration with other programs in North Carolina, the United States and countries around the world will continue to advance the evidence and knowledge in the field of health care transition. In the end, expanding our HCT program to those with varying medical conditions, and linking to innovative programs at other centers, will allow us all to develop useful and valid HCT-specific tools and reliable outcome measures to decrease morbidity/mortality of our youth with chronic health conditions/disabilities and to improve their health-related quality of quality of life.

Acknowledgments

Funding (present and past): The North Carolina Children's Hospital, The Renal Research Institute, The American Society of Nephrology, K.B. Reynolds Charitable Trust, UNC Center for Education Research and Therapeutics, The UNC Departments of Medicine, Pediatrics and Kidney Center.

We would like to thank our adolescent/young adult patients, their parents/families and our team of volunteers. We also would like to thank Ms. Jennifer Hoskins, Ms. Regina Andreoni, Sandra Kim, MD; Maureen Kelly, NP; Patricia Jones, MD; Elisabeth Dellon, MD; Elizabeth Champion, MD; Benjamin Harris, MD, Laura Robinson, MD; Mary Campion, MD; Amanda Cartee, MD; Jim Belsante, MD; Bradley Layton, MPH, PhD; Ahinee Amomoo, PhD; Susan Hogan, PhD; Karina Javalkar, Angie Johnson, MS3, Sarah Cohen, BS, Alexandra Phillips, Mia Lassiter, MPH, Ali Annaim, MS3, Diane Pozefsky, PhD; Sohini Sengupta, PhD; Ms. Rebecca Ferris, Alexander Ferris, Mike Ferris; Alan Stiles, MD; Marschall Runge, MD; Sue Tolleson-Reinhart, PhD; Ms. Janet Hadar, Heather Ansede, MSW, David Tauer, RN, Carol Ford, MD; Victoria Pham, MD; Sarah Massie, MPH; Sandy Grubbs, RN, CNP; Debbie Gipson, MD, MS; William Primack, MD, William Conley, MD; Clara Neyhart, RN; Lynn McCoy, RN; Caroline Jeannette, MSW; Ms. Trina Pugh, Ms. Jean Brown; Elizabeth Prata, FNP, Ms. Claudia Rojas, Lauren Kerns, RN, Cecily Betz, RN PhD*[1]; Patience White, MD*, David Wood, MD, MPH; Greg Sawicki, MD; Mara Medeiros, MD; Melvin Bonilla-Felix, MD, Mary Carter, PhD; Nathan Levine, MD; Peter Kotanko, MD, PhD; Geri Matsoon, MD, MPH; Monique Winslow, MPH, Irene Jurczyk; Tejas Desai, MD, Susan Massengill, MD, the North Carolina CHAT Program, Lorraine Bell, MD*; John Reiss, PhD*, Nikki Becker, MD*, Betty Presler, RN, PhD*, Roberta Williams, MD*, Megumi Okumura, MD, Peter Scal, MD, Mary Ciccarelli, MD, MPH, Sophie Jan, MD, Jason Woodward, MD, Peter Sim, MD, the UNC Transition Team; the Renal Research Institute, K.B. Reynolds Charitable Trust; the American Society of Nephrology, the Victory Junction Camp Staff; the UNC Kidney Center, Center for Faculty Development and the Odum Institute, the Mountain Area Health Education Center in North Carolina, the Midwest Pediatric Nephrology Consortium and the members of the International and Interdisciplinary Health Care Transition Research Consortium.

REFERENCES

[1] Blum RW, Garell D, Hodgman CH, Jorissen TW, Okinow NA, Orr DP, et al. Transition from child-centered to adult health-care systems for adolescents with chronic conditions. A position paper of the Society for Adolescent Medicine. J Adolesc Health1993;14(7):570-6.

[2] Ferris ME, Mahan JD. Pediatric chronic kidney disease and the process of health care transition. Seminars Nephrology 2009;29(4):435-44.

[3] A consensus statement on health care transitions for young adults with special health care needs. Pediatrics 2002;110(6 Pt 2):1304-6.

[4] Rosen DS, Blum RW, Britto M, Sawyer SM, Siegel DM. Transition to adult health care for adolescents and young adults with chronic conditions: position paper of the Society for Adolescent Medicine. J Adolesc Health 2003;33(4):309-11.

[5] Bell LE, Ferris ME, Fenton N, Hooper SR. Health care transition for adolescents with CKD-the journey from pediatric to adult care. Adv Chr Kidney Dis 2011;18(5):384-90.

[6] Cooley WC, Sagerman PJ. Supporting the health care transition from adolescence to adulthood in the medical home. Pediatrics 2011;128(1):182-200.

---

[1] Those with the * at the end are published/field experts consulted prior to our program's inauguration.

[7]   Watson AR, Harden PN, Ferris ME, Kerr PG, Mahan JD, Ramzy MF. Transition from pediatric to adult renal services: a consensus statement by the International Society of Nephrology (ISN) and the International Pediatric Nephrology Association (IPNA). Kidney Int 2011;80(7):704-7.

[8]   Wang G, McGrath BB, Watts C. Health care transitions among youth with disabilities or special health care needs: an ecological approach. J Pediatr Nurs 2010;25(6):505-50.

[9]   Schwartz LA, Tuchman LK, Hobbie WL, Ginsberg JP. A social-ecological model of readiness for transition to adult-oriented care for adolescents and young adults with chronic health conditions. Child Care Health Dev 2011;37(6):883-95.

[10] Betz CL. Transition of adolescents with special health care needs: review and analysis of the literature. Issues Comprehensive Pediatr Nurs 2004;27(3):179-241.

[11] Bickford K, Ford C, Bozik K, Tolleson-Rinehart S, Chin H, Gipson D, et al. Measuring readiness for transition in adolescents and young adults with chronic kidney disease [Abstract]. 4th Congress of the International Pediatric Transplant Association, Cancun, Mexico, 2007.

[12] Sawicki GS, Lukens-Bull K, Yin X, Demars N, Huang IC, Livingood W, et al. Measuring the transition readiness of youth with special healthcare needs: validation of the TRAQ--Transition Readiness Assessment Questionnaire. J Pediatr Psychol 2011;36(2):160-71.

[13] Ferris M, Ford C, Gipson D, Tolleson-Rinehart S, Bickord K, Chin H. The UNC TR$_x$ANSITION Scale^{TM} among adolescents with chronic kidney disease [Abstract]. American Society of Nephrology Renal Week, San Francisco, CA, 2007.

[14] Doan M, Fenton N, Iglesia E, Bickford K, Ferris M. Baseline TR$_x$ANSITION Scale^{TM} scores across multiple health conditions [Abstract]. Pediatric Academic Societies Annual Meeting, Boston, MA, 2012.

[15] Sengupta S, Bickford K, Ferris M. Psychometric validation of the UNC TRxANSITION Scale^{TM} version 3 to measure health care transition among adolescents and emerging adults with chronic disease [Abstract]. Pediatric Academic Societies Annual Meeting, Denver, CO, 2011.

[16] Ferris ME, Harward DH, Bickford K, Layton JB, Ferris MT, Hogan SL, et al. T A clinical tool to measure the components of health-care transition from pediatric care to adult care: the UNC TR(x)ANSITION scale. Ren Fail 2012;34(6):744-53.

[17] Ferris M, Kelly M, Martin N, Freeman K, Kim S, Gipson D. Sustained use of a practical tool to assist adolescents with disease self-management [Abstract]. Society for Adolescent Medicine Annual Meeting, 2008.

[18] Ko Z, Fenton N, Benton M, Hancock L, Haberman C, Ferris M. Social media use and adolescents' transition readiness [Abstract]. Pediatric Academic Societies Annual Meeting, Boston, MA, 2012.

[19] Kratz L, Uding N, Trahms CM, Villareale N, Kieckhefer GM. Managing childhood chronic illness: parent perspectives and implications for parent-provider relationships. Fam Systems Health 2009;27(4):303-13.

[20] Kieckhefer GM, Trahms CM. Supporting development of children with chronic conditions: from compliance toward shared management. Pediatr Nurs 2000;26(4):354-63.

[21] Modi AC, Pai AL, Hommel KA, Hood KK, Cortina S, Hilliard ME, et al. Pediatric self-management: a framework for research, practice, and policy. Pediatrics 2012;129(2):e473-85.

[22] Iglesia E, Fenton N, Bickford K, Doan M, Ferris M. Parent and adolescent concordance on transition readiness among adolescents with chronic conditions [Abstract]. Pediatric Academic Societies Annual Meeting, Boston, MA, 2012.

[23] Fenton N, Ferris M, Baucom D, Bickford K, Gibson K, Primack W. How resilience factors influence adjustment in adolescents with chronic kidney disease [Abstract]. 13th International Conference on Dialysis, Advances in CKD 2011, Miami, FL, 2011.

In: Disability and Chronic Disease
Editors: J. Merrick, S. Aspler and M. Morad

ISBN: 978-1-62948-288-0
© 2014 Nova Science Publishers, Inc.

Chapter 21

CLINICIAN PERCEPTIONS OF TRANSITION OF PATIENTS WITH PEDIATRIC-ONSET CHRONIC DISEASE TO ADULT MEDICAL CARE

Susan M Fernandes, MHP, PA-C, Michael J Landzberg, MD,*
Laurie N Fishman, MD, Paul Khairy, MD, PhD,
Gregory S Sawicki, MD, MPH, Sonja Ziniel, PhD,
Patrice Melvin, MPH, Joanne O'Sullivan-Oliveira, PhD, FNP, BC,
Peter Greenspan, MD and Ami B Bhatt, MD

Departments of Cardiology, Medicine and Surgery, Children's Hospital Boston,
Department of Pediatrics, Harvard Medical School, Boston and the Massachusetts
General Hospital for Children, Boston, Massachusetts, US

We sought to determine if the delivery of transitioning education/assessment and barriers to transfer to adult centered care differed across two types of pediatric institutions. Design: A web-based, multiple-choice, cross-sectional survey was distributed to 195 outpatient clinicians at a pediatric facility integrated within an adult institution. Results were then compared to previously reported data from a free-standing children's hospital. Results: Overall, the response rate was 56% (109/195) with 81/109 (74%) respondents providing outpatient care to patients >11 years of age. The majority of clinicians (67%) stated that their patients receive transitioning education/assessment, usually informally (90%), between the age of 11 and 16 years (44%). Older age (74%) and the presence of adult co-morbidities (70%) were the most common triggers to transfer. The patient's (95%) and parent's (91%) emotional attachment to the pediatric provider was perceived to be the most common barriers to transfer. In comparison with previous data from a free-standing children's hospital, there were no significant differences in the report of delivery of transitioning education/assessment, triggers to transfer and barriers to care and desire for departmental and hospital support for transitioning programs. Conclusion: Delivery of transitioning education/assessment for patients with pediatric onset chronic disease is often inconsistent and informal regardless of the type of pediatric institution. Age and

* Correspondence: Susan M Fernandes, MHP, PA-C, Department of Cardiology, Children's Hospital Boston, 300 Longwood Avenue, Boston, MA 02115, United States. E-mail: Sue.Fernandes@cardio.chboston.org.

adult co-morbidities appear to be the most common triggers to transfer while emotional attachment remains the most common perceived barrier to transfer. Clinicians overwhelmingly favor hospital based resources for the development of transitioning programs and resources to streamline the transfer process.

INTRODUCTION

Medical and surgical innovation for the treatment of complex pediatric diseases has increased survival into adulthood for diverse patient populations, including those with cystic fibrosis, congenital heart disease, diabetes, sickle cell disease, inflammatory bowel disease, childhood cancers and organ transplantation (1-7). As these patients enter adolescence and young adulthood they will require skills to become independent adults capable of managing their own healthcare needs. Despite this, transitioning programs have not become universally accepted, with the majority of such existing programs being condition-specific and informal (5, 7-11).

In the United States many adults with pediatric origin chronic disease continue to receive care at pediatric facilities (12). The lack of a standard approach to transitioning education/assessment may inhibit the successful transfer of these patients to an adult-oriented health care system. In a recent study, we found that at one of the largest free-standing children's hospitals, patients are not routinely provided with this transition related education and assessment. Attachment of the patient and parent to the pediatric provider and facility emerged as significant barriers to adult-oriented care (13).

The objective of this study was to determine if the delivery of transitioning education/assessment and barriers to transfer to adult-centered care differ at a pediatric facility that is integrated within an adult institution compared to a free-standing children's hospital. We hypothesized that many of the barriers to adult-centered care in free-standing children's hospitals would not exist in a pediatric facility intimately aligned with an adult healthcare institution.

OUR STUDY

We conducted a cross-sectional web-based survey of health care clinicians at a pediatric facility that is integrated within an adult institution (IPF) and a free-standing children's hospital (FSCH), as previously reported (13). In the IPF, we identified 195 clinicians, including physicians, nurses and social workers who were likely to provide care to patients over the age of 11 years in outpatient settings. Clinicians not actively seeing patients over the age of 11 in outpatient settings were excluded from further questioning. The survey was approved by the local institutional review board and administered in July of 2010.

Survey design

The survey tool has been previously described in detail (13). It was developed over a 12-month time frame, through a working group of 10 clinicians and researchers with an interest in health care transition. The working group included physician, nursing, physician assistant and social worker representation. The clinicians had a wide range of outpatient clinical expertise including cardiology, pulmonology, gastroenterology, adolescent medicine, general surgery and hematology/oncology. Questions were developed based on a review of the health care transition literature and guided by a survey methodologist. The final survey included a total of 25 questions within the following six categories: 1) inclusion criteria; 2) transitioning education/assessment; 3) transfer to an adult-oriented health care system; 4) demographics; 5) age appropriate care; and 6) resources.

Transitioning was defined as the "tools required by patients to become independent adults capable of managing and self-directing their healthcare" and encompassed disease knowledge, understanding of medication use and side effects, symptoms requiring urgent care, congenital/genetic anomalies in offspring, impact of high risk behaviors and disease impact on education and insurability. Transfer was defined as the "movement of adolescents and young adults with chronic physical and medical conditions from child-centered to adult-oriented health-care systems" (14).

Statistical analysis

Descriptive analyses of provider demographics were summarized using means and standard deviations for continuous variables and proportions for categorical variables. Demographic differences across the four provider sub groups were analyzed using Pearson's chi-square or Fisher's Exact test for categorical variables and one way analysis of variance (ANOVA) for continuous variables. Barriers to and impetus for the transitioning of patients into adult care were ranked and differences in clinician beliefs were assessed using chi square analysis. In order to evaluate differences between clinicians that care for adult patients, we dichotomized age into over 25 years versus all other age groups. Chi square analysis was used to assess differences in clinician characteristics between these two groups. Survey results were reported in aggregate so that clinician confidentiality was ensured. Comparisons between responses at the two institutions (i.e., FSCH versus IPF) were performed using independent sample t-tests for continuous variables and Fisher's Exact tests for categorical variables. All analyses were performed using SAS software version 9.2 (SAS, Cary, NC), and a 2-sided p value <0.05 was considered to indicated statistical significance.

FINDINGS

A total of 195 outpatient clinicians (135 physicians, 52 nurses, 8 social workers) at an IPF were invited to participate in the web-based survey. The response rate was 56% (109/195). Overall, 81/109 (74%) provided outpatient care to patients >11 years of age and were, therefore, eligible for analysis: 55 physicians, 19 nurses and 7 social workers. Clinician characteristics are presented in table 1.

Table 1. Clinician Characteristics

		Clinician Role			
	Overall	MD	RN	SW	p value
Total Responses	N= 81	N=55	N=19	N=7	
Number of Years in Practice					0.535
Mean ± SD		19.0 + 11.6	17.7 + 12.0	13.9 + 10.6	
Number of Years at Facility					0.021
Mean ± SD		15.5 + 10.4	14.2 + 11.9	3.7 + 3.3	
Gender					<0.001
Female	60.5%	44.3%	94.1%	100.0%	
Hispanic Ethnicity					0.258
Yes	3.9%	3.8%	0.0%	14.3%	
Race					
White	94.5%	91.8%	100.0%	100.0%	0.355
Black	0.0%	0.0%	0.0%	0.0%	
Asian	16.7%	23.3%	0.0%	0.0%	0.187
Age Group Currently Caring For					
Providing care for patients ≥25 years	23.0%	26.4%	12.5%	20.0%	0.504
Department					<0.001
Medicine	54.3%	69.1%	21.1%	28.6%	
Cardiology	21.0%	14.6%	47.4%	0.0%	
Surgery	9.9%	9.1%	15.8%	0.0%	
Other	6.2%	0.0%	0.0%	71.4%	
Not Specified	8.6%	7.3%	15.8%	0.0%	

Transitioning education/assessment

The majority of clinicians (67%) at the IPF stated their patients receive transitioning education/assessment (65% physicians, 74% nurses and 57% social workers, p= 0.690). A substantial number of clinicians (33%) stated their patients did not receive this type of assessment/education or were unsure if they were receiving it. The overwhelming majority of clinicians (90%) indicated that transitioning education/assessment was usually provided informally between the ages of 11 and 16 years (44%).

Reasons for transfer to an adult-oriented health care system

The most common patient characteristics cited by clinicians as reasons to transfer a patient to an adult-oriented health care system included age (74%), presence of adult co-morbidities (70%), and graduation from college (69%). Marriage (64%) and pregnancy (47%) were also common reasons to prompt transfer. The use of alcohol or illicit drugs (19%) and graduation from high school (14%) were less likely to prompt transfer.

Physicians at the IPF were more likely to consider adult co-morbidities (81%) as a reason to transfer compared to nurses and social workers (p=0.017). Nurses (61%) were more likely to indicate pregnancy as a reason for transfer compared to physicians and social workers (p=0.038).

Barriers to transfer to an adult oriented health care system

Clinicians at the IPF tended to agree on barriers to transfer. They listed the patient's (95%) and parent's (91%) emotional attachment to the pediatric provider as the most common barriers to transfer. Patient's emotional/cognitive delay (87%) was a common perceived barrier as well as the pediatric provider's attachment to the family (81%). The lack of qualified adult clinicians in specialty (73%), patient non-compliance with transfer (68%), and unstable medical conditions (57%) were also identified as barriers by more than half the clinicians. Only 17% indicated that insurance issues were a barrier to adult-oriented health care.

Adult-oriented healthcare within a pediatric setting

Most of the clinicians at the IPF felt that they (97%) and their department (94%) could provide age appropriate care to patients under the age of 18, with decreasing percentages as patient age increased. Only 43% thought that they could provide age appropriate care to patients >25 years and only 33% felt their department could provide age appropriate care for patients >25 years. However, 26% of clinicians stated they could provide age-appropriate care for patients >40 years and 25% for patients >50 years, while only 19% thought their department could provide age appropriate care for patients >40 years of age.

Resources for transitioning and transfer

Clinicians at the IPF were in agreement regarding the need for departmental and hospital resources for the development of transitioning programs and resources to streamline the transfer process (p= 0.682, p=0.340, p=0.569 respectively). Many clinicians (68%) felt there should be a specific program within their department to provide transitioning education/assessment and 83% of clinicians thought their institution should provide this resource. The majority of clinicians (88%) felt that their institution should provide resources to streamline the transfer process.

Free-standing pediatric hospital versus pediatric institution integrated within an adult hospital

Survey results from the FSCH have been previously reported (13). The response rate was higher at the FSCH compared to the IPF (368/479, 77% versus 109/195, 56%, p=<0.001). Demographics of the respondents were similar, except that physicians constituted a greater proportion of respondents at the IPF (68% versus 37%, p= <0.001) and more women participated in the survey at the FSCH (75.2% versus 60.5%, p=0.011). Comparisons of clinician characteristics are summarized in Table 2.

Table 2. Comparison of Clinician Characteristics

	Pediatric facility integrated within an adult institution	Free-standing children's hospital	p value
Total Responses	N=81	N=368	
Response Rate			
Overall	109/195 (56%)	368/479 (77%)	<0.001
Provide outpatient care for patients ≥11years	81/109 (74%)	329/368 (89%)	
Clinical Role			
MD	55/109 (67.9%)	123/329 (37.4%)	<0.001
RN	19/109 (23.5%)	141/329 (42.9%)	
SW	7/109 (8.6%)	40/329 (12.2%)	
PA	0/0 (0.0%)	25/329 (7.6%)	
Number of Years in Practice			
Mean ± SD	18.3 + 11.5	17.5 + 11.7	0.615
Number of Years at Institution			
Mean ± SD	14.2 + 10.7	12.5 + 10.2	0.222
Gender			
Female	60.5%	75.2%	0.011
Hispanic Ethnicity			
Yes	3.9%	5.0%	1.000
Race			
White	94.5%	95.8%	0.635
Black	0.0%	2.4%	1.000
Asian	16.7%	15.3%	0.835
Age Group Currently Caring For			
Providing care for patients ≥25 years	23.0%	32.5%	0.112

A similar proportion of clinicians at the FSCH (72%) and IPF (67%) stated that their patients receive transitioning education/assessment (p= 0.281). Both centers overwhelmingly indicated that these services were provided informally (92% versus 90%, p=0.910) and both centers indicated that this assessment/education typically begins between the ages of 11 and 16 years (48% versus 44%, p=0.509).

A comparison of the two institutions with regard to the most common patient characteristics that prompted transfer of a patient to an adult-oriented health care system are presented in Table 3. There were no significant differences. The top five most important characteristics were common to both.

Clinicians at both institutions tended to agree regarding the most common barriers to adult-oriented health care, as presented in Table 4. More than 90% of clinicians at both institutions identified the patient's and parent's emotional attachment to the pediatric provider as a significant barrier to adult-oriented health care (p=0.987 and p=0.140 respectively). Clinicians at the FSCH were more likely to state that insurance issues were a barrier to adult-oriented health care than clinicians at the IPF (p=0.001).

Table 3. Characteristics requiring transfer to an adult oriented healthcare system

Requirements for Transfer	Pediatric facility integrated within an adult institution	Free-standing children's hospital	p value
Age	74.4%	78.7%	0.412
Adult co-morbidities	69.7%	78.5%	0.105
College graduation	68.8%	67.1%	0.773
Marriage	63.6%	56.3%	0.241
Pregnancy	46.8%	58.0%	0.075
Alcohol/Illicit drug use	18.7%	29.2%	0.067
High school graduation	14.5%	15.9%	0.755

Table 4. Perceived barriers to transfer

Barriers to Transfer	Pediatric facility integrated within an adult institution	Free-standing children's hospital	p value
Patient's Emotional attachment to Pediatric Provider	94.7%	95.1%	0.897
Parent's Emotional attachment to Pediatric Provider	90.7%	95.7%	0.140
Patient's Emotional/Cognitive Delay	86.8%	85.6%	0.777
Provider's attachment to family/patient	81.1%	78.6%	0.631
Lack of qualified adult providers in specialty	73.0%	65.7%	0.231
Patient's Non-Compliance with Transfer	68.5%	78.1%	0.085
Patient's Unstable Medical Condition	57.3%	68.2%	0.075
Insurance Issues	16.7%	36.9%	0.001

The regular provision of care of patients over the age of 25 years was not uncommon in both institutions (33% versus in 23% in the FSCH and IPF, respectively, p=0.112). Clinicians at both institutions often continued to provide care for patients over the age of 40 years (23% versus 26%, p= 0.583) and a similar percentage of clinicians continued to care for patients over the age of 50 years (21% versus 25%, p=0.574).

The overwhelming majority of clinicians at both institutions favored departmental or hospital based programs to improve the delivery of transitioning education/assessment, with no significant differences between the two institutions (p=0.527 and p=0.127, respectively). Clinicians at the FSCH felt more strongly about the need for resources to streamline the transfer process (95% versus 88%, p=0.038).

DISCUSSION

The care of adolescent and adult survivors with pediatric onset chronic disease poses a significant challenge for the healthcare system. Successful transition to independent self-care and transfer to an adult-oriented health care system are dependent on numerous factors that may be impacted by the type of health care setting. In this study, we evaluated clinicians' perceptions for transition education /assessment at an IPF, assessed perceived characteristics that prompt transfer to an adult-oriented health care system, and explored perceived barriers of transfer. Comparisons were made to our previously conducted survey in a FSCH.

Our key findings include: 1) while the majority of clinicians at both institutions perceive that their patients receive transitioning education/assessment, it is most often reported as informal; 2) age and adult co-morbidities are the most frequently quoted triggers for transfer in both types of institutions; 3) the overwhelming majority of clinicians perceive the patients' and parents' attachment to the provider to be the most common barriers to transfer; 4) clinicians at both institutions favor institutional support for the development of transitioning programs, but clinicians at the FSCH were more likely to indicate the additional need for resources to streamline the transfer process.

Transitioning programs have been recommended by numerous organizations (15-17). Reasons for the lack of institutional commitment to such programs is unclear but is likely multi-factorial, including costs, lack of reimbursement for such programs and a lack of evidence demonstrating improved outcomes as a result of such programs. The timing of transfer is likely determined by a clinician's perceived ability to provide age appropriate care to a particular patient, as well as patient and family readiness for transfer and departmental and institutional policies regarding adult care (18). Of interest, the majority of clinicians at both institutions felt that they and their department could provide age appropriate care to patients 25 years of age and younger, with support for this statement decreasing beyond 25 years of age. There is some evidence that transfer is more successful at older ages (19) after the late adolescent years therefore it may be reasonable for pediatric providers to be involved in their care until a patient's early 20s. Patients, parents and clinicians appear more likely to support care transfer to an adult-oriented health care system at an older age cut-off.

The presence of adult co-morbidities was a commonly perceived trigger to transfer by clinicians at both institutions. The ability to manage adult co-morbidities may place the pediatric trained clinician beyond their level of comfort in care provision. If transfer is prompted by the onset of an adult co-morbidity, that transfer may then occur during clinical instability. The relationship between patient and family and the new adult provider may be strained in this acute setting, which may put adult providers and institutions at risk for litigation (20). Formal processes of transitioning education/assessment, partnered care between pediatric and adult clinicians, and elective transfer (4) when clinically stable should mitigate these risks.

Many clinicians believe that the patients and parents' emotional attachment to the provider and institution leads to resistance to transfer. This has been previously observed by Clarizia and colleges in Canada, although at a lower prevalence, 69% versus 95%, likely secondary to cultural and healthcare system differences (21). This perception may be biased by the clinician's own admission that their own attachment to patient and family is a barrier to transfer (22). Departments and institutions, therefore, may choose to address the emotional needs not only of their patients and families but also of their affected clinicians. Implementation of transitioning programs may help provide the necessary skills and confidence for patients and parents to overcome this emotional hurdle while educational programs for clinicians may provide support and guidance on successful transition and termination of direct care relationships.

The lack of qualified adult clinicians in specialty was considered a common barrier to adult centered care for patients with pediatric onset chronic disease by a large number of clinicians. A collaborative effort towards patient care, training of providers to care for this adult population, establishment of quality outcomes and reporting of such may contribute to overcoming of this barrier. Caring for the needs of the growing number of patients with pediatric onset chronic disease likely to reach adulthood over the next decade is likely to exhaust resources in pediatric facilities (7). Collaborative efforts between pediatric and adult facilities so as to accomplish these stated goals are to be encouraged.

The practitioners in this study stated the overwhelming desire for departmental and hospital-based programs to improve the delivery of transitioning education/assessment, although more clinicians favor hospital-based rather than departmental based programs. This sentiment is in accord with the success that has been seen at the institutional level in other forms of transition programming, where such has been shown to reduce hospital admissions and increase patients' ability to reach self-identified personal goals in the geriatric population (23). Adolescent and young adults with complex childhood onset disease face many of the same challenges, as do elder patients with chronic conditions. Healthcare institutions may therefore benefit from hospital-wide programs that encourage self-care management for all persons, including adolescents and young adults, with chronic disease. Such institutional based transition programs have the potential to result in improved patient satisfaction and decreased overall health care costs and resources. Establishment of quality measures regarding transition outcomes will assist in the validation of reimbursement strategies for these services.

Clinicians at the FSCH were more likely to indicate the need for resources to streamline the transfer process. If patients stay within an IPF, rather than shift to an entirely new healthcare system, the facility, hospital culture and medical record system may not change. Regardless of whether patients transfer within an institution to a new set of providers or to an entirely new system, care transfers places patients at increased risk for medical errors, duplicate testing, inappropriate testing and loss to care (24). Healthcare institutions are encouraged to develop strategies to mitigate this risk; such may be assisted by ensuring that the patient who is transferring care has the necessary transitioning skills to improve the direction and implementation of their health care.

Our study has several limitations. The characteristics and geographic location of the two institutions within this study may not allow for generalizability to other institutions. In addition, results reflect self-reporting. Social desirability response bias may have overestimated the actual percentage of clinicians who perform transitioning education/assessment and the lack of open-ended survey questions may result in leading question bias.

Contrary to our hypothesis, few differences in the perception regarding delivery of transitioning education/assessment, triggers to adult-oriented care, or barriers to transition were identified between clinicians in IPF and FSCH. We recognize the complexities of testing perceptions, which may not reflect actual practice. Given this, further study examining actual practices and exploration of the impact of care organization and clinician demographics on transition and transfer practices is indicated. An assessment of the patients' and their parents' perceptions in comparison to the clinicians' perception/practice is also indicated.

In conclusion, as individuals with pediatric onset chronic disease mature to adult age, the preparation of these individuals to manage and participate in their health care appears to have components that lie with parents, patients and providers. Regardless of the type of pediatric institution, the delivery of transitioning education/assessment often appears as inconsistent and informal. Older age and new onset adult co-morbidities are stated as the most common triggers to transfer, and may lead to risk to patient-caregiver relationship formation at an extremely vulnerable phase of development. In the clinician's perspective, parental and patient emotional attachment to the provider and institution is a major barrier to transfer, in addition to their own attachment to the patient and family. Transitioning programs should, therefore, address patient and family-related and clinician-related barriers. Clinicians overwhelmingly favor hospital-based resources for the development of transitioning programs and resources to streamline the transfer to adult oriented health care.

ACKNOWLEDGMENTS

The authors would like to acknowledge the efforts of Handan Titiz, Ed. M. and Meera Midha. Research funded by the Dunlevie Foundation. There are no relationships with industry.

REFERENCES

[1]   Scal P, Evans T, Blozis S, Okinow N, Blum R. Trends in transition from pediatric to adult health care services for young adults with chronic conditions. J Adolesc Health 1999;24(4):259-64.

[2]   Fernandes SM, Landzberg MJ. Transitioning the young adult with congenital heart disease for life-long medical care. Pediatr Clin North Am 2004;51:1739-48.

[3]   McDonagh JE, Kellya DA. Transitioning care of the pediatric recipient to adult caregivers. Pediatr Clin North Am 2003;51(6):1561-83.

[4]   Sawicki GS, Lukens-Bull K, Yin X, Demars N, Huang IC, Livingood W, Reiss J, Wood D. Measuring the transition readiness of youth with special healthcare needs: Validation of the TRAQ--Transition Readiness Assessment Questionnaire. J Pediatr Psychol 2011;36(2):160-71.

[5]   Lotstein DS, McPherson M, Strickland B, Newacheck PW. Transition Planning for youth with special health care needs: Results from the National Survey of Children with Special Health Care Needs. Pediatrics 2005;115(6):1562-8.

[6]   Baldassano R, Ferry G, Griffiths A, Mack D, Markowitz J, Winter H. Transition of the patient with inflammatory bowel disease from pediatric to adult care: recommendations of the North American Society for Pediatric Gastroenterology, Hepatology and Nutrition. Pediatr Gastroenterol Nutr 2002;34(3):245-8.

[7]   Betz CL. Approaches to transition in other chronic illnesses and conditions. Pediatr Clin North Am 2010;57(4):983-96.

[8]   Bell L. Adolescent dialysis patient transition to adult care: a cross-sectional survey. Pediatr Nephrol 2007;22(5):720-6.

[9]   McLaughlin SE, Diener-West M, Indurkhya A, Rubin H, Heckmann R, Boyle MP. Improving transition from pediatric to adult cystic fibrosis care: Lessons from a national survey of current practices. Pediatrics 2008;121(5):e1160-6.

[10]   Hilderson D, Saidi AS, Van Deyk K, Verstappen A, Kovacs AH, Fernandes SM, Canobbio MM, Fleck D, Meadows A, Linstead R, Moons P. Attitude toward and current practice of transfer and transition of adolescents with congenital heart disease in the United States of America and Europe. Pediatr Cardiol 2009;30(6):786-93.

[11]   De Beaufort C, Jarosz-Chobot P, Frank M, De Bart J, Deja G. Transition from pediatric to adult diabetes care: smooth or slippery? Pediatr Diabetes 2010;11(1):24-7.

[12]   Okumura MJ, Campbell AD, Nasr SZ, Davis MM. Inpatient health care use among adult survivors of chronic childhood illnesses in the United States. Arch Pediatr Adolesc Med 2006;10:1054-60.

[13]   Fernandes SM, Fishman L, O'Sullivan-Oliviera J, Ziniel S, Melvin P, Khairy P, O'Brien R, Webster R, Landzberg MJ, Sawicki GS. Current practices for the transition and transfer of patients with a wide

spectrum of pediatric-onset chronic diseases: Results of a clinician survey at a free-standing pediatric hospital. Int J Child Adolesc Health 2011;4(3):507-15.

[14] Blum RW. Improving transition for adolescents with special health care needs from pediatric to adult-centered health care. Pediatrics 2002;110(6):1301–3.

[15] American Academy of Pediatrics, American Academy of Family Physicians, American College of Physicians-American Society of Internal Medicine. A consensus statement on health care transitions for young adults with special health care needs. Pediatrics 2002;110(6):1304-6.

[16] Blum RW, Garell D, Hodgman CH, Jorissen TW, Okinow NA, Orr DP, Slap GB. Transition from child-centered to adult health-care systems for adolescents with chronic conditions : A position paper of the Society for Adolescent Medicine. J Adolesc Health 1993;14(7):570-6.

[17] Rosen DS, Blum RW, Britto M, Sawyer SM, Siegel DM. Transition to adult health care for adolescents and young adults with chronic conditions : Position paper of the society for adolescent medicine. J Adolesc Health 2003;33(4):309-11.

[18] Patel MS, O'Hare K. Residency training in transition of youth with childhood-onset chronic disease. Pediatrics 2010;126(Suppl 3):S190-3.

[19] Reid GJ, Irvine MJ, McCrindle BW, Sananes R, Ritvo PG, Siu SC, Webb GD. Prevalence and correlates of successful transfer from pediatric to adult health care among a cohort of young adults with complex congenital heart defects. Pediatrics 2004;113(3):e197-205.

[20] Lester G, Smith S. Listening and talking to patients. A remedy for malpractice suits? West J Med 1993;158(3):268-72.

[21] Clarizia NA, Chahal N, Manlhiot C, Kilburn J, Redington AN, McCrindle BW. Transition to adult health care for adolescents and young adults with congenital heart disease: Perspectives of the patient, parent and health care provider. Can J Cardiol 2009;25(9):317-22.

[22] Fox A. Physicians as barriers to successful transitional care. Int J Adolesc Med Health 2002;14(1):3-7.

[23] Coleman EA, Boult C. Improving the quality of transitional care for persons with complex care needs. J Am Geriatr Soc 2003;51(4):556-7.

[24] Parry C , Mahoney E, Chalmers SA, Coleman EA. Assessing the quality of transitional care: further applications of the care transitions measure. Med Care 2008;46(3):317-22.

In: Disability and Chronic Disease
Editors: J. Merrick, S. Aspler and M. Morad

ISBN: 978-1-62948-288-0
© 2014 Nova Science Publishers, Inc.

Chapter 22

ASSESSING THE SATISFACTION OF TEENS WITH KIDNEY TRANSPLANTS

*Cheryl Belair, CCLS[1], Jordan Gilleland, PhD[*2] and Sandra Amaral, MD, MHS[3]*

[1]Department of Transplant Services, Children's Healthcare of Atlanta, Atlanta
[2]Children's Healthcare of Atlanta and Emory University, Atlanta
[3]Department of Pediatrics, Emory University, Atlanta, Georgia, US

Adolescents with kidney transplants are at increased risk for allograft rejection and loss. These negative health outcomes are likely multifactorial, but seem to be exacerbated during the time of transition from pediatric to adult healthcare providers. In June 2007, our center initiated an adolescent-focused transition clinic for adolescent kidney transplant recipients with the goal of improving adolescent healthcare self-management and easing adolescents' transition to adult health services. We conducted a telephone survey of 21 young adult kidney transplant recipients who had attended this transition clinic to assess their satisfaction with receiving adolescent-specific, multidisciplinary care. Eleven patients (52%) had transitioned within the prior 2 years and 10 patients (48%) were pending transition in the coming year. All 21 patients felt that being seen independently was beneficial. Nineteen patients (90%) believed that the adolescent clinic helped them prepare for transition to the adult center and 18 patients (86%) felt more knowledgeable about their medical condition and disease after attending the clinic. Those that did not feel that the clinic helped them stated that they already felt knowledgeable about their medications and condition prior to the clinic. Nine of the eleven patients (82%) who had transferred noted that they felt fully prepared at time of transition. These results suggest that adolescents with kidney transplants perceive benefit from attending an adolescent-focused transition clinic. Whether improved health knowledge and improved ability to communicate with providers independently leads to better long-term health outcomes and smoother transition deserves further exploration.

* Correspondence: Jordan Gilleland, PhD, Postdoctoral Fellow, Emory University School of Medicine, Children's Healthcare of Atlanta, 1405 Clifton Rd. NE, AFLAC Cancer and Blood, Disorders Center, 4th floor, Atlanta, GA, 30322-1060 United States. E-mail: Jordan.Gilleland@choa.org or jgilleland@gmail.com.

INTRODUCTION

Children who undergo kidney transplantation at less than 18 years of age experience excellent one-year allograft survival rates of 93-94%, however these statistics alarmingly change at 5 years status post transplant. The 5-year allograft survival rate for patients who receive a transplanted kidney between the ages of 11 and 17 years drops to a disappointing 63% (1). The only other age group to experience such a low allograft survival rate (59%) is comprised of patients over 65 years of age. In the North American Pediatric Renal Trials and Collaborative Studies (NAPRTCS) registry, adolescents had the poorest graft survival among all pediatric age groups, and once diagnosed with rejection, they did not respond as well to treatment, exhibiting fewer complete rejection reversals and greater residual allograft dysfunction (2).

These negative health outcomes in adolescents are likely multifactorial, but seem to be exacerbated during the time of transition from pediatric to adult healthcare providers (3-4). The transition of adolescents to adult medical services adds to the risk of allograft loss because of discontinuity in care combined with the complex and challenging psychosocial issues faced by adolescents with chronic illness. In a study of 20 young adults with kidney transplants in the United Kingdom who had been transferred from pediatric to adult transplant centers, 8 transplants failed within 36 months of transfer (40%) (4). In 2007, the United States Government Accountability Office published a report that examined the frequency of transplant failures and subsequent cost to Medicare from 1997 through 2004 (5). Three age groups were defined: pediatric recipients were those younger than 18 years old, transitional recipients were those younger than 18 at the time of transplant and at least 18 at the end of the study interval, and adult recipients were those at least 18 at the time of transplant. Transitional recipients experienced the highest rate of transplant failures compared with pediatric or adult recipients illustrating the challenges present during the adolescent years.

Medication nonadherence is a major risk factor for allograft rejection and loss in both adults and pediatrics and results in poor long-term kidney transplant outcomes and subsequent devastating medical and economic consequences on individual and societal levels. Ettenger et al. (6) found that nonadherence led to rejection with subsequent kidney allograft loss or dysfunction in 71% of patients who had received deceased donor kidney transplants (N=70). The UNOS registry has reported that 13% of allograft loss in adolescent kidney transplant recipients is due to nonadherence.[7] In a recent study of the USRDS database, Chisholm et al. (8) found that pediatric kidney transplant recipients who experienced allograft failure were twice as likely to be nonadherent (OR 2.07, 95% CI 1.12-4.06) and greater adherence to immunosuppressive medication was significantly associated with longer time to graft failure (P=0.009).

Although transition programming for adolescents with chronic illness is purported to be necessary, there is little evidence to support their utility. Two years after designing and implementing an Adolescent Kidney Transplant Transition Clinic (AKTTC), we performed survey of patients who attended our transition clinic and transitioned to or are pending transition to an adult healthcare setting within the year to assess patient satisfaction with such a comprehensive program. In the current investigation, we review participants' surveys to explore patient satisfaction with the AKTTC.

OUR STUDY

In June 2007, we initiated a novel Adolescent Kidney Transplant Transition Clinic (AKTTC) as a healthcare self-management program at Emory-Children's Healthcare of Atlanta. Healthcare self-management and the provision of transitional care are inextricably linked with medication adherence and are necessary components of caring for adolescents with chronic illness. At least one study in adolescent liver transplant recipients has demonstrated that an intervention designed to facilitate transition of healthcare responsibility from parent to patient can result in improved medication adherence (9). The Society for Adolescent Medicine, maintaining the belief that adolescents can be empowered to effect positive health-related outcomes, proposed transition principles for optimal health care services to facilitate the transition of adolescents with chronic illness to adult health care providers. These principles include providing age-appropriate care, enhancing autonomy, addressing adolescent-specific health issues, and designating particular health professionals to facilitate this process of development (10). In the development of the AKTTC at Emory-CHOA, we have modeled a unique healthcare self-management program that implements the principles of adolescent transition. Patients join the program when they turn 14 years old or reach one year post-transplant, when laboratory monitoring and visit frequency become less frequent and allograft survival rates begin to decline (11). The intensive multidisciplinary care team sees patients every three months. Patients rotate through 15-minute encounters with six different care providers, including the transplant coordinator, psychologist, social worker, pharmacist, nutritionist or child life specialist and a designated nephrologist. The nutritionist and child life specialist alternate seeing patients every other visit. Importantly, to reinforce the concept of the adolescent's autonomy and responsibility for self-care, patients are seen alone, while parents wait in the waiting room. Parents are then consulted at the end of the visit. Patients receive more one-on-one time for communication and counseling with each healthcare provider. Care providers incorporate several approaches to address adherence, including behavioral modification strategies and patient education. In our program, each provider asks the patient a pre-specified set of questions to identify facilitators and barriers to adherence. The patient interviews encourage frank discussion about the impact of individual behavior and environmental influences on overall health status and specifically allograft function. The clinical programming focuses on encouraging a development progression of responsibility of healthcare by the patient.

Each member of the care team has a specific role designed to achieve a 21-item checklist of healthcare self-management skills that we recommend patients achieve prior to transition to adult medical care, including such tasks as calling in one's own medication refills and carrying a medication list in one's wallet. This checklist is given to patients at their first clinic visit; the patient is assigned up to three tasks from this checklist as homework at the end of each visit and his/her progress toward achievement of these tasks is assessed at the next visit. The pharmacist is responsible for assessing the patient's medication knowledge, including medication indications and doses, as well as medication adherence and barriers to adherence. The pharmacist and patient develop a plan for improvement in knowledge and adherence between visits. The transplant coordinator and physician deal with any medical issues as well as assess the patient's knowledge of his/her diagnosis, address sexual health, substance and alcohol use, and the impact of behavior on transplant function. The psychologist identifies and addresses any psychosocial co-morbidities which may impact adherence, such as depression or family conflict. The process of transition to adult services is discussed with the patient at each visit. Positive reinforcement is provided for improvements in healthcare self-management skills. To make further gains in healthcare self-management, behavioral strategies, such as programming medication reminder alarms into one's cell phone, are individually developed with each patient.

Patient survey

For this survey, we telephoned any patient who was seen at least twice in the AKTTC program and who had transitioned to the adult healthcare setting or who was pending transition to the adult healthcare setting within the upcoming year. Patients were telephoned from January 11, 2010-February 11, 2010.

We based our clinic model on the principles of transition recommended by Rosen et al. (10), such as providing opportunities to enhance autonomy, increase personal responsibility and facilitate self reliance. Our survey questions were directed toward learning more about which components of our model were of most and least benefit from the patient perspective. The purpose was to assess our current efficacy in improving the transition of care from the patient's viewpoint and using the data to improve our multidisciplinary cared model beyond its current form. A preliminary review of this study was conducted by the Children's Healthcare of Atlanta/Emory University School of Medicine IRB Board and was deemed exempt from a full review due to its quality improvement nature.

Table 1. Demographics by group

Demographics	Pre-Transition Patients (N=10)	Post-Transition Patients (N=11)
Mean Age (years)[*] Age difference: t=-3.95 (p=.002)	20.60 (± .302)	21.57 (± .744)
Gender (N)		
Male	8 (80.0%)	6 (54.4%)
Female	2 (20.0%)	5 (45.5%)
Ethnicity (N)		
Caucasian	8 (80.0%)	6 (54.4%)
African American	2 (20.0%)	5 (45.5%)
Diagnosis (N)		
Cystic/Hereditary/Congenital	1 (10%)	2 (18.2%)
Glomerulonephritis	5 (50%)	4 (36.4%)
Secondary GN/Vasculitis	2 (20%)	2 (18.2%)
Interstitial Nephritis/Pyelonephritis	2 (20%)	1 (9.1%)
Miscellaneous	0 (0%)	2 (18.2%)
Mean Time since transplant (years)	6.30 (± 3.50)	5.65 (± 2.63)
Mean Age at transplant (years)	14.22 (± 3.38)	15.94 (± 2.69)
Mean Number of AKTTC visits[*] Visit number difference: t=4.69 (p=.001)	8.70 (± .1.41)	4.64 (± .2.38)

The AKTTC satisfaction survey asked a series of twelve questions. Participant responses to questions 1-6 are detailed in table 2. To assess patients' opinions on clinic design and programming we asked: "Was meeting with the multidisciplinary team members independently, without parents, beneficial?", "Was seeing each team member at each clinic visit beneficial?", and "Where the homework assignments that you received in clinic beneficial?" To gauge perceptions of potential clinic benefits we asked: "Do you feel that the AKTTC helped prepare you for transition to the adult center?" and "Did you feel more knowledgeable about your medical condition and medication after attending the AKTTC?" and "Where there any differences between the pediatric transplant clinic and the adult clinic that you did not feel prepared for?"

The results of Questions 7-12 are not listed in table 2, but are listed in the body of this study. These questions asked patients to explain what part of the AKTTC helped them the most and least, changes to the AKTTC that they would recommend, how their kidney function is doing now, and what they are doing with their time. Clinical and medical characteristics, including age, race, gender and kidney transplant status were collected from the medical chart and are detailed in table 1. Survey responses were recorded verbatim.

Table 2. Comparison of post-transition patient and pre-transition patient responses to the AKTTC satisfaction survey

Question		Responses			Total
		Yes	No	Somewhat	
1. "Was meeting with the multidisciplinary team members independently, without parents, beneficial to you?"	Post-transition group	8	-	3	11
	Pre-transition group	7	-	3	10
2. "Was seeing all of the team members at each clinic visit beneficial to you?"	Post-transition group	10	1	-	11
	Pre-transition group	8	2	-	10
3. "Where the homework assignments that you received at each clinic visit beneficial to you?" **	Post-transition group	4	-	2	6
	Pre-transition group	5	-	5	10
4. "Do you feel that the clinic helped prepare you for transitioning to the adult transplant center?"	Post-transition group	7	1	3	11
	Pre-transition group	6	1	3	10
5. "Did you feel more knowledgeable about your medical condition and medications after attending the ATTC clinic?"	Post-transition group	5	2	4	11
	Pre-transition group	9	1	-	10
6. "Where there any differences between the pediatric transplant clinic and the adult clinic that you did not feel prepared for?"	Post-transition group	2	9	-	11
	Pre-transition group	NA	NA	NA	NA

Note: ** Five participants did not remember the homework assignments

FINDINGS

Twenty-five patients were eligible to participate in the survey. We were able to contact 22 patients by phone and 21 completed the telephone survey (95%). One patient declined participation. Of the patients who completed the survey, 33% were Black, 67% White, 67% male. Mean age was 21.1 years (± .75 years). Patients were seen on average 6.57 times (± 2.84 visits) in the AKTTC prior to transfer. Eleven patients (52%) had transferred to adult services. Ten (48%) will be transferring to adult services within the next year. Independent samples t-test were used to compare the pre- and post- transition participants. The pre-transition participants were significantly younger than the post-transition participants (t=-3.95, p=.002) and had attended significantly more AKTTC visits (t=4.69, p=.001).

Among the 21 subjects who completed the survey, eighteen (86%) still had a functioning kidney transplant at the time they were surveyed. Two patients lost their transplant due to nonadherence but both cases occurred prior to transition to adult services. One additional patient lost allograft function after transition, however allograft loss occurred secondary to other medical complications, not related to adherence.

Table 2 provides a summary of survey responses. There were no significant differences in the survey answers of the pre- and post-transition groups. All 21patients found attending the AKTTC without his/her parents to be beneficial. The most common reasons for this were that the adolescents felt like they could share more information when the parents were not in the room and that they felt like they had more responsibility for their healthcare management. A few teens stated that they felt they had to change their answers to questions when their parents were present.

As part of the clinic programming, patients received homework assignments as detailed in the methods section. Sixteen patients (76%) remembered their homework assignments. Of those patients, the assignments that were believed to be most beneficial were learning medications and learning details about insurance.

Five patients (45%) toured the adult healthcare facility to which they would be transferring prior to their transfer. All 5 patients found this to be helpful because they knew where to go for clinic appointments and where able to meet the new staff. Four patients also remembered receiving a transition packet and contact info for the adult setting. Patients reported this to be beneficial and an easy place to find contact information when needed.

Eighteen patients (86%) felt that the AKTTC helped them prepare for transition to the adult center, by "learning to become independent in a step by step process". The three subjects who did not feel the AKTTC helped them be more prepared reported feeling well-prepared for transition prior to enrollment in the AKTTC. Eighteen patients (86%) reported that they felt more knowledgeable about their medical condition and their medications because of participation in the AKTTC program. Patients reported that the most helpful component of the program was meeting with all of the providers one on one, homework assignments, seeing the doctor independently and going on the tour. Of the eleven patients who had transferred to the adult setting, the biggest differences between the pediatric and adult settings were reported to be longer clinic visits and wait times, more responsibilities, and having to initiate concerns. Nine patients (81%) stated that they felt prepared to transition to the adult center at time of transfer. Of the 2 that did not feel prepared, they felt unprepared for "people's lack of helpfulness" at the adult center and "nurses are not as hands on" at the adult center.

CONCLUSION

Long-term allograft survival in adolescents with kidney transplants is poor and likely due to a myriad of reasons, including the complex developmental issues of adolescence with changes in independence, exacerbated by the transition of healthcare responsibility and transition of medical care from pediatric to adult healthcare settings. Transitional care is purported to be necessary to improve long-term health outcomes for adolescents with chronic illness but little is known regarding whether such programs are actually perceived to be beneficial by the patient. We initiated a multidisciplinary, adolescent-focused transitional care program based on the recommended principles of transition suggested by the Society for Adolescent Medicine. Patients who participated in this programming were surveyed and overall reported satisfaction with the AKTTC program. They also found it useful to meet the adult healthcare team in advance of their transfer. Further, both groups of patients pre-and post- transition reported experiencing equal benefits from the AKTTC programming which indicate that the advantages offered by the program are evident during the process of transition and after transfer of care. Our findings suggest that this type of program is worthwhile. Specifically, patients perceived benefit in meeting with providers independently, receiving adolescent specific education and being given more responsibility for management of their healthcare.

Our findings are consistent with those reported in other adolescent chronic illness populations. Several studies have reported the importance of patients being seen independently in the pediatric healthcare setting prior to transfer. Being seen independently has been associated with successful transfer in young adults with congenital heart disease, juvenile idiopathic arthritis, cystic fibrosis and other solid organ transplants (12-15). Patients with chronic illness have reported that the keys to successful transition include having transition be a stepwise process, having a trusting, reciprocal relationship with the healthcare team, including discussions about insurance and bridging differences between adult and pediatric healthcare settings (16). In addition, patients with varied chronic illnesses have reported that it is helpful to discuss transition early and to meet the adult healthcare team before transfer (17,18). Taken together, the data suggest that it is likely a dynamic balance between adolescent healthcare responsibility and parental involvement during the transition process in which teens take on increasing amounts of responsibility and parents become less involved over time as teen's approach transfer to adult care.

Of the eleven patients that transitioned to the adult transplant clinic, only one patient (9%) returned to dialysis after transition and this was not related to nonadherence or loss to follow-up during transition. Of the patients who are impending transition to adult services from the pediatric setting, all feel more prepared for the transition as a result of receiving adolescent-focused and healthcare self-management focused care. Further study is warranted to assess long-term health outcomes of patients who attend an adolescent-focused transition clinic compared with those who do not receive such services.

ACKNOWLEDGMENTS

The adolescent kidney transplant transition clinic at Emory-CHOA has been supported by The Mason Trust, The Georgia Transplant Foundation, Emory Healthcare and Children's Healthcare of Atlanta.

REFERENCES

[1] US Dept of HHS. UNOS: Organ Donation and Transplantation. 2010. Accessed 2013 Aug 01. URL: http://www.unos.org/data.

[2] Smith J, et al. Renal transplant outcomes in adolescents: A report of the North American Pediatric Renal Transplant Cooperative Study. Pediatr Transplant 2002;6(6):493-9.

[3] Annunziato R, et al. Adherence and medical outcomes in pediatric liver transplant recipients who transition to adult services. Pediatr Transplant 2007;11(6):608-14.

[4] Watson A. Non-compliance and transfer from paediatric to adult transplant unit. Ped Nephrol 2000;14(6): 469-72.

[5] General Accountability Office. End-stage renal disease: Characteristics of kidney transplant recipients, Frequency of transplant failures, and cost to medicare. September 2007. GAO-07-1117.

[6] Ettenger R, et al. Improved cadaveric renal transplant outcomes in children. Pediatr Nephrol 1991;5(1):137-42.

[7] Cecka J, et al. Pediatric renal transplantation: a review of the UNOS data. Pediatr Transplant 1997;1(1):55-64.

[8] Chisholm-Burns MA, Spivey CA, et al. Immunosuppressant Therapy Adherence and Graft Failure Among Pediatric Renal Transplant Recipients. Am J Transplant 2009;9(11):2497-504.

[9] Annunziato R, et al. Transitioning health care responsibility from caregiver to patient: a pilot study aiming to facilitate medication adherence during this process. Ped Transpl 2008;12(3):309-15.

[10] Rosen D, et al. Transition to adult health care for adolescents and young adults with chronic conditions: Position paper of the Society for Adolescent Medicine. J Adolesc Health 2003;33(4):309-11.

[11] US Dept of Health and Human Services. United States OPTN/SRTR 2006 Annual Report. Accessed 2013 Aug 01. URL: http://www.optn.org/

[12] Reid GJ, Irvine MJ, McCrindle BW, Sananes R, Ritvo PG, Siu SC, Webb GD. Prevalence and correlates of successful transfer from pediatric to adult health care among a cohort of young adults with complex congenital heart defects. Pediatrics 2004;113(3):e197-205..

[13] Shaw KL, Southwood TR, McDonagh JE. Transitional care for adolescents with juvenile idiopathic arthritis: a Delphi study. Rheumatology 2004;43(8):1000-6..

[14] Boyle MP, Farukhi Z, Nosky ML. Strategies for improving transition to adult cystic fibrosis care, based on patient and parent views. Pediatr Pulmonol 2001; 32(6):428-36..

[15] Stabile L, Rosser L, Porterfiled KM, McCauley S, Levenson C, Haglund J, Christman K. Transfer versus transition: success in pediatric transplantation brings the welcome challenge of transition. Prog Transplant 2005;15(4):363-70.

[16] Reiss JG, Gibson RW, Walker LR. Health care transition: youth, family and provider perspectives. Pediatrics 2005;115(1):112-20.

[17] Tuchman LK, Slap GB, Britto ML. Transition to adult care: experiences and expectations of adolescents with a chronic illness. Child Care Health Dev 2008; 34(5):557-63.

[18] Anthony SJ, Kaufman M, Drabble A, Seifert-Hansen M, Dipchand AI, Martin K. Perceptions of transitional care needs and experiences in pediatric heart transplant Recipients. Am J Transplant 2009;9(3):614-9.

SECTION FOUR: ACKNOWLEDGMENTS

In: Disability and Chronic Disease
Editors: J. Merrick, S. Aspler and M. Morad

ISBN: 978-1-62948-288-0
© 2014 Nova Science Publishers, Inc.

Chapter 23

ABOUT THE EDITORS

Joav Merrick, MD, MMedSci, DMSc, is professor of pediatrics, child health and human development affiliated with Kentucky Children's Hospital, University of Kentucky, Lexington, Kentucky, United States and the Division of Pediatrics, Hadassah Hebrew University Medical Center, Mt Scopus Campus, Jerusalem, Israel, the medical director of the Health Services, Division for Intellectual and Developmental Disabilities, Ministry of Social Affairs and Social Services, Jerusalem, the founder and director of the National Institute of Child Health and Human Development in Israel. Numerous publications in the field of pediatrics, child health and human development, rehabilitation, intellectual disability, disability, health, welfare, abuse, advocacy, quality of life and prevention. Received the Peter Sabroe Child Award for outstanding work on behalf of Danish Children in 1985 and the International LEGO-Prize ("The Children's Nobel Prize") for an extraordinary contribution towards improvement in child welfare and well-being in 1987. E-mail: jmerrick@zahav.net.il

Shoshana Aspler, RN, BScN, MPH, is Chief Community Nurse, Health Services, Office Medical Director, Division for Intellectual and Developmental Disabilities, Ministry of Social Affairs and Social Services, Jerusalem and affiliated with the National Institute of Child Health and Human Development in Israel. She is a specialist in disaster medicine and has published in the areas of disaster medicine, intellectual disability and public health issues. E-mail: shoshiasp@walla.com

Mohammed Morad, MD, FRCP (Edin), MRCPS(Glasg) is specialist in family medicine, now working as the medical director of the Yaski Community Medical Center, Ben Gurion University of the Negev, Clalit Health Services, Beer-Sheva, a university affiliated community medical center. He is a senior lecturer in family medicine affiliated with the Department of Family Medicine, Division of Community Health and Center for Multidisciplinary Research in Aging at the Faculty of Health Sciences, Ben Gurion University of the Negev, Beer-Sheva, Israel. Associate director of the National Institute of Child Health and Human Development in Jerusalem, Israel, professor of pediatrics at the Department of Pediatrics, University of Kentucky, Lexington, Kentucky, United States and 2011-2012 he spend a year as the leading general practitioner responsible for out-of-hours primary care service in the NHS Lanarkshire area in Scotland. Before Scotland he worked as the medical director of a large medical specialist center for the south of Israel in the city of

Beer-Sheva operated by the Clalit Health Services (150 medical specialists, 300 support staff and 250,000 annual visits). Publications on Bedouin health, health aspects, spiritual health and aging in persons with intellectual disability, and presenter on public health topics, health policy and services for the disadvantaged at national and international conferences. E-mail: morad62@gmail.com

In: Disability and Chronic Disease
Editors: J. Merrick, S. Aspler and M. Morad

ISBN: 978-1-62948-288-0
© 2014 Nova Science Publishers, Inc.

Chapter 24

ABOUT THE NATIONAL INSTITUTE OF CHILD HEALTH AND HUMAN DEVELOPMENT IN ISRAEL

The National Institute of Child Health and Human Development (NICHD) in Israel was established in 1998 as a virtual institute under the auspicies of the Medical Director, Ministry of Social Affairs and Social Services in order to function as the research arm for the Office of the Medical Director. In 1998 the National Council for Child Health and Pediatrics, Ministry of Health and in 1999 the Director General and Deputy Director General of the Ministry of Health endorsed the establishment of the NICHD.

MISSION

The mission of a National Institute for Child Health and Human Development in Israel is to provide an academic focal point for the scholarly interdisciplinary study of child life, health, public health, welfare, disability, rehabilitation, intellectual disability and related aspects of human development. This mission includes research, teaching, clinical work, information and public service activities in the field of child health and human development.

SERVICE AND ACADEMIC ACTIVITIES

Over the years many activities became focused in the south of Israel due to collaboration with various professionals at the Faculty of Health Sciences (FOHS) at the Ben Gurion University of the Negev (BGU). Since 2000 an affiliation with the Zusman Child Development Center at the Pediatric Division of Soroka University Medical Center has resulted in collaboration around the establishment of the Down Syndrome Clinic at that center. In 2002 a full course on "Disability" was established at the Recanati School for Allied Professions in the Community, FOHS, BGU and in 2005 collaboration was started with the Primary Care Unit of the faculty and disability became part of the master of public health course on "Children and society". In the academic year 2005-2006 a one semester course on "Aging with disability" was started as part of the master of science program in gerontology in our collaboration with the Center for Multidisciplinary Research in Aging. In 2010 collaborations with the Division of Pediatrics, Hadassah Hebrew University Medical Center, Jerusalem, Israel around the National Down Syndrome Center and teaching students and residents about intellectual and developmental disabilities as part of their training at this campus.

RESEARCH ACTIVITIES

The affiliated staff have over the years published work from projects and research activities in this national and international collaboration. In the year 2000 the International Journal of Adolescent Medicine and Health and in 2005 the International Journal on Disability and Human Development of De Gruyter Publishing House (Berlin and New York) were affiliated with the National Institute of Child Health and Human Development. From 2008 also the International Journal of Child Health and Human Development (Nova Science, New York), the International Journal of Child and Adolescent Health (Nova Science) and the Journal of Pain Management (Nova Science) affiliated and from 2009 the International Public Health Journal (Nova Science) and Journal of Alternative Medicine Research (Nova Science). All peer-reviewed international journals.

NATIONAL COLLABORATIONS

Nationally the NICHD works in collaboration with the Faculty of Health Sciences, Ben Gurion University of the Negev; Department of Physical Therapy, Sackler School of Medicine, Tel Aviv University; Autism Center, Assaf HaRofeh Medical Center; National Rett and PKU Centers at Chaim Sheba Medical Center, Tel HaShomer; Department of Physiotherapy, Haifa University; Department of Education, Bar Ilan University, Ramat Gan, Faculty of Social Sciences and Health Sciences; College of Judea and Samaria in Ariel and in 2011 affiliation with Center for Pediatric Chronic Diseases and National Center for Down Syndrome, Department of Pediatrics, Hadassah Hebrew University Medical Center, Mount Scopus Campus, Jerusalem.

INTERNATIONAL COLLABORATIONS

Internationally with the Department of Disability and Human Development, College of Applied Health Sciences, University of Illinois at Chicago; Strong Center for Developmental Disabilities, Golisano Children's Hospital at Strong, University of Rochester School of Medicine and Dentistry, New York; Centre on Intellectual Disabilities, University of Albany, New York; Centre for Chronic Disease Prevention and Control, Health Canada, Ottawa; Chandler Medical Center and Children's Hospital, Kentucky Children's Hospital, Section of Adolescent Medicine, University of Kentucky, Lexington; Chronic Disease Prevention and Control Research Center, Baylor College of Medicine, Houston, Texas; Division of Neuroscience, Department of Psychiatry, Columbia University, New York; Institute for the Study of Disadvantage and Disability, Atlanta; Center for Autism and Related Disorders, Department   Psychiatry, Children's Hospital Boston, Boston; Department of Paediatrics,

Child Health and Adolescent Medicine, Children's Hospital at Westmead, Westmead, Australia; International Centre for the Study of Occupational and Mental Health, Düsseldorf, Germany; Centre for Advanced Studies in Nursing, Department of General Practice and Primary Care, University of Aberdeen, Aberdeen, United Kingdom; Quality of Life Research Center, Copenhagen, Denmark; Nordic School of Public Health, Gottenburg, Sweden, Scandinavian Institute of Quality of Working Life, Oslo, Norway; The Department of Applied Social Sciences (APSS) of The Hong Kong Polytechnic University Hong Kong.

TARGETS

Our focus is on research, international collaborations, clinical work, teaching and policy in health, disability and human development and to establish the NICHD as a permanent institute at one of the residential care centers for persons with intellectual disability in Israel in order to conduct model research and together with the four university schools of public health/medicine in Israel establish a national master and doctoral program in disability and human development at the institute to secure the next generation of professionals working in this often non-prestigious/low-status field of work.

Contact

Joav Merrick, MD, MMedSci, DMSc
Professor of Pediatrics, Child Health and Human Development
Medical Director, Health Services, Division for Intellectual and Developmental Disabilities, Ministry of Social Affairs and Social Services, POB 1260, IL-91012 Jerusalem, Israel.
E-mail: jmerrick@zahav.net.il

In: Disability and Chronic Disease
Editors: J. Merrick, S. Aspler and M. Morad

ISBN: 978-1-62948-288-0
© 2014 Nova Science Publishers, Inc.

Chapter 25

ABOUT THE BOOK SERIES "DISABILITY STUDIES"

Disability studies is a book series with publications from a multidisciplinary group of researchers, practitioners and clinicians for an international professional forum interested in the broad spectrum of disability, intellectual disability, health and human development.

- Reiter S. Disability from a humanistic perspective: Towards a better quality of life. New York: Nova Science, 2008
- Knotkova H, Cruciani R, Merrick J, eds. Pain. Brain stimulation in the treatment of pain. New York: Nova Science, 2010.
- Prasher VP, ed. Contemporary issues in intellectual disabilities. New York: Nova Science, 2010.
- Lotan M, Merrick J, eds. Rett syndrome: Therapeutic interventions. New York: Nova Science, 2011.
- Satgé D, Merrick J, eds. Cancer in children and adults with intellectual disabilities: Current research aspects. New York: Nova Science, 2011.
- Knotkova H, Cruciani RA, Merrick J, eds. Neural plasticity in chronic pain. New York: Nova Science, 2011.
- Prasher VP. Down syndrome and dementia. A comprehensive and historical review. New York: Nova Science, 2012.

Contact

Professor Joav Merrick, MD, MMedSci, DMSc
Medical Director, Health Services, Division for Intellectual and Developmental Disabilities
Ministry of Social Affairs and Social Services, POBox 1260
IL-91012 Jerusalem, Israel
E-mail: jmerrick@internet-zahav.net

SECTION FIVE: INDEX

INDEX

B

C

D

F

G

J

K

L

M

P

Q

T

U

V

W

Y